Reiner Labitzke, Manual of Cable Osteosyntheses

Springer-Verlag Berlin Heidelberg GmbH

Reiner Labitzke

Manual of Cable Osteosyntheses

History, Technical Basis, Biomechanics of the
Tension Band Principle,
and Instructions for Operation

With contributions by
A.J. Weiland, New York, K.-P. Schmit-Neuerburg, Essen
Frei Otto, Stuttgart, A. Richter, Darmstadt
D.M. Dall, Hermanus, SA, and A. Miles, Bath, UK

With 156 Figures in 400 Parts

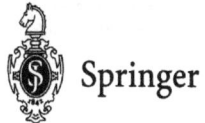

Springer

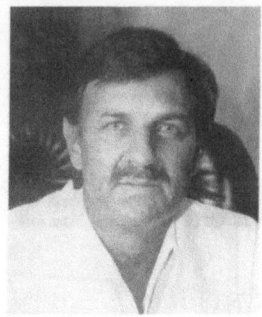

Univ.-Prof. Dr. med. habil. Reiner Labitzke
Chair of Surgery of Private University of Witten/Herdecke
Director of the Clinic for general surgery and traumatology of UWH at Evangeli-
sches Krankenhaus, D-58239 Schwerte, Germany
Studies of human medicine at Humboldt-University and Free University Berlin and
University of Vienna. Specialist for visceral surgery and traumatology. Fields of scientific work in traumatology: Biomechanics; Development of methods of operations
and implants, e.g. elastic rib clamps for the flail-chest stabilisation (1976); the cable
osteosynthesis system (1978) for tension bandings and related operations; the Endo-
Helix (1989), an atraumatic screwed-in intramedullary stabilisator for biological
osteosyntheses of humerus and childlike fractures of tubular bones.

ISBN 978-3-642-63059-0

Cataloging-in-Publication Data applied for

Die Deutsche Bibliothek – CIP-Einheitsaufnahme
Labitzke, Reiner : Manual of cable osteosyntheses / R. Labitzke. – Berlin ; Heidelberg ;
New York ; Barcelona ; Hong Kong ; London ; Milan ; Paris ; Singapore ; Tokyo :
Springer, 2000
ISBN 978-3-642-63059-0   ISBN 978-3-642-57167-1 (eBook)
DOI 10.1007/978-3-642-57167-1

© Springer-Verlag Berlin Heidelberg 2000
Originally published by Springer-Verlag Berlin Heidelberg New York in 2000
Softcover reprint of the hardcover 1st edition 2000

Cover design: E. Kirchner, D-69121 Heidelberg
Typesetting: FotoSatz Pfeifer GmbH, D-82166 Gräfelfing
Printed on acid-free paper – SPIN: 10718532   24/3135 – 5 4 3 2 1 0

This book is dedicated to all those who step by step helped in the creation, development and application of cables with their imagination, vision and drive and who in many cases have remained anonymous, as well as to Netti, Tini, Nina and Niki

Foreword

Professor Reiner Labitzke has authored a manual which focuses on the application of cable osteosyntheses. This technique is an integral part of the orthopaedic and trauma surgeon's armamentarium for the treatment of fractures and non-unions.

The manual describes osteosynthesis techniques which can be performed with cables after an introduction which includes a brief history of wires and cables in medicine. Biomechanical data comparing tensile strengths, cerclage wire and wire cables provide a scientific basis for the use of this technique.

The main section of the text describes the application of cables in the treatment of patella and olecranon fractures, in addition to its use in ankle joint and pilon fractures. This technique has also been used by the authors for the treatment of acetabular fractures and in performing osteotomies at the knee level.

The manual is well illustrated and contains explanatory illustrations and photographs for each of the techniques described. For orthopaedists and trauma surgeons not familiar with the many applications of cable osteosyntheses, this text will be a welcome addition to their library.

Andrew J. Weiland, MD, Professor of Orthopaedic and Plastic Surgery
at Cornell University Medical College, Attending Orthopaedic Surgeon,
Hospital for Special Surgery, New York, NY, USA

Foreword

FOREWORD

Reiner Labitzke had completed his surgical training at the time he applied for the vacant position of a senior registrar at the Department of Trauma Surgery in March 1976, 1 year after I had been elected chairman of the Traumatology Department and Director of the University Clinic in Essen. Being an "AO clinic" we followed strictly the AO philosophy with regard to clinical application of the newly developed operative methods for fracture fixation as well as to basic research and scientific analysis of fracture healing and bone remodeling under modified biomechanical conditions.

While interviewing Reiner Labitzke I was attracted by his enthusiastic dedication to biomechanical research projects. His constructive criticism of the classic tension band technique of fracture fixation had led him already to a new concept of bipolar compression by lateral tension banding. Disappointed by a high rate of instability and delayed union of olecranon fractures treated with the AO technique of placing the prestressed wire furthest from the load axis, we changed to Labitzke's technique of bilateral cable tension banding, which proved to be the perfect solution to our instability problems.

During the following years, from 1976–1980, Reiner Labitzke successfully studied the fields of biomechanics and metallurgy. Besides his daily work as a surgeon, his valuable conceptional input was rightly felt to merit recognition. He developed a new method of plate stabilization of flail chest injuries, introduced a "sleeve-rope closure" of median sternotomy in open heart surgery, modified bone instruments and implants in accordance with biomechanical results from the basic laboratory, and evaluated the methods developed by careful clinical evaluation of the patients during their initial treatment and follow up.

The "Manual of Cable Osteosyntheses" is an abstract of his biomechanical research and a comprehensive report of the remarkable clinical results he achieved within 20 years of operative fracture fixation. It can be recommended to surgeons specialized in trauma and orthopedic surgery, for their routine work and as advice in special cases.

Univ.-Prof. (em.) Dr. med. K.-P. Schmit-Neuerburg, Essen

Foreword

I find this book by Reiner Labitzke on the use of steel cables to repair bone defects fascinating because it shows how the excellent options for using steel cables in the field of technology can be implemented in medicine. It is about nature and human beings and the use of technical devices in life.

It says in the Bible: "And God saw everything that he had made, and, behold, it was very good."

But is nature always good and always effective? Is bone good? It breaks if it is subjected to extreme overloading. It is not ideal. No one would ever design the shock strut of an aeroplane or a bicycle frame using artificial bone.

Human beings cannot exist without nature, both animate and inanimate, and nature is therefore good, at least for human beings. However, we can also ask the opposite question, one that is quite rightly a central issue in our day and age: Are human beings good for nature? We invent houses, weapons, vehicles for use on land, in the air and in space without any relation to nature. We are afraid of the forces of nature.

If nature is very good, why not imitate it? It is now very popular to say that we should take nature as our guide. Of course, we may imitate nature, but it requires skill. "Our new design was inspired by nature" is something you often read, or even "Frei Otto studied spider webs and was thus able to build his wide-span roofs with thin nets of steel cables, such as the roof for the Olympic Stadium in Munich." Such statements are frequently made in books about bionics, but they are usually wrong.

Spider webs did not serve as a model, not even subconsciously. My roofs were built using the particular features of steel wire cables and the existing techniques used to construct cranes and suspension bridges, combined with the age-old production methods for tents and sails, and improved on the basis of new theoretical models of how to minimise the amount of material and energy required.

In the 1960s, when the first extremely thin, very wide-span nets hung in the air, the biologists involved in spider research recognised the similarity. Zoologists, architects, engineers and cable specialists compared ropes, knots, foundations and anchor points and did in fact discover real similarities between the webs spun by spiders and the nets constructed by architects. Both bear loads, are elastic, relatively fixed, are made of very thin, high-tensile, flexible elements and have a similar shape.

However, spiders spin their webs to catch insects as they always have done according to genetically anchored construction plans, while we continue to improve the construction of large net roofs to protect us against the rain and cold using the knowledge obtained in technology and architecture. Little has changed in reality, but all those involved have learned from each other. The zoologists have increased their understanding of human technology, while the architects have increased their understanding of the constructions found in nature. That is the first step towards regarding nature as a whole.

Bone is a part of nature, a part of human beings. It is neither very good nor bad. It has the outstanding feature that it can adapt by internal modification and, to a limited extent, is able to repair itself. In the case of complicated fractures, the help given by the treating physician is good, sometimes even very good, and often saves lives.

Instead of using the thick bonding wires that have commonly been used up to now, Reiner Labitzke repairs bone using fine, thin cables, high-performance products from the field of high-grade steel/fine-wire technology – at long last, a method that is heading in the right direction. The bonding wires that have been used up to now are too stiff and take all the load instead of forming an elastic, mechanical unit with the bone.

It is a logical method that has been thought through very well and is based on knowledge at the exact border between technology and biology, i.e. wire cable constructions that are subject to tensile stress, but also at the limits of our biological understanding of bone. Bones are bundles of fibres and three-dimensional nets containing gaps filled with hard substance. There is no equivalent to bone in the field of technology, although there are certain similarities to timber-frame construction, pre-stressed concrete and construction using fibre-strengthened plastics.

By introducing steel cables into medicine, I believe that Reiner Labitzke has opened up the way for the surgical treatment of fractures to be further developed, also in terms of the materials used. I can also imagine that instead of individual cables, for example, whole networks may be used. Extremely soft or particularly hard types of steel or elastic wires twisted like spirals that extend and stretch, forming a transition to screws, can be used as required. I can also imagine other materials being used that either remain in the bone or can be removed, and material that, although initially required to be very strong, is degradable without leaving any residue.

The present level of technological knowledge is high and developments are rapid. Knowledge about bone has also grown in the past decade. However, bone remains the same. It cannot be improved. It merely changes in the course of an organism's life from being soft to being hard, it alters its shape, and it may break and grow together again.

But do we know how its shape and fine structure arise, how the fibres really bear loads in conjunction with the hard substance and what the significance of the internal pressure is, for example?

In the course of our work on living constructions, we discovered that, although the hard substance of bone primarily reduces deformation under load, its weight-bearing capacity depends above all on the network of high-tensile connective tissue fibres that organise growth, determine the shape and also, in conjunction with the internal pressure, reshape, repair and even continually improve in relation to the load.

It is the structure of the connective tissue fibres and the adapted internal pressure that are behind the secret of how the shape and adjusted weight-bearing capacity of bone arise. The fine, load-dependent deformations that continually occur in the hard substance stored between the connective tissue also apparently allow the fine structure to adapt to altered load. This would appear to be a very particular role of the hard substance.

Great progress could be achieved in bone surgery if the self-repair mechanisms could be stimulated not only to heal fractures, but also to restore entire bones.

There are still a number of open questions for the generations to come and a range of details that doctors, architects and engineers ought to discuss and work on together in the near future. Unfortunately, this is something that has only occurred in exceptional cases up to now.

For me, the introduction of elastic steel cable constructions not only marks the beginning of a considerable improvement in surgical techniques, it also reflects our improved understanding of the weight-bearing behaviour of bone.

I hope that Reiner Labitzke is able to make good progress in further developing the surgical treatment of bones, and I hope that this book is very successful. It is, I believe, a particular milestone on a long road.

Univ.-Prof. (em.) Dr.-Ing. Dr. h.c.mult. Frei Otto
Director of Institute for Leightweight Structures (IL)
University of Stuttgart, Germany

Foreword

It is common practice for the author of a new scientific book to ask one of his academic teachers to write a foreword so as to give the book a good start and to generally facilitate its acceptance in the scientific community for which it has been written. In this case, the situation is somewhat different: I am neither one of Professor Reiner Labitzke's academic teachers nor even an academic in the field of medicine. I am an experimental physicist who is writing this short foreword to the book of a friend and esteemed colleague from another field, a man who certainly does not need any extra help from an outsider like me in promoting something that has turned out as well as the piece of work that now lies before us.

Professor Labitzke and I met – perhaps not surprisingly – in a hospital in the summer of 1973. As a young professor at the Ruhr University in Bochum my Achilles tendon ruptured after playing soccer with my students and I was operated on immediately at the most renowned hospital in town, „Bergmannsheil," by the famous surgeon Professor Rehn. Reiner Labitzke was one of his young interns, who, after having found out that I was a physicist, spent every free minute of his time at my bedside asking me questions about physics. I noticed at that time already that besides his dedication to the medical profession, he was always curious, the basic drive which motivates a scientist to want to understand nature and which may even lead to new discoveries. We became friends and I recall that, after being released from the hospital, Professor Rolf Niedermayer, my late colleague in the physics department at the university, and I designed and built, upon request of Reiner Labitzke, a small apparatus in our mechanical workshop which was able to adjust and measure by a simple method the torque given to a single wire when it is distorted, a problem typically encountered by a surgeon working on the osteosyntheses of fracture and dislocation using monofilament wires. In 1974 I took a chair in physics at the Technical University in Darmstadt and so our direct involvement in discussions and experiments relevant to problems of physics and engineering naturally ceased. Over the years, though, I have taken a personal interest in what Professor Labitzke, who already for some time now has been director of the Surgical Clinic of the University of Witten/Herdekke, has achieved in this field. About 2 years ago, I also had the opportunity and pleasure to give him some final advice on the physics and engineering topics presented in this book.

It goes without saying that the principles of physics and engineering also hold in medicine, and as a physicist I can very well judge that Professor Labitzke has cleverly, convincingly, and in terms of physics completely correctly transformed the well-known principle of flexible multistrand cable systems into applications for osteosynthesis. When he pioneered the introduction of cables into the surgical treatment of bone fractures instead of the hitherto generally used technique of employing rigid cerclage wires in 1978, I already wondered why this had not been done before. The former principle has so many more advantages – not least of guaranteeing much higher stability – than the latter, and it is hoped that something that is so obvious in physics and engineering will also become accepted in medicine. Therefore, may Professor Labitzke's clearly structured and intelligently and, also from the point of view of a physicist, didactically well-written book pave the way to acceptance of this technique, become widely distributed, and soon be a standard text in modern osteosynthesis.

Professor Dr. rer.nat. Dr. h.c. mult. Achim Richter
Director of the Nuclear Physics Institute
Technical University Darmstadt, Germany

Foreword

In the late 1960's, one of us was trained by Sir John Charnley in the philosophy and practice of total hip arthroplasty. The Charnley method of low friction arthroplasty was designed with a small 22,25 mm head and, as a result, conventional approaches had a high incidence of dislocation. For this reason John Charnley insisted on the trochanteric osteotomy approach to the hip joint as an integral part of the technique of low friction arthroplasty. The advantages of this approach were, increased exposure, and increased stability of the prosthetic joint post-operatively, due to the fact that the abductor muscles could be tensioned by the distal advancement of the greater trochanter.

The major disadvantage of this approach was due to a relatively high incidence of trochanteric detachment. Fixation techniques at that time involved the use of monofilament stainless steel wire. It was this single clinical problem which led us to the realization of the advantages of multifilament cables over monofilament wires. In this excellent manual of cable osteosyntheses, Professor Labitzke has kindly referred to our first clinical results which were published in the *Journal of Bone and Joint Surgery* in 1983.

At more or less the same time as we were developing enthusiasm and excitement about the use of multifilament cables in orthopaedic surgery, Professor Labitzke was doing exactly the same thing on another continent – as is so often the case in science. In the practice of orthopaedic surgery and traumatology it is always exciting to find a colleague with directly similar interests and views.

Professor Labitzke has indeed provided an authentic manual covering the historical, experimental and clinical aspects of the use of multifilament cables in orthopaedic surgery and traumatology. His in-depth bibliography, especially in the historical section, and the wealth of information that he has presented on the subject is highly commendable. The strength issues of monofilament wire are compared with the superior mechanical properties of multifilament cable. In this context, we could add our own realization of the importance of the superior fatigue strength of multifilament cable compared to monofilament wire. He goes on to present an in-depth analysis of tension banding and convincing arguments in favour of bi-lateral tension banding with cables. The clinical sections discuss in depth the techniques that he has developed for treatment of fractures of the patella, olecranon process, medial malleolus, and osseous prominences including the greater trochanter, acetabulum and that of the pelvic ring. In addition he has developed techniques using multifilament cables for valgus osteotomy of the proximal tibia, ankle arthrodesis and certain soft tissue injuries. There is also a brief section on the treatment of shattering of the femur shaft following total endoprosthesis insertion. The Dall-Miles cable system, which is similar in principle to the system developed by Professor Labitzke, has been used in many of these applications, but has probably been used most extensively in revision total hip arthroplasty – especially for allograft fixation in deficient femoral bone stock, periprosthetic fractures of the femur and re-attachment of the greater trochanter. The system has been used extensively in North America and world-wide with very gratifying clinical results.

For this reason, we are particularly delighted to find that our successful experience with multifilament cable is shared by Professor Labitzke, not only in principle, but also in his clinical results.

We are in full agreement with the author when he says "Now, however, the time has come for wire to be replaced ... the future, indeed, belongs to cables".

Desmond M. Dall, M. Ch(Orth), F.R.C.S,
Emeritus Professor of Clinical Orthopaedic Surgery
University of Southern California, Los Angeles, Calif., U.S.A.

Anthony W. Miles MSc(Eng), Reader in Biomechanics
University of Bath, Bath, England

Preface

Tension bandings are a principle with which technology has been able to tame great forces. Nobody would even dream of using rigid wire, a fact that one would readily acknowledge upon examining suspension bridges that today span many of the world's largest rivers. This principle, transferred to the comparatively small forces existent in bone surgery, has always fascinated me. It is for this reason that I have never really understood why one of the best tools that engineers have at their disposal should not also be put to good use within the operating theatre.

This treatise deals to a large extent with the biomechanics of the tension band. Here it was necessary – with the aid of engineering science – to newly define the theoretical concept of operative tension banding, which to date has raised a few erroneous assumptions within the medical community.

Consequently, the necessity arose to adapt wire cables for operative use and to develop a practical system with appropriate tools. Twenty years of experience have shown that this attempt indeed has been successful. Since 1978, I have been using supple wire cables designed in accordance with my own specifications for osteosyntheses, a process which throughout the past decades has usually been reserved for cerclage wire. In stark contrast to rigid wire, wire cables have many advantages which are reflected in a broadening of indications as well as in an improvement of results. Many colleagues, who have been using this method for almost as long as I have, and indeed several large companies have come to value these advantages. Despite a patent protection different types of cables, ranging in price, have been steadily entering the German as well as the international market, a fact that will undoubtedly be beneficial to the success of the wire cable.

With this book, richly illustrated with 400 single descriptions and 5 diagrams, I would like to pass on my knowledge. It seemed inappropriate to publish these findings at an earlier stage, simply because the euphoria that is often present when implementing a new idea should eventually give way to a certain level of objectivity.

I set to work with realistic expectations, and a conviction that is possibly best summed up by Max Planck in his "Wissenschaftliche Selbstbiographie" of 1955 – a scientific autobiography: "A new scientific truth does not usually establish itself in a way that its opponents are convinced and declare themselves converted, but rather due to the fact that they gradually demise, thus allowing the new generation to grow up with the truth."

This book is designed to appeal not only to the experienced surgeon but also to younger doctors with a questing attitude to medical life. It offers an overview of the historical and technical facts. The reader is also given the opportunity to thoroughly study the principles of tension banding as well as the ideal material to realise it – wire cables.

Despite the scientific proof of the theories underlying the following explanations it would be inappropriate to dismiss possible reservations or criticisms. Within this respect, allow me to quote from Theodor Billroth's preface, published in 1876 in "Über das Lehren und Lernen" (On Teaching and Learning): "One might choose to judge me, but one will not succeed in diminishing the value of my work, which is characterised by the accurate compilation of pertinent facts, many of which will be as new to my colleagues as they were to me upon stumbling across them" [273].

I extend my thanks to all those who have accompanied and supported this work – for their consideration, assistance and patience. To my wife and children, who in the last years saw me spending more time in my study than anywhere else. To my hospital colleagues, especially to Dr. Hahn for supporting me when it came to studying databases, retrieving and sorting X-ray bags and outpatient clinic notes, as well as the call-up of patients. My friends T. Redelings, Dr. G. Conrad and Dr. M. Mielsch gave me interesting stimuli during the writing of the book. My thanks also go to Mrs. B. Klett and Mrs. H. Bongert for dealing with the paperwork; St.Clair Bull Consulting translated the text into English. My daughter, Mrs. N. Labitzke, was a great help in proofreading and in drawing up the subject index. Mr. Schilling from the *Zentralbibliothek für Medizin* in Cologne helped me in tracking down long-lost original works. Mr. Bowe, the former head of the workshop of the Institut für Werkstoffkunde at the *Ruhr University Bochum*, performed trials on the stability of wires and cables as well as operative procedures. This work was updated thanks to Mr. Grünewald and Dr. Partz of the board of directors of the *Stahlwerk Ergste Westig GmbH* in Schwerte. Mr. Könnecke of *Feinseilerei Engelmann* in Hanover promoted the development of wire cables from the start and assisted me in word and deed. Mr. Bahmüller, Team Design Schwerte, took the photographs of the implants and the tools and Mrs. B. Rosigkeit provided the sketches. I would also like to thank Mr. Runkel, chief engineer of the *Rheinische Brückenbauamt*, for the graphic demonstrations and many technical details about suspension bridges. I also thank Prof. Dr. Schmit-Neuerburg of the *Klinikum der GHS Essen*, my former surgical chief, for his much appreciated medical input, and Prof. Dr. rer. nat. Dr. h.c. mult. Richter of the *Technische Universität Darmstadt* for the technical foreword. My gratitude also goes to Mr. Dall, M.D., South Africa, and Mr. Miles, Engineer, from Bath, GB – who were the first using cables after my own publications – as well as to Professor Weiland, M.D., New York and past President of the American Orthopaedic Association for their contributions. My thank also goes to Prof. Dr.-Ing. Dr. h.c. mult. Otto, the former director of the Institute for Leightweight Structures of the *University of Stuttgart*, who applies cables for his visionary architectural constructions, and who has emphasized "how the excellent options for using steel cables in the field of technology can be implemented in medicine". Not least, I thank Mrs. G. Schröder and Mrs. M. Himberger from *Springer-Verlag* for their support.

Univ.-Prof. Dr. Reiner Labitzke
Schwerte, Germany

Contents

CHAPTER 1

Introduction

This book focuses on wire cables, and includes a description of their origins, their development and diverse uses in technology, as well as their possibilities and advantages in surgical medicine. In the latter, the main indication is for tension banding. However, because this principle has – very one-sidedly and from a technical point of view incorrectly – been viewed as dynamic-eccentric, it stands to reason that its mechanism should be described in detail. The mathematical formula, as a vehicle of scientific thought, is not sufficient however when dealing with medical aspects, due to the fact that it frequently lacks the desired level of lucidity. All details discussed in this book, which at times are relatively complex, will therefore be expressed as simply as possible.

Following a publication on this subject in 1997 [220], the director of a trauma surgery clinic phoned out of the blue to tell me that he had at last understood the principles of tension bands. Since his time as an assistant, he had been using the accepted technique and, despite some failures, he had never had doubts about the efficacy of its underlying principle, so deeply was it ingrained. Apparently a widespread phenomenon!

Impressed by their versatility, I soon realized that the standard criteria used in textbooks or academic publications were hardly adequate to capture fully and convey the level of enthusiasm generated during a lengthy study of the properties and possible uses of wire cables. So many once forgotten historical and technical details have been brought to light that they deserve to be included in what essentially is a surgical treatise; they will give further insight into the subject.

> ▶ This publication comprises three parts: historical, experimental, and clinical. The latter is the most substantial section and is intended as a "surgical atlas" for general and orthopedic surgeons.

He who propagates things new without delving into past *history* and without honoring those who have gone before him would paint an incomplete and abstract picture. For every invention has undergone its unique form of evolution. F. Müller [263], Emeritus for plastic surgery at *Bergmannsheil Bochum*, the oldest trauma clinic worldwide, was correct when – as part of his retirement speech in 1990 – he stated: "The speed with which time elapses also shortens our memory of what has preceded, of great names and great deeds. We are quick to forget that we stand on the shoulders of those whom have gone before us."

A lot of time was devoted to composing a *chronicle* of wires in bone surgery. The quest to find the origins led to the very roots of trauma surgery.

During the research stage of this book I soon became aware of the fact that it would be impossible to reconstruct perfectly the exact first use of wire, an implant often disregarded as such, and the beginnings of the first trauma surgery. Various developments are to be observed in different clinical centers. It remains unknown who actually was the first to have had the idea of using wire. Occasionally, it was also impossible to judge who was the first to have proposed a new procedure and it was often difficult to ascertain who was the first to have standardized procedures. "One can see," wrote Pletzer [302], a student of Trendelenburg in Bonn, in his dissertation on patella fractures, "how in this area too, arguments about priorities made agreement impossible."

As surgery began to develop with the discovery of general anesthesia and antiseptics, wire also benefited. It was used sporadically to begin with, later systematically and more frequently, in the healing of broken bones. It was the basis for trauma surgery and to this day has contributed much to its development. Now, however, the time has come for wire to be replaced.

In the second section, data compiled on the basis of *experiments* are listed with the aim of evaluating and comparing wires and cables from a mechanical point of view. The outstanding properties of a wire cable are, however, not only reflected in mere figures but also in the overwhelming clinical evidence and thus ultimately in the well-being of patients, the most important yardstick to be judged by. Results ascertained independently of each other [13, 104, 135, 145, 220, 356] speak for themselves – or should we say, for cables. Rigid, homogeneous wire, i.e., the cerclage wire that we have been accustomed to for so many decades and that is still eulogized throughout the world, does not even come close to the excellent results of materials testing achieved by supple cables. Moreover, cables are much easier to handle and are more effective than wires. The future, indeed, belongs to cables.

The versatility of wire cables is described and discussed in detail in the third section, the *clinical part*. Even a fleeting glance at X-rays reveals the higher surgical quality achieved by this approach (Fig. 1):

Owing to the fact that these are operating methods using new forms of implant (which have often developed automatically), the indications and the detailed technical implementation of osteosyntheses are just as important as the results, with which, in turn, these methods can be evaluated conclusively. The statistical analysis includes over 1200 cases – at the time of printing, this figure had increased to 1600. Frequent indications are ideally suited to define the cables' main area of use. It is, however, the rarer cases that reveal the true strengths of cables. One will acknowledge that cables ensure results that remained unattainable in the era of cerclage wires.

Many of the problems occurring are portrayed in X-rays of the patella and olecranon. That is due to the fact that, since my early days as an assistant to Jörg Rehn in Bochum, I have kept most of these X-rays. Naturally, all statements made based on these X-rays are valid for all applications discussed in this publication.

For easier reading, long quotations have been shortened without highlighting the omitted subordinate clauses. It goes without saying that the meaning of the quotation remains unaltered.

International distribution of the ostheosynthesis set, System Labitzke, is by ABAmed Express, P. O. Box 5131, D-58239 Schwerte, Fax: 0049-2304-70728, E-mail: www.abamedexpress.de

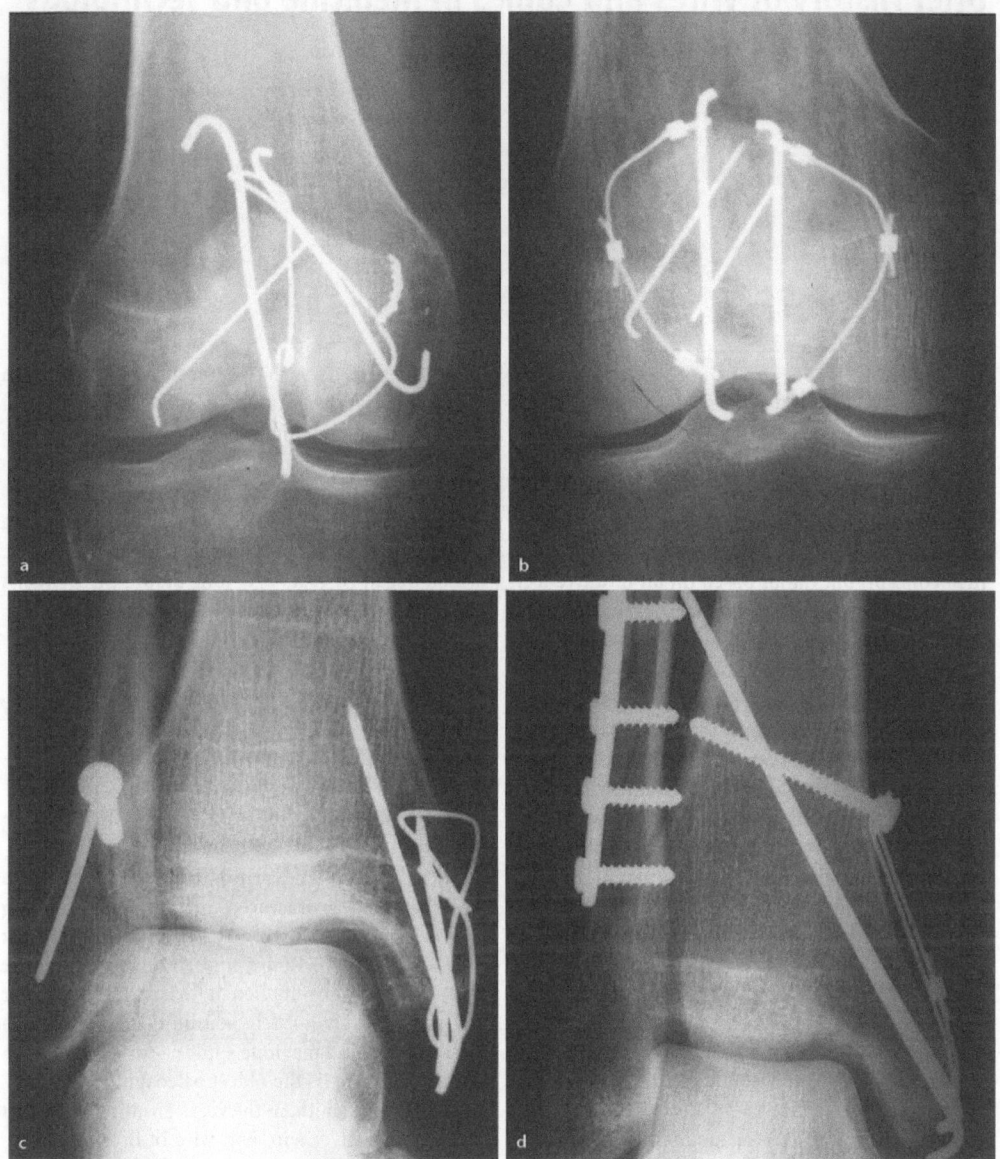

Fig. 1. High biomechanical quality of cable osteontheses in comparison with cerclage wire techniques

CHAPTER 2

Brief History of Wires and Cables in Medicine and Technology

History is a jungle, and no path that one cuts into it
opens up the whole forest

Sebastian Haffner

2.1
Conventional Binding Wire

Binding wire gave surgery new impetus. As long ago as 150 years it facilitated the transition from the age of conservative treatment of trauma to the era of surgery. At first, wires were used without a system or firm concept, but rather based on an intuitive feeling for "bone sutures," by which everyone understood his own method of holding fragments together. From 1870 onwards, Lord Lister – with aseptic precautions – adapted bone fragments systematically using wires. It was thanks to him that know-how became more focused, thus leading to a few generally acknowledged procedures, one of the main examples of which was Payrs' method of patella wiring – very popular for a long time – cf. Fig. 53. Bone suture became an all-embracing term, and was in common use from around 1860 until 1960. Everything that we call osteosynthesis today would be referred to as bone suture by older authors [183]. Even in 1944, R. Zenker [168] understood bone suture in the broadest sense of the word to be any protection of the fragments against a renewed displacement. In the narrower sense it is a metallic suture [238] and has always been seen as such.

Bone surgery took a tremendous step forward thanks to the systematic work of Willeneggeret al. [264, 266] from Switzerland, who in 1957 formed a working party for questions relating to osteosynthesis, in short the AO/ASIF (Arbeitsgemeinschaft für Osteosynthesefragen). Later it opened its doors to trauma surgeons from many other countries. It assimilated known operating procedures and standardized them as AO techniques. Its merits lay on the one hand in the development of operating techniques using standardized implants and on the other hand in the advancement of basic research. However, only that which changes and adapts will continue to exist. As such, the recent departure from rigid osteosynthesis to a more dynamic way of thinking and operating must be seen as a return to medical values. This transition from rigidity to flexibility also affected cerclage wire. Its gradual replacement with supple wire cables can be seen as the dawn of a new age of "biological" osteosyntheses, which began 20 years ago, long before the Zeitgeist made an official introduction.

2.1.1
Bone Suture: The Original Form of Osteosynthesis

It is virtually impossible to determine when the first sporadic use of wire began, because it had been utilized in ancient times. Hippocrates is supposed to have splinted a fractured mandible by binding neighboring teeth with gold wire. Celsus brought this knowledge to Rome, and Arabian doctors are supposed to have applied it to shattered tubular bones [360]. It can safely be said that wire was the first implant and the bone suture – for a long time a technical term – is the oldest osteosynthesis procedure. At their zenith, in the years around the turn of the century, silver wire and wire of bronze, aluminum, or fired iron were preferred; later Krupp stainless steel wire was introduced [64, 167, 223, 338, 388].

Bone suture as a term was first associated with Wilhelm Busch [43], Bonn 1857. Up to this time teachings relating to fractures were – with occasional exceptions – purely conservative [56, 93, 105, 125]. The almost incurable non-union first promoted open procedures, namely the fixation of debrided fracture ends with foreign material. "This principle," wrote Busch, "forms the basis of the bone suture, in which after a performed resection one pierces the fragments completely and ties them together with a rustproof wire so that the sawed surfaces of the bone are pressed together."

The first successful bone suture in pre-antiseptic and pre-anaesthetic times was achieved by Rodgers [321] at New York Hospital on 31 July 1827. He sutured a non-healing humerus fracture in a 15-year-old boy with silver wire: "I drilled the ends of the ununited fragments and brought them into apposition by means of a silver wire loop."

In 1775, Lapuyade and Sicre from France had been less successful. They attempted an open reduction of a humerus fracture, and "brass or iron wire was used to fasten the fragments together" says Robinson [319, 94]. The patient died and the case led to legal proceedings. According to Zierold [436], Icart in the same year also united a fracture with iron wires. However, that is incorrect. In the original work [143] Icart defended the two accused Toulouse surgeons – without ever actually having done it himself – by saying that "...this thread of brass, of silver or of lead *would be* applicable in certain cases."

In an era when antisepsis and asepsis were unknown, the idea of a fracture surgically opened and the fragments reduced with bare hands and held together with wires must have been thought of as sacrilege. According to Ceci [46], Genoa, as early as "three hundred years ago an Italian, Severino, mentioned the direct suture of a broken piece of the patella, for which he was considered to be deranged." Wahl [402] in 1883 doubted the practical implementation because "...a case history of a performed patella suture is not available in writing."

According to Ravoth, as one will find upon reading the secondary literature, Dieffenbach has the patent rights on the first suturing of the patella [90, 139, 171, 252, 264, 338, 402]. Pletzer [302] believed that this was not correct: "According to Jalaguier the glory belongs to the Englishman Rhea Barton (1834). The first written notes about a patellar suturing seem to stem from Cooper, San Francisco, who in 1861 first recommended the bone suture as one of his successfully applied methods." This information was soon confirmed [162, 402].

However, the heyday of the bone suture was in the middle of the nineteenth century, "which was an inspired era for medicine" [176]. Two fundamental requirements, which are based on the most beneficial discoveries of mankind, were met – general anesthesia and antisepsis: in 1844 the American dentist Horace Wells initiated the first laughing gas narcosis, and in 1846 the US dentist William Morton, a pupil of Wells, carried out the first ether narcosis with

John Warren, the famous surgeon at Massachusetts General Hospital, Boston. In the same year Ignaz Semmelweis, a German-Hungarian gynecologist in Vienna, became aware that post-partum death occurred due to sections with unclean hands. He introduced hand disinfection with chlorinated water. Louis Pasteur recognized that microbes produced fermentation, Robert Koch pinpointed many of them (most importantly the tubercle bacillus) and Joseph Lister, then professor of surgery at Glasgow University, found that the use of phenol or carbolic acid, was a useful measure against microbes [1, 238, 379, 380]. Despite long and stubborn ignorance of this knowledge, his first publication in the Lancet in 1867 heralded the dawn of a new "antiseptic age" [237].

Lister also brought about a more systematic approach to bone sutures – "his second great achievement after carbolic acid, alas often forgotten" [219]. Thus, he should be regarded as the true founder of wire osteosynthesis. Even prior to 1880 he had discovered "that the use of a metallic suture, antiseptically applied, which we had employed in ununited fractures of the shafts of the long bones, ought, in suitable cases, to be extended to the olecranon and patella" [238].

Since Lister, it had become possible to operate without the constant, often fatal, risk of infection – without pain and even in cases that were not deemed an emergency, but rather an attempt at restoring "quality of life." His techniques spread quickly throughout Europe, where Trendelenburg and Lucas-Championiere became the leading protagonists [377].

The successor to Lister's technique, direct bone suturing, also an openly performed osteosynthesis with wires, was almost certainly developed by Erwin Payr. It dates back to before the turn of the century and was often performed beyond the second half of the twentieth century [90, 130, 171, 338].

Cerclage is attributed to Paul Berger, Paris 1892 [14]. It is not as such a bone suture due to the fact that the bone is not pierced. Today it is still used around the patella as an extensor tension band near the joint in order to prevent its dorsal gaping. It also holds together a split femur during prosthesis replacement procedures.

Bernhard Weber's work (St. Gallen 1963 [408]) on the fundamentals and possibilities of tension band osteosynthesis almost did away with previous wire sutures at one fell swoop – a new era of fracture treatment began, with treatments that could be adapted for use on the whole skeleton. His idea consisted of neutralizing distracting muscle forces through pre-stressed wires and, in doing so, pulling together widely displaced fractures. This is described in more detail in Chap. 4.4.

The implementation of technical recommendations, i.e., to produce *static* interfragmentary compression by means of pre-tension in the resulting forces [195–198], as well as the introduction of highly durable, flexible wire cables as suitable tension devices [200, 202, 203, 206] have greatly improved the results of tension banding.

2.1.2
Chronology of Osteosyntheses

In the search for the origins of cerclage wire a few hidden treasures of other types of osteosyntheses came to light. These were published in 1995 [219]. In this case a short chronological overview will suffice (Fig. 2).

There are five osteosynthesis principles: listed in chronological order they are:

1. Wire osteosynthesis – the modern version with wire cables
2. External fixation
3. Plates and screws
4. K-wires
5. Medullary cavity stabilizers

In 1843, Carl Wutzer, Bonn, introduced a "screw device" which had the feature of an external fixator, but unfortunately this was not successful. In 1851, Bernhard von Langenbeck, Dieffenbach's successor at the *Charité*, Berlin, had success with an improved version [103, 279], but it was Lambotte 1902 [222] who achieved a breakthrough with the fixator. Several modern versions have proved to be successful, as has the internal fixator for the spine.

Carl Hansmann, Hamburg 1886 [37, 120, 430], is heralded as the inventor of the bone plate, although in the same year Themistocles Gluck, a pupil of von Langenbeck, also reported on osteosyntheses with plates and screws [420]. The plate was eventually successful after improvements by Lane [264, 360]. As a point of interest – the renowned Halstedt himself took the Hansmann plate to the United States: "I happened to be in Hamburg when Hansmann, Schede's first assistant, was perfecting this method."

These achievements were never completely forgotten [94, 171], but it was not until recently that they were brought to the fore [37, 279, 430].

The forerunner of the K-wire was the wire extension (Codivilla and Steinmann 1907 [365]) and is attributed to Kirschner [166], Heidelberg 1909. Despite relative instabilities it is still in frequent use for pediatric fractures and fractures of the radius loco typico [160] as well as in the Ilisaroff device [331].

In 1939 Küntscher [191–193] developed the fifth principle of osteosynthesis, the intramedullary nail. Vehemently rejected at first, it is presently used worldwide and experiencing a renaissance as interlocking and compact ("unreamed") nails.

Fifty years later, the spiral-shaped "EndoHelix" [213, 214, 216, 218] is showing good results. Screwed in atraumatically, not hammered in, kind to the endosteal vascular system and the osteoblasts, it almost conforms to the ideal of a biological osteosynthesis – cf. Fig. 106.

2.1.3
Experiences with Cerclage Wire: A Critique

How cerclage wire is used was and is common surgical knowledge. It was never very popular because it is difficult to handle and the results are rarely satisfactory. In 1905, Thiem [377] found it troublesome, Vorschütz [400] not ideal, Shaw [356] in 1988 saw ill-fated results, Labitzke and Towfig [205] and von Issendorff et al. [145] found it unsuitable. According to von Brunn [31] and Brill and Hopf [29], it did not establish adequate stability or interfragmentary compression; rather, according to Shaw, only inadequate bone stabilization. Its ends are twisted or occasionally turned into a loop. Both types of fixation provide little resistance and were soon criticized.

Zur Verth 1925 [395]: "It is not the unsatisfactory torsion knot alone that in the latter years have made the wire suture in bone surgery less popular. Still one cannot deny that the knot of the wire suture is unmanageable and unsatisfactory. Using the wire flexes it is possible to avoid loosening; however, the wire may well rupture once pulled too tight. The suture has to be repeated, an often time-consuming procedure that is hardly a salutary experience for the patient".

Kirschner 1925 [167]: "The fastener recommended by M. Borchardt, created by bending one end of the wire, pulled through the loop of the other end of

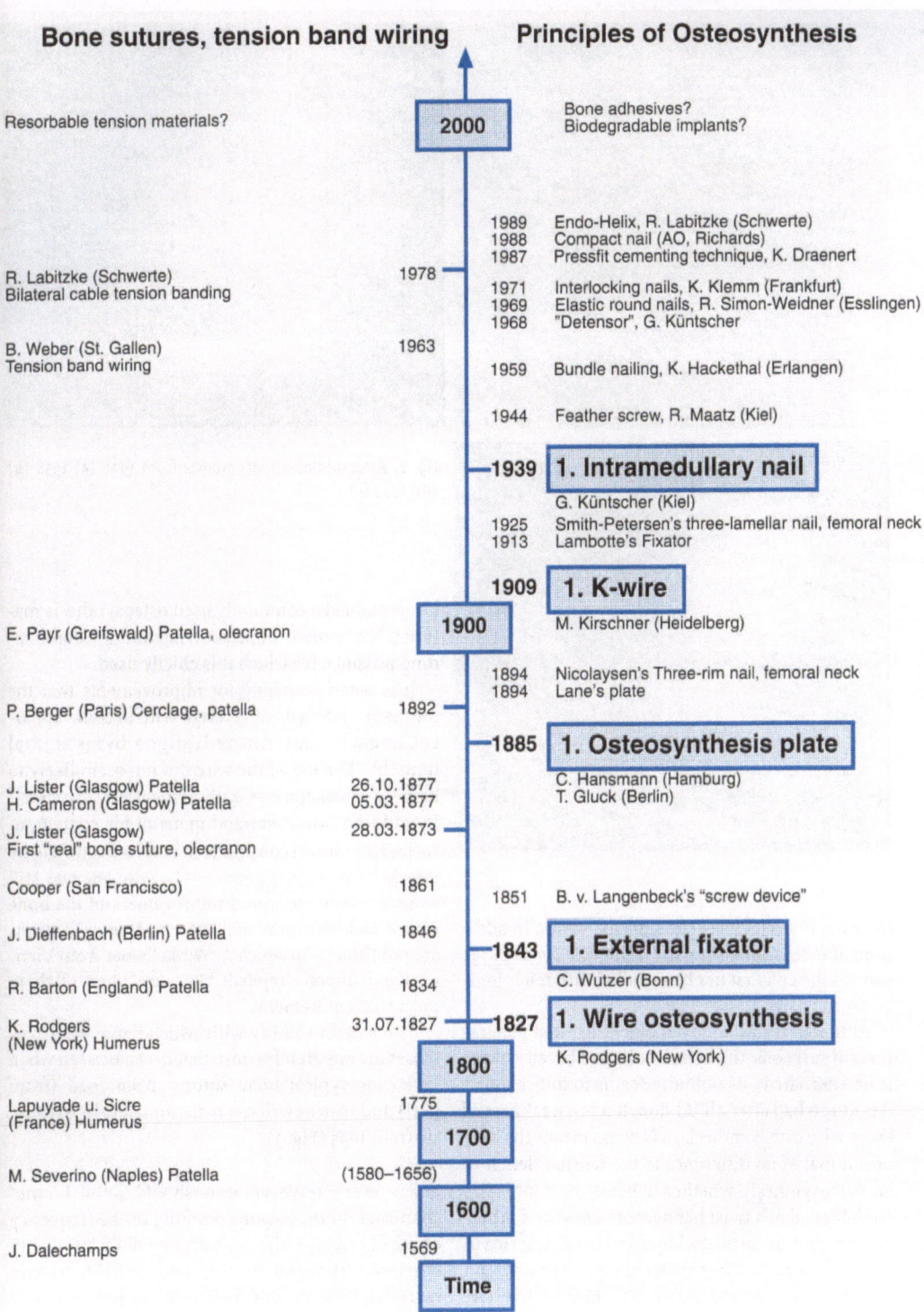

Fig. 2. Chronogram of the Development of Osteosynthesis

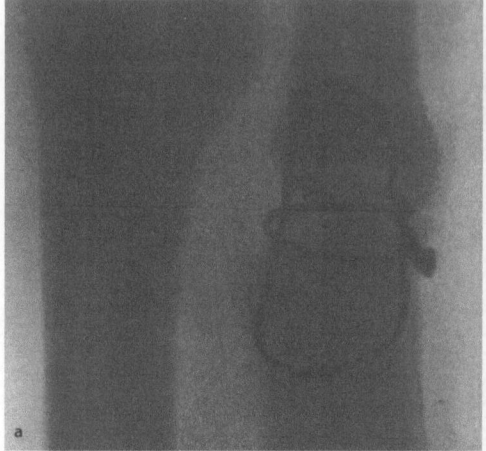

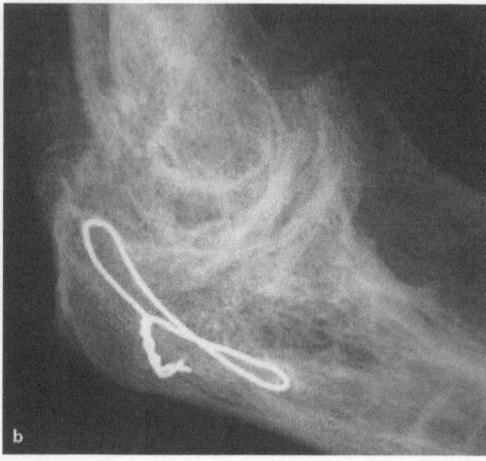

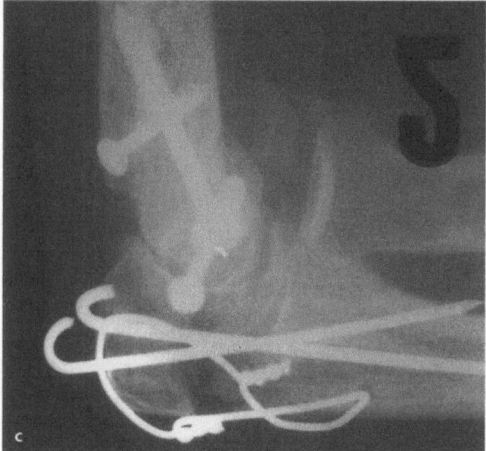

Fig. 3. Attempts of osteosynthesis from 1926 (**a**) 1958 (**b**) and 1995 (**c**)

the wire, is stretched at the slightest strain. In addition, the tension originally achieved slackens as soon as the end that has been pulled through is folded down."

Although it has annoyed and frustrated generations of surgeons, the twist is still used because there is no alternative. Its ubiquity seems to indicate that it is not so bad after all. Although it is a weakness of every wire osteosynthesis, it is by no means the only one: it makes no difference to the tension deficit of an osteosynthesis whether a bend or a loop has straightened or a twist has become untwisted. Alternatives, such as the ideas imported from America in the 1920s, include wires soldered together [395], and new introductions such as the wire plug for the sternum [381] and a screw lock [95, 96] are merely slight improvements because they retain the rigid cerclage wire, the cause of all problems. Irrespective of this, it

has remained a commonly used osteosynthesis material. It has made bone suturing and tension banding possible, for which it is chiefly used.

It is when searching for improvements that the mechanical deficits of cerclage wire become apparent. Its quality was criticized early on, by Lister [239] himself: "The use of the wire did not seem likely to be very satisfactory as a permanent arrangement." In addition, Kirschner and many of his contemporaries (see above) considered it and its fixation to be inferior. Demel [63] pondered "...why one was still working on the technical improvement of the bone suture and why more and more new modifications are published." To which A. Winkelbauer from Vienna [423] directly replied: "Because none of them meet the requirements."

The lack of solidity with which some osteosyntheses are apparently constructed, can be seen when reviewing typical bone sutures from 1926 (from [64]) and 1958 as well as an attempt at osteosynthesis from 1995 (Fig. 3).

Today every osteosynthesis should fulfill biomechanical criteria. Anyone pointing to the frequency of use of cerclage wire as an argument for its quality overlooks, above all, that it is not a suitable tension material, because it is impossible to produce controllable interfragmentary compression. That is because of its unfavorable material properties, especially due to the plastic elongation which occurs

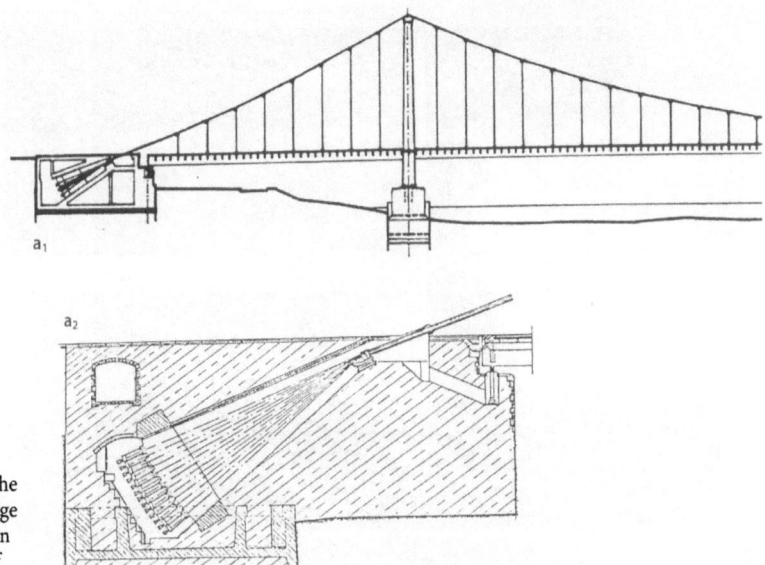

Fig. 4. Firm foundation of the cables of a suspension bridge (**a**). So called simple tension band without anchorage of the cerclage wire (**b**)

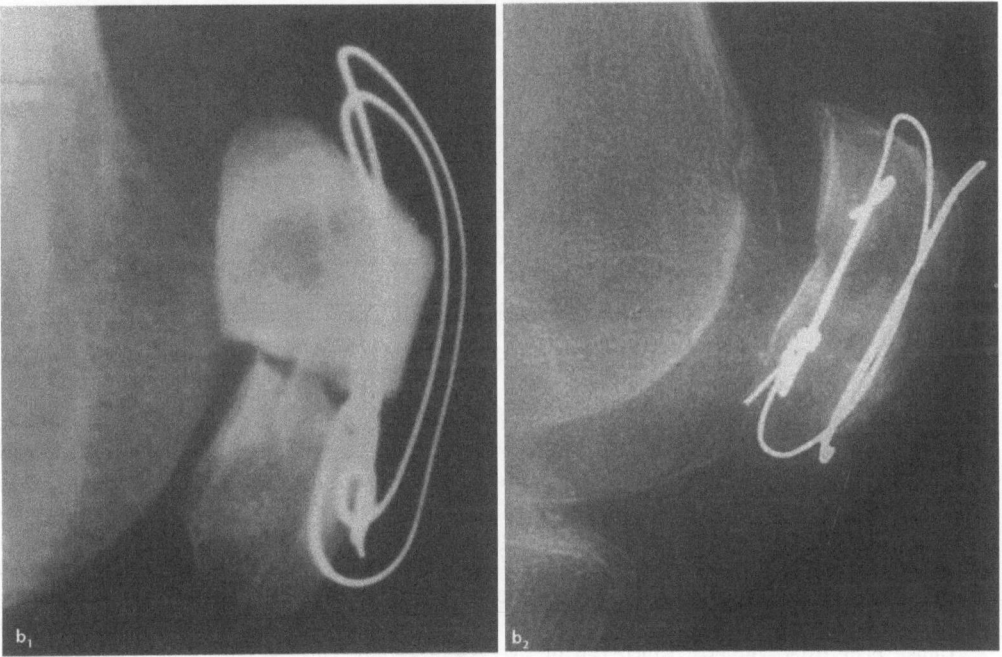

at an early stage and the high level of rigidity which paradoxically leads to a low degree of resistance to tearing. That is why cerclage wire is not suitable as a material for osteosynthesis.

In order to be applicable to more than mere fragment adaptation the tension band wire must be pre-stressed. In this respect it is necessary to anchor it to auxiliary points – Kirschner wires, screws, or transosseously into a bore canal. This is not universally acknowledged. There are still those to whom going "around the tendon insertion" seems quite sufficient [41, 266, 434]. Suffice it to say that the supporting ca-

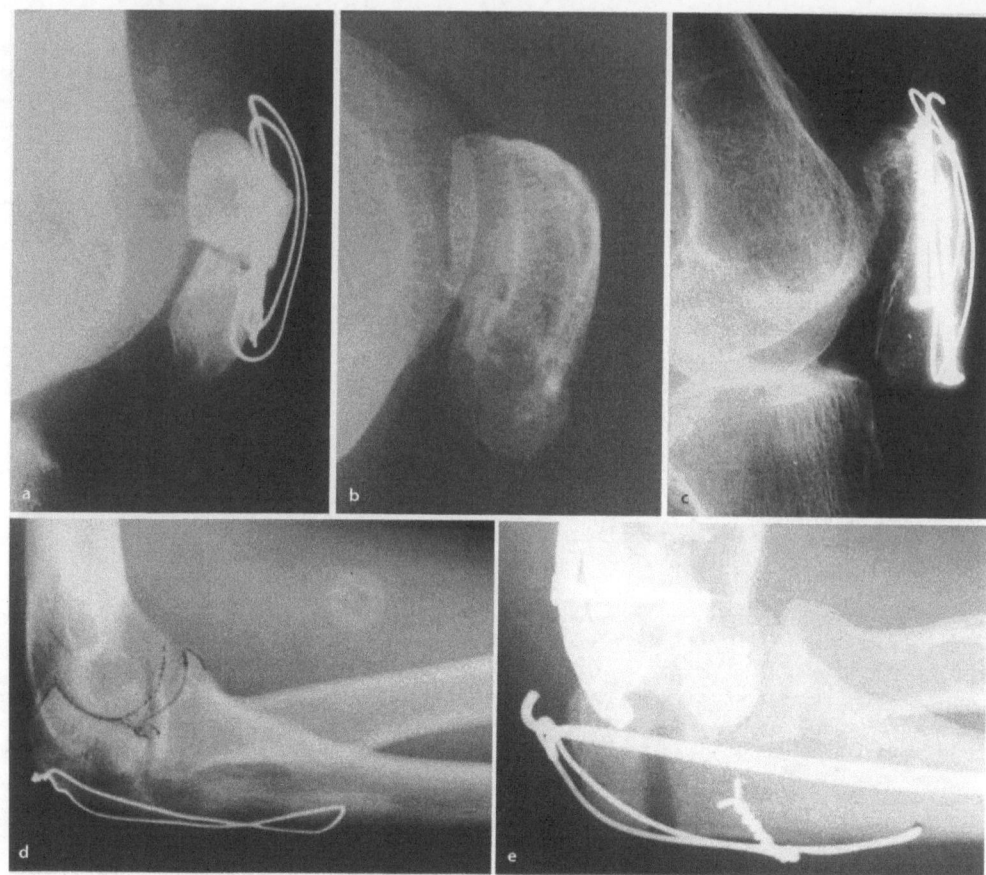

Fig 5. Disadvantages of wire osteosyntheses: step formation (**a, b**) angulation (**c**), incongruency of the joint surface (**d**), dislocation (**e**)

ble of a suspension bridge is not merely buried in loose sand at the bank of the river, but is attached to thick concrete foundations which lie protected in sturdy chambers. The sketch of the Rhine bridge, built in Köln-Rodenkirchen in 1941, with its bridge chamber, reveals the firm anchorage of the suspension cable, an element that is missing in surgical wire tension bands illustrated (Fig. 4).

Unlike plate osteosynthesis, which can be assessed radiologically without too many difficulties, the wire maze of a tension band disguises the fact that the fragments are only loosely fitted together. Because bends and loops are so typical of each of these operations, we accept them as being inevitable. They *are* indeed in-built problems and visible proof of never-attained solidity, of imminent or even existent loosening. The typical consequences

of wire osteosyntheses – step formation, angulation, shifting and lengthening of the joint surfaces, as well as dislocation – are to be feared (Fig. 5).

Non-unions in spongy bones are rare and so bony reconstruction can easily be seen as a positive result. However, the late incongruent arthrosis is attributed to the accident itself, i.e., a post-traumatic consequence, rather than the result of a poor osteosynthesis procedure. This may seem understandable, as recurrent failures are not always easy to cope with. However, one must remain adamant: the discrepancy between the tremendous demands on the "great" osteosynthesis and the comparatively low expectancies which are attached to the tension band is a traumatological paradox. Anyone wanting to reserve osteosyntheses with wire for beginners [53, 153] – and according to general opinion as cited by Roesgen and Koch [323] people regard "the tension band oste-osynthesis as a simple procedure of surgical treatment of bone fractures," a method that, as Ansorge [5] puts it, requires "neither particular technical nor special instrumental expertise," hampers the progress of implants and improved operative methods.

Disregarding the composition of the material, which has been adapted to today's standards for implants, the common flexion-resistant round wire is still the same bulky structure as before, with which the biomechanically-orientated operator, as Shaw and Daubert wrote in 1988 [356], has serious difficulties: "The use of cerclage wire or tension band fixation techniques is frequently indicated but uniformly difficult to perform. Broken wires or inadequate fixation are all too often the ill-fated results of these techniques."

In 1990, von Issendorff et al. [145] also discovered after an experimental examination of the wire tension band osteosynthesis that a permanent tautness with a monofilament wire could not be achieved despite all efforts. Also, in our experience, tension bandings with cerclage wire can only be surgically realized in a few cases [195, 207, 220], because it depends on chance as to whether the forces are produced by the rigid implant and are then transferred to the surfaces of the fracture. Permanent tautness is however a prerequisite for the stability of osteosynthesis. In the world of technology the usage of a material with deficient mechanical traits would not even be considered, let alone simply "tried out." Surgeons however only had this type of wire, whose unmanageable characteristics are often detrimental and whose mechanical applicability is questionable. Its rigidity and its propensity to break just as one is about to carry out the twist, one of the most important moments of osteosynthesis, are highly disruptive. "The wire does not tolerate the tension, it tears, and goes back into distraction and what had been laboriously achieved is lost", so Winkelbauer 1925 [423]. The entire procedure has to be repeated. Successful repositioning and stability cannot always be achieved again. During the post-operative treatment there is a tendency towards secondary loosening because kinks and loops in the wire straighten themselves out. Thus, the initial adaptation turns into distraction, inducing dislocation. This leads to unsatisfactory results. Regarding this point, people often claim results could have been far better had this or that been considered during the operation. "Possibilities of mistakes present themselves on three levels with direct consequences on the biomechanics. Owing to tactical mistakes the adaptation of fragments is not possible. Technical failures usually result in breaks in the material. Incorrect calculations in the assessment of the bony scaffold result in collapse of the osteosynthesis" according to Roesgen [323]. Such an argument remains without effect if the essentials – in this case the biomechanics – are not heeded. Irrespective of how much effort one puts into it, use of cerclage wire will always lead to merely average results. "Every surgeon who performs bone suturing knows very well that the effort spent at trying to obtain a successful operation is often lost and the expected result does not materialise" said Orsos on 1925 [286].

This is proved by thousands of X-rays and the experience of hundreds of surgeons.

▶ Only he who has fully comprehended that twisted, bent forms and wire loops are evidence for an imperfect bonding of the bone will realize that conventional cerclage wire is unsuitable as an implant.

If one considers how much the modern forms of osteosynthesis plates differ from Hansmann's *prototype* of some 100 years ago, and how many elements of today's implants have been adapted to our requirements regarding biomechanics, handling, and patient comfort, it is quite astonishing that in the passing of time wire has remained almost totally unchanged. Neither its poor mechanical features nor its troublesome application initiated a wave of research into the matter. Instead, one attempted to make it softer and more pliable, and – with the help of improved tools – more effective, as we know, without success.

The search for optimal results calls for fundamental changes. Instead of the stiff wire a new implant is needed, one that is satisfactory in every respect – from handling through to the biomechanics. Currently, this is the wire cable; in time we may be using a synthetic material which is reabsorbed by the body or perhaps even something else.

The polyfilament cable is commonly seen as the next step. It found its way into medicine in the form of the round-stranded cross lay cable (Labitzke 1978 [203, 207]). As shown in the two cross-sections of Fig. 6, its structure and properties make it a completely new product that far outshines cerclage

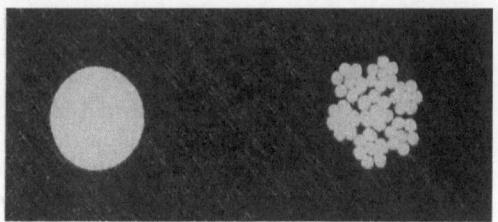

Fig. 6 Cerclage wire – cable

wires. On the left is the conventional cerclage wire, on the right the cable that is the focus of this publication, consisting of seven strands, each in turn with seven super-fine wires (diameter of each 1 mm; magnification 18×).

Within this context A. Dwyer and co-workers from Sydney can be cited as one example [79, 80]. Since 1964 they have been using a titanium cable in the anterior correction of scoliosis. It consists of 7 strands each comprising 19 wires. At a diameter of 1/8 in. (3.18 mm), it is very thick and spans the convex side of the scoliosis with a special attachment to every vertebra. It was neither suitable nor indeed intended for general traumatological applications.

2.2
Wire Cables – State-of-the-art Solution

Wire cables have been known and used for a long time. Their exact age and origin remain unknown. However, cables are much younger than wire which, as is shown in pieces of jewelry that have been found, dates back to a time before the Bronze Age.

Cave paintings found in Spain dating back to the Mesolithic period (approx. 20,000 years ago) clearly show the structure of ropes twisted from natural fibers, which were used to climb trees and rocks. The pontoon bridge across the Dardanelles, 1350 m in length, was built by Xerxes during the war in 480 B.C. between Persia and Greece, and is looked upon as one of the most famous engineering feats of antiquity. Two ropes made of white flax and four ropes made of papyrus had held the ships together. The Greek historian Heredot had calculated that the ropes had to have a thickness of 22 cm [410].

Since 1834, wire cables have been used as a traction mechanism on a large scale, thanks to Albert [2]; in operative medicine they have only been in use for a few years [79, 206]. Although some facts remain unclear, enough details are known within the history of technology to draw a fairly complete picture of the development of cables. Unfortunately inconsistent recording has caused a certain degree of confusion with regards to details of the early history of the wire cable [412]. According to Dickmann [69], "...towards the end of the eighteenth century and during the first decades of the nineteenth century, wire cables were classified as a welded or braided chain or as a cluster of single strands running parallel and held together by clamps or wire braces and eventually as the cable made of twisted wire strands we know today. This confusion is the reason why the actual invention of the wire cable has been contested for many years."

2.2.1
A Brief Introduction, Including Valuable Technical Data

"The cable can be seen as one of the oldest mechanical components. The fact that by twisting or braiding single pliable and elastic strands, made of strips cut from animal skins or plant fibres, it became possible to create cables which by far surpass the strength of those made of single strands arranged parallel to each other, as well as achieving an even strain on all strands, was obviously recognized by man at a very early stage" wrote Dieterich [71] in 1908.

To begin with, let us look at wire cables – which were produced much later – along more general lines and not just from the familiar surgical viewpoint. Wire cables are extremely diverse, and can be applied almost universally. Therefore they were predestined

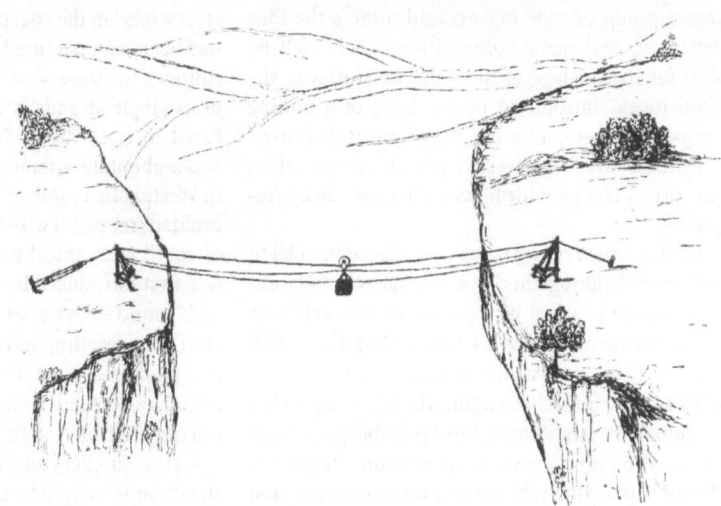

Fig. 7. Early cable railway [from 71]

to find their way into the operating theaters. Learning about their technical properties, one comes to appreciate their value even more.

In Northern Mythology, the three Norns, goddesses regarded as the dispensers of fate, attempt to pull eternal wisdom from the very depths of Mother Earth. They use a flexible cable spun and twisted from many single strands, an allegory outlining that only thus may wisdom be gained and held. A single rigid wire would not hold the very force embedded in wisdom everlasting – the flexibility of a cable was the solution. The fact that eventually it was torn, bringing about the collapse of order, may symbolize that even wire cables can be strained only so far and should be looked upon as an interim solution only.

Miners were the first to use wire cables systematically. But Leonardo da Vinci had already visualized cables for the movement of loads. In his description of a paternoster lift he states: "The cable for the above instrument must be of wires of fired iron or copper, otherwise it will soon collapse" (quoted from [71]).

The wire cable has revolutionized technology. As a hard-wearing material it is used in many sectors, including surgery where it has been in use for some years. Some expositions on the history of technology dating back to the turn of the century touch upon the fact that cables were already utilized by the Romans and even earlier in Egypt [257, 360]. Reference is made to a cable 4.10 m in length found during excavations at Pompeii in 1590 [69, 411]. The Deutsche Drahtmuseum (German Wire Museum) in Altena/ Westphalia has dated this oldest known cable back

to the year 79 B.C. It is on exhibition in the Museo Nazionale in Naples. It is made of bronze and consists of 3 strands each made of 19 wires. The wires have a diameter of 0.7 mm, stranded in cross lays (as shown in Fig. 8).

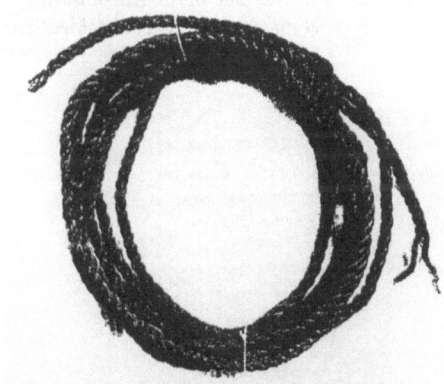

Fig. 8. The oldest-known cable, found 1590 in Pompeii

In 1750, the American physicist Benjamin Franklin came to the conclusion that it was possible to arrest lightning by using metal leads; this was the beginning of the production of lightning conductors made of a multi-stranded copper compound. Although these conductors were constantly referred to as wire cables, they were simply strands of combined wires, which were not designed for the hauling or transport of heavy loads [411]. Nevertheless, it gave a group of rope makers and miners the idea that these new metal compositions could well be used for the haulage of heavy loads. However, the "iron ropes" introduced by the head of a mining company, Christoph Sander, as early as 1568, proved to be too heavy. They were in actual fact not cables but forged chains with links which tore away frequently.

Cables, where round wires were placed parallel to each other held together by a cordage of thin circular wires, also cannot be regarded as wire cables in the modern sense. They lack the true bonding which is achieved by twisting the strands (the *Schlag*), resulting in the impact strength, which is what makes a common transmission of force possible [413]. Such cables, also known as suspension boom, bearer cables, or supporting cables, carry famous suspension bridges such as the bridge across the River Gala constructed in England by Richard Lee in 1816, the *East River Bridge* linking New York and Brooklyn built by the German-American John A. Roebling in 1878, and the *Golden Gate Bridge* in San Francisco built by Joseph Strauss in 1889 [45, 315, 369].

In 1777, Epp described a wire cable made of steel, in 1798 the Englishman Hancock referred to drawn cables made of strong steel. In 1822, Combes (author of the well-known "Manual on the Art of Mining"), claimed to have come across a "cable braided from

steel wires" in the coal pit of the Rive de Gier, which had been manufactured in Lyon. In 1831, a 30 *Lachter* (miner's measure = 57.60 m) long steel cable made of 45 single strands is said to have been manufactured in Halsbrügge, Saxony. In 1927, Vogel [396] spoke about the attempt by the coal mining industry in Westphalia in 1818 to "introduce ropes and cables braided from steel wire for the hauling of large loads of coal." Mechanical manufacturing of wire cables was first introduced by the Frenchman Regnier. He had "found a device, which made it possible to twist steel wire resulting in cables which were as perfect and pliable as those made of hemp," Weber quoted from Hildts Handelszeitung (Trade Journal) in 1784 (all quoted from [411]).

Carl Henschel from Kassel, famous for the construction of railroads, conceived the idea of "moving loads by using a stationary steam engine and cables." He passed this idea on to Albert, senior official in the Clausthal mining industry, and within mining circles regarded as the inventor of the wire cable [65, 66, 228, 267, 411] (Fig. 9).

As one might expect, because revolutionary innovations are rarely an overnight affair, Albert had had forerunners. He had four wires twisted into one strand; three strands were made into a cable with a diameter of 17 mm (Fig. 10). Because the twisting direction of the strands coincides with the cable, it is referred to as long lay, or, following the old style, the *Albertschlag*. Where the wires in the strand are laid to the left and the strand is laid to the right (or vice versa), the method is referred to as cross lay, developed by Theodor Guilleaume in 1840 [28, 392].

According to Weber [411], credit must mainly go to Albert, because he recognized the quality of wire cables as an ideal means for haulage, tested them, and introduced them to the mining industry [2].

The development of wire cables is closely connected with the world-famous manufacturers *Felten and Guilleaume* of Cologne. They also developed

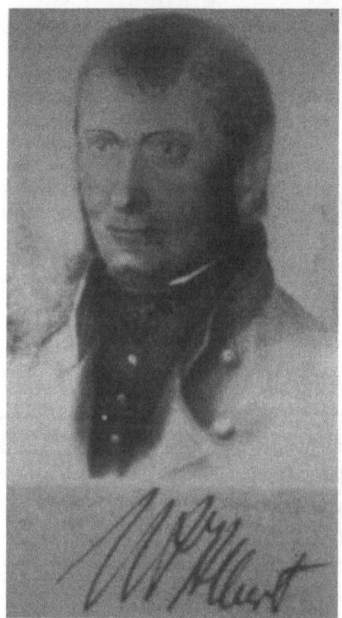

Fig. 9. Wilhelm A.J. Albert (1787–1846; from [65])

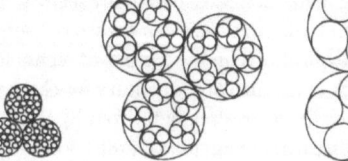

Fig. 10. Cross-section of historical wire cables: on the left the cable from Pompeii, ∅ 8 mm; in the centre the cable from Saxony, ∅ 16 mm; and on the far right Albert's cable ∅ 17 mm [from 411].

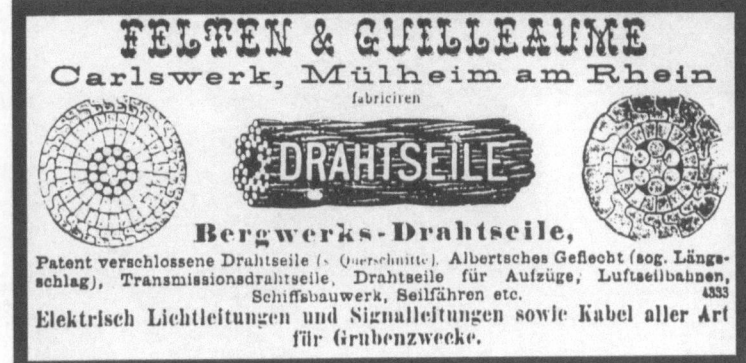

Fig. 11. Advertisement dating back to 1835 in "Glückauf", a well-known journal for miners [from 23]

fully sealed cables [267], which, because their strands are shaped geometrically, do not show any free space in their cross-section. Thus the inside is protected against corrosion, which makes them particularly stable and suited for the construction of bridges (Fig. 11).

The main advantage of cable wires lies in the fact that, in spite of their enormous solidity, cable wires retain a high degree of flexibility. Because of its structure wire cable is predestined to carry loads [392]. Depending on the requirements, they are made of a varying number of different single wires. Wire cables are the most effective tractive force known in technology. They are used for many different purposes. Wire cables support bridges, haul loads from the very depths of coal mines, and draw cable cars, lifts, and conveyances of various types. In the aviation sector, wire cables transfer control signals via a set of rollers to the rudders. Ropes and cables are used in shipbuilding. In Low German they are referred to as *Reep*. In Hamburg it was the tradition to twine ropes on a long track which ran through the city in a straight line. It has become world famous as the *Reeperbahn*.

The four-mast bark *Pamir*, built in 1905 and sunk in a hurricane in the Atlantic in September 1957, had 22 km of ropes and wire cables on board in order to secure its 54 m high rigging against the force of the winds.

In hilly San Francisco with its extreme gradient, *cable cars* are used as public transport, where all other means of conveyance failed. They are pulled with wire cables via a set of wheels which are installed below street level. The electric drive is located in a central engine house. The system was constructed in 1873 by the Scottish engineer Andrew Hallidie (his father held the first English patent for the manufacture of wire cables). It was overhauled a few years ago and, according to information given in a brochure, it will last for another 100 years.

A construction with cables offers an elegant solution, using only a minimum of materials. If the enormous weight of a suspension bridge could not be supported by slim wire cables, the structure would have to be carried by units made of steel or concrete with the result that the general proportions would be massive. The weight of such a construction would of course also limit the length of the bridge and not even vaguely reach the fantastic span of suspension bridges constructed with wire cables. Building bridges without wire cables would not only mean an increase in cost; it would also mean that bridges would lose their aesthetic charm. The elegant lines of a bridge built with wire cables are a joy to behold (Fig. 12).

The photograph taken by Jean Gaumy of the construction of the *Pont de Normandie*, a diagonal cable bridge across the River Seine near Le Havre, officially opened in 1995, documents the boldness of mankind and the craftsmanship, with both skill and attention to detail – a cluster of cables cascading from the pylon, giving the entire structure an air of strength and power.

The *Verrazano-Narrow-Bridge* connecting Brooklyn with Staten Island was built by Oskar Amman from Switzerland. Completed in 1964, it was his "last great masterpiece" [369]. With its span of 1298 m it was then the longest suspension bridge in the world.

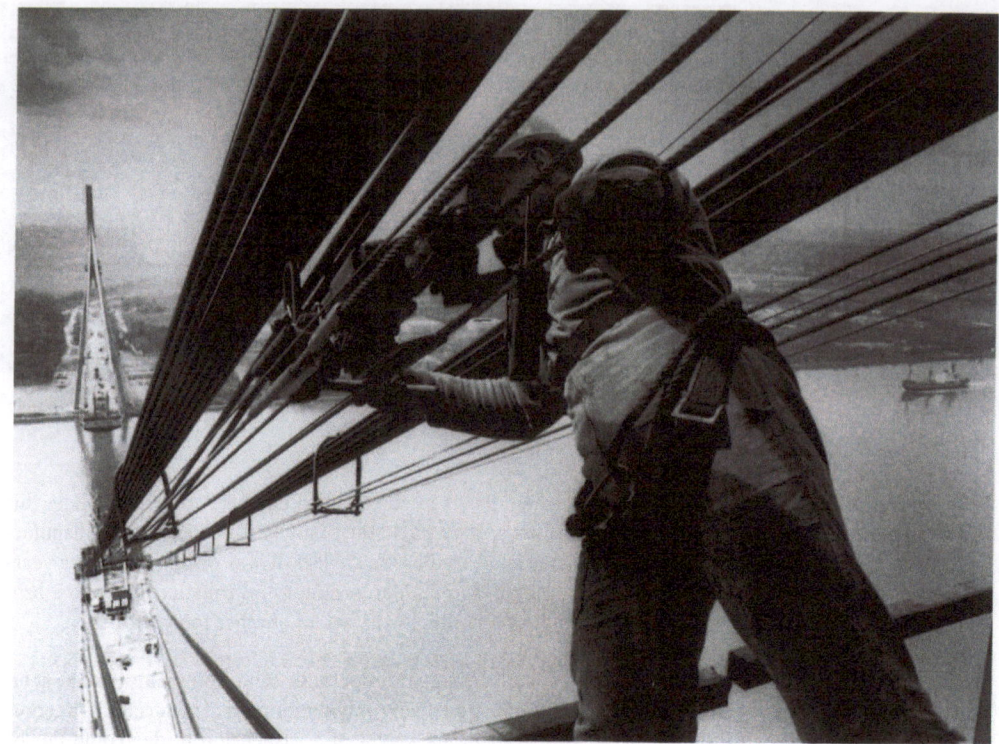

Fig. 12. The *Pont de Normandie* under construction (with kind permission of FOCUS Agency, Hamburg)

According to Amman's calculations, the attainable qualities of steel are such that a suspension span of a maximum of 1500 m can be achieved. The *Humber Bridge* in Kingston-upon-Hull in England with its span of 1410 m comes extremely close to the set limit. In April 1998 the Japanese officially opened the *Akashi-Kaikyo "Pearl Bridge"* and broke the existing record with a proud 1991 m. This unbelievable achievement shows that the quality of steel can obviously still be improved.

"These few examples clearly demonstrate the quality of wire cables as an outstanding means of tension. Their development surely has earned at least as much of our admiration as the soaring cable railway constructions or the epitome of the perfected suspension bridges" stated Regensburger [315].

By using different patterns, it is possible to achieve specific advantages suited to the task in hand. The characteristics of cables with identical cross sec-

tions strongly depend on the number of components used. Cables with a small number of thicker wires tend to be stiff and hardly pliable. Just as a glass fiber cable becomes more transparent the greater the number of strands used, a cable with a large number of strands becomes stronger and more pliable. Griffith [115] outlined a fact that may come as a surprise: a solid round wire with a fully compact cross section tears more easily and has a lower loading capacity, or expressed in another way, an aeriferous cable gains in strength with a greater number of single strands. His mathematically substantiated theory is based on the fundamental concept that both solid and fluid bodies have the same surface tension, which counteracts energy caused by tearing. The surface tension increases dramatically with the number of single strands resulting in the increase of the cable surface. This property, *strength through multiplicity*, is put into effect by nature time and time again; as fiber composites it is used in lightweight constructions [124, 288, 289]. The greatest effect of reinforcement is achieved by laying fibers in the direction of the actual tension, i.e., with the cable.

▶The architects and structural engineers Frei Otto and partners utilized these properties for example in the boldly conceptualized construction of the roofs of the Olympic tent in Munich and the German Pavilion during the World Exhibition 1967 bin Montreal. The entire weight of the transparent glass skin is carried by a filigree network of cables. Note the similarity with the natural construction of cartwheel spiders which is linked to a central hub and anchored on blades of grass and twigs with supporting links [188, 189, 272] (Fig. 13).

With such properties, wire cables can of course also be utilized as an implant. Technical criteria also apply to living matter. Especially where certain fractures are concerned, the wire cable has proved to be an outstanding osteosynthesis material, as experience during the last 20 years has shown. In spite of this fact, it is not being used exclusively. The technical commission of the AO which was asked, at that time, to give an opinion on the wire cable and to weigh up all the pros and cons was "unable to recognize the interesting idea of a wire cable being used as an implant." Based on this, several surgeons decided

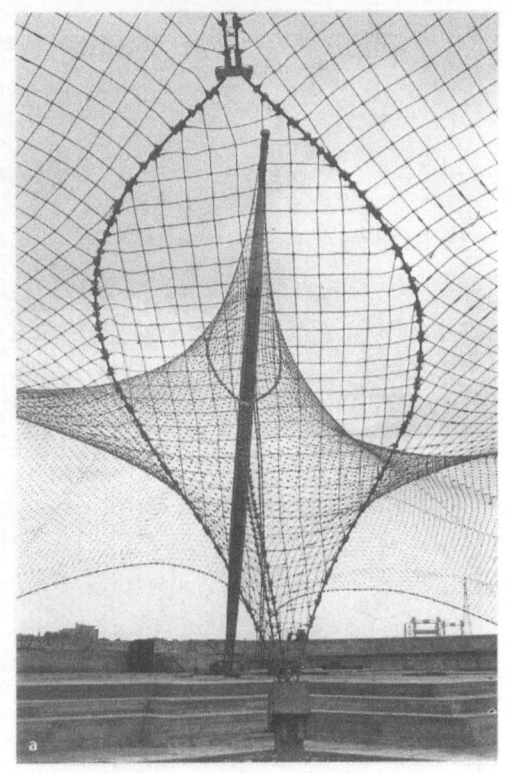

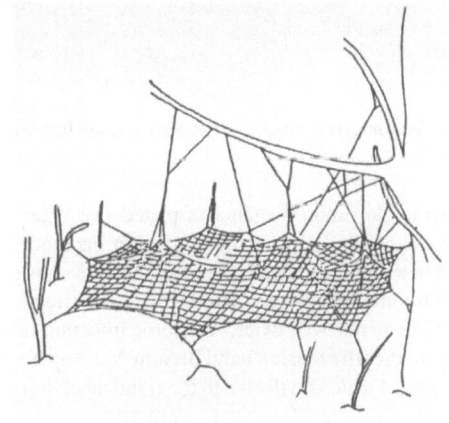

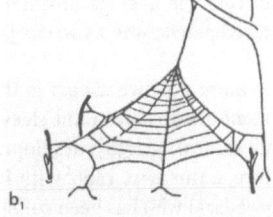

Fig. 13. Networks in architecture (by courtesy of Frei Otto) and in nature [from 189]

against using cables, not wanting to test yet another implant. They predicted that wire cables would never be accepted because the seal would be too obtrusive. In a letter addressed to the author personally, it was also pointed out that such "tractive wires" could easily be obtained from any DIY-store. Discussions based on scientific evidence and free of emotion

would definitely have been beneficial. American companies were quicker to recognize the qualities of the wire cable and started production some years ago.

Just one glaring example of the problems which can arise with rigid cerclage wires (Fig. 14): H. K., a 26-year-old tiler sustained a comminuted fracture

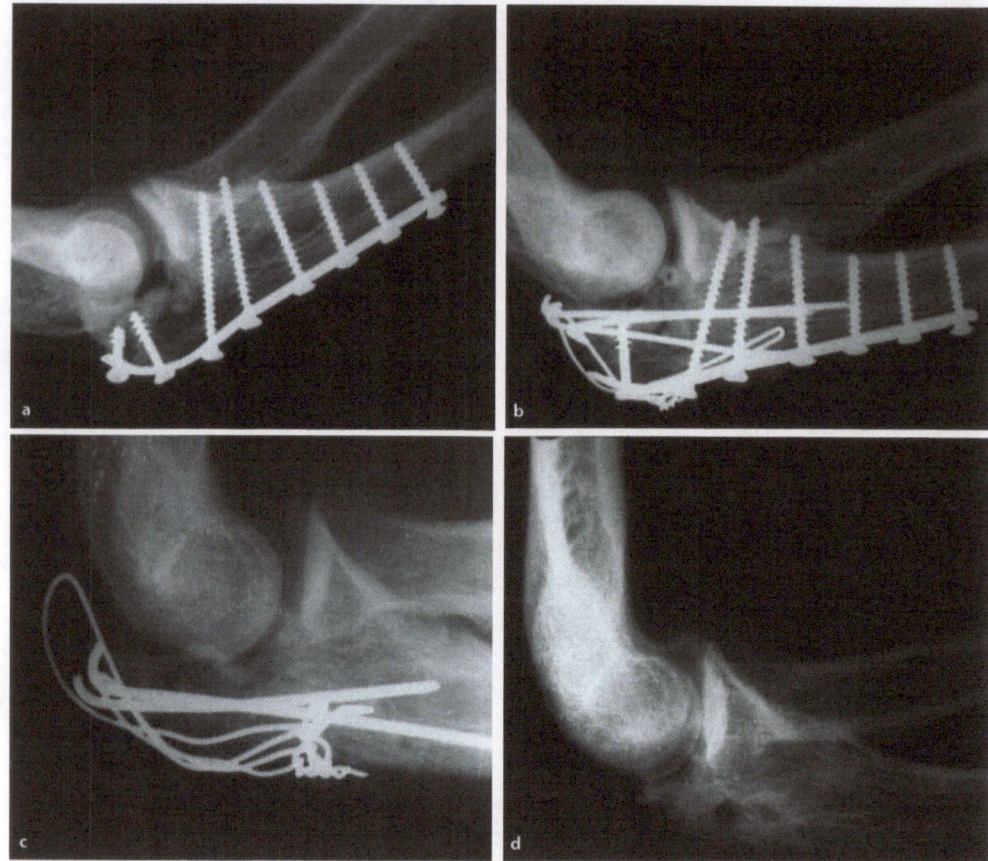

Fig. 14 A not very untypical rigid wire tension banding casuistry

of the olecranon, which was plated (**a**). After two weeks an avulsion on the olecranon occured. The plate was not removed, the olecranon was given an additional wire tension band (**b**). The tension band had to be renewed twice. A chronic infection developed, the wire tension band became loose again and again (**c**) which finally led to the removal of the olecranon which had become necrotic (**d**).

After a total of 11 opertions in 5 admissions, a defect-healing was attained by replacement of the triceps insertion with the palmaris longus tendon.

Loss of strength and movement restriction of 0 – 20 – 100 ° / 60 – 0 – 60 ° after 110 days of hospitalization and 21 months of inability to work, led to job loss and 20% permanent disability.

This is not an isolated case; Kiviluoto and Santavirta [169] indicated sick leave of up to 236 days and an average of 77 days – cf. Fig. 66. (As a point of interest, in 1921 the average hospital admission for a fractured patella was 7.5 weeks [361].)

A more positive aspect is the fact that the above-mentioned cables (and sleeves) have inspired new ideas: Towfigh [383] developed the flexor tendon suture, a fine wire cable with two spurs; Kluger et al. [172, 275] who has been combining them successfully with Harrington instrumentation since 1982, outlined their strengths, acknowledging Labitzke as the initiator. Reck et al. [314] altered the sleeves for percutaneous anchorage of the Lengemann suture.

▶ Cables are now well regarded for their reliability and are seen as state of the art.

2.2.2
Principle of Cable Osteosyntheses

Anyone who thinks and works in a biomechanical framework will want to discard unwieldy wire cerclage; only a cable is able to stabilize fractures with enough security. For practical reasons the diameter of cables, like wire, has been set at 1 mm. That is certainly enough for the forces which are desirable for tension banding. Of course, cable ends must not be knotted together like threads, nor is twisting used. Cables are securely brought together whilst taut using a crimp, the dimensions of which are very small. They are therefore easy to squeeze, do not create bulk, and are not disruptive. Naturally the size of the tools has been adapted to these measurements and they have been designed to ensure a firm grip.

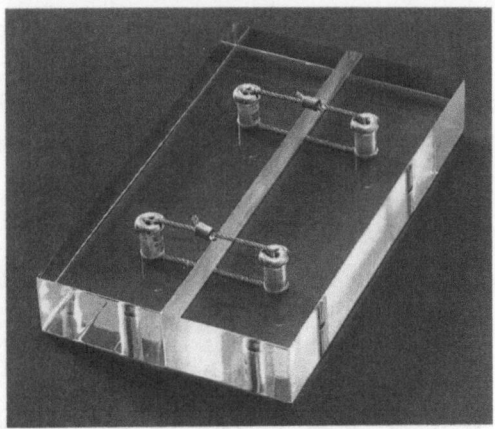

Fig. 15. Principle of sleeve-cable osteosynthesis

Wire cables allow an osteosynthesis technique to be realized which has nothing in common with cerclage wiring. Properties that distinguish wire cable as an implant are the following: it is as pliable as it is strong and resistant. Thus it is suited to every anatomical situation. Loops and kinks, characteristics of rigid wire, are totally eliminated. The cable is enormously strain resistant and may be optimally tightened and fixed so that osteosyntheses remain stable and resistant to load. Cable does not cut into the living bone (as clarified by Brill and Hopf [29] following experiments on cadavers – see Chap. 4.4). During post-operative treatment secondary dislocations need not be feared, provided everything has been safely anchored and the cables correctly squeezed together.

Ready-made wire cables 15 cm in length are particularly suitable for *tension bandings*. With their loops at one end, they are ready to be hooked onto Kirschner wires or screws. With such a firmly made foundation they can easily be pre-stressed, thus giving osteosyntheses a high degree of stability.

For a *cerclage*, a cable is cut to the appropriate length from a 10 m roll and guided around the bone using an instrument.

Cables combined with sleeves are very useful – of course it only makes sense to anchor cables to bone with a strong cortical layer or to devices that can stand up to the forces resulting from cable tension. Cancellous bones would give under the pressure of cables laid trans-osseously if they were not protected using special cable anchorages. Self-tapping polyethylene sleeves with an external diameter of

5 mm, which are screwed into the soft bone, make a foundation for the pull of the cable and reduce its pressure on the bone to a tolerable level (Fig. 15). There are two forms of sleeve-cable combinations: for static osteosynthesis the closure of the longitudinal sternotomy in cardiac surgery is a clear example, see Chap. 4.13; flexible joint bridge banding is dealt with, using Malgaigne's injury as an example, in Chap. 4.12.

2.2.3
The Osteosynthesis Set

Special instruments have been developed for the safe handling of the cable. They are available either in the container or as additional trays to those available in the operating theater. The tools required up to now – repositioning forceps, curved pins, hammers, Kirschner wires, side cutters, raspatories, etc. – are still needed; cerclage wires and wire spanners can be discarded. Instead, wire cables, crimps, and PE-sleeves are included with the new instruments (Fig. 16).

2.2.3.1
Wire Cables

Wire cables are made from high-grade stainless steel, 1.4441 ISO standard, corresponding to the latest international standards for implants and are authorized for long-term implantation. This material

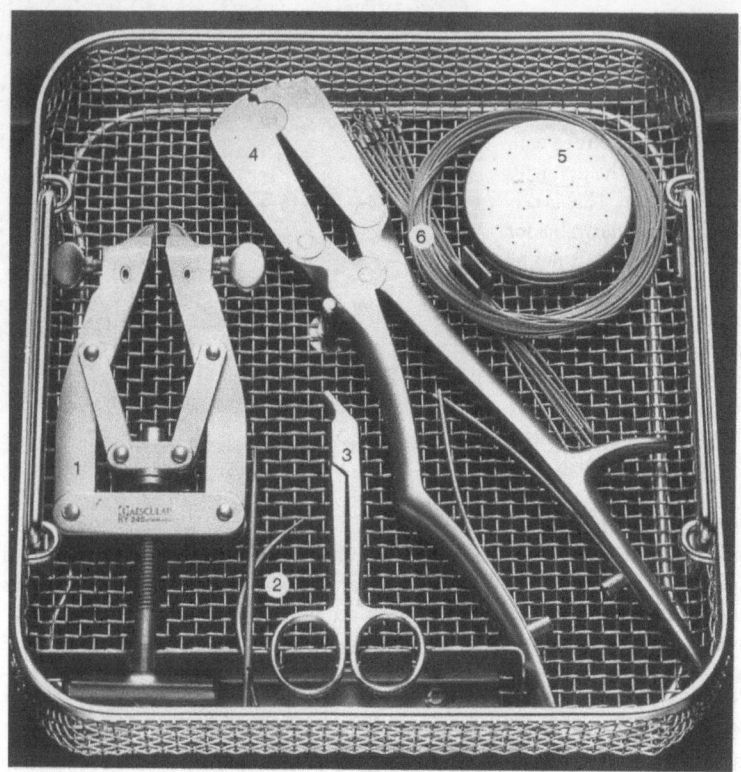

Fig. 16. The osteosynthesis set: *1* Cable tensioner, *2* two awls, *3* cable scissors, *4* crimp pliers, *5* crimp box, *6* several cables

has a resistance to breakage of 1770 MPa. The decision in favor of so-called cross-lay-cables was made because they offer particular advantages for surgical purposes. Their surface is mat and easy to grip. They are twisted to the right, made taut for increased strength with very low give, take up little space, and are unstressed. These properties account for their high resistance to breakage and make possible smooth cutting with special cutters without the tendency to unwind or fray upon cutting. This construction also fulfills our requirement for slight elasticity which is desirable for bone healing. A cable consists of 49 individual filaments, that is 7 strands with 7 super-fine wires each – 6 of which are wound around a core strand – cf. Figs. 6 and 18. This structure makes the cables supple and break-resistant and accounts for their especially high quality [115], characteristics which cerclage wire does not even begin to match. The clean cross-section of the material has an area of 0.4489 mm^2, only 58% of that of round wire whose cross-section measures

0.7678 mm^2. Despite the surface area being almost halved the resistance to strain is many times higher, see Chap. 3.

Cables come in three versions: on a continuous roll, 10 m in length, and ready-made as single pieces 15 cm in length with an end loop. The latter are particularly suitable for tension bandings as they can be attached extremely well to screws and Kirschner wires. For special applications – the lengthening of a limb and the vertebral column – cables 60 cm and 120 cm in length are available either with a loop or with one end piece made of soft round wire or laser-welded. They can be easily guided around the vertebral arches. For normal trauma use, this version is not to be considered as it is unnecessary and somewhat expensive; instead awls are used (Fig. 17).

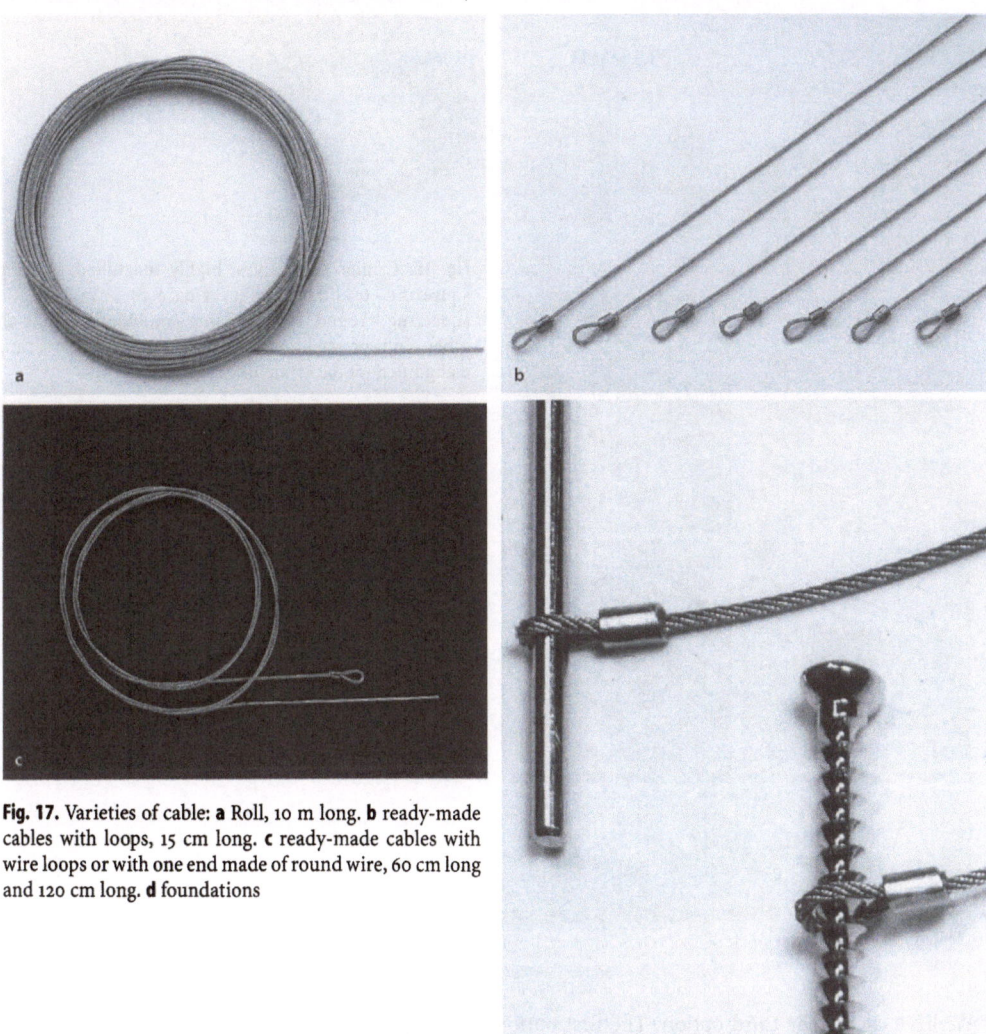

Fig. 17. Varieties of cable: **a** Roll, 10 m long. **b** ready-made cables with loops, 15 cm long. **c** ready-made cables with wire loops or with one end made of round wire, 60 cm long and 120 cm long. **d** foundations

2.2.3.2
Crimps

Crimps are also made of high-grade stainless steel, 1.4441 ISO standard. They hold the taut cables permanently and firmly together. Crimps, a technical term, are a type of seal, with the difference that they are *squeezed into shape*. This results in optimal cohesive strength through the interlocking of cable and crimp. Upon squeezing, the cables are gently brought together and embedded in the applied crimp. Compared with others, this type of fixation is the most secure. It fulfills the technical quality requirement DIN 3093, which calls for 85% of the breaking strain of the cables for the crimp connection.

Technicians distinguish between three different ways of connecting materials [426]:

1. Substance cohesion (cohesion by union of the materials, for example by soldering or welding)
2. Closure by force or friction (cohesion of the surfaces by friction)
3. Closure by molding together (cohesion through two components interlocking with each other)

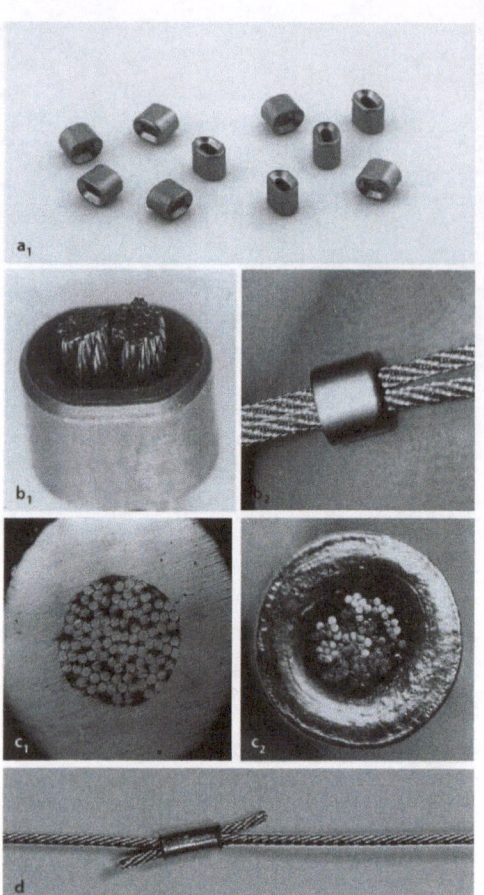

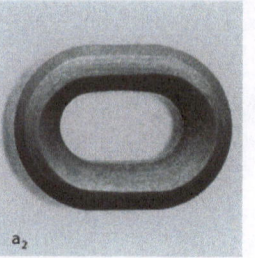

Fig. 18. Crimps and cables, highly magnified: **a** before squeezing – oval, **b** before squeezing, across 2 cables, **c** after squeezing – round. Both cables are moulded into one another and pressed into the inner wall of the crimp, **d** alignment of the crimp under cable tension

We have chosen the third option. The first option proved to be impractical because of the high temperatures involved, and the second lacks stability.

Before squeezing, the crimps are oval, in order to be able to accept two cables lying next to each other. They are 3.0 mm long, 3.8 mm high, and 2.7 mm wide; the wall is 0.8 mm thick. They are widened on the inside forming a funnel shape at both ends. Thus the possibility of damaging the cables with sharp edges is eliminated (Fig. 18).

Crimps and wire cables are made of exactly the same material. Cables are hard and elastic, the crimps are soft. They have to have plastic properties so that they can be easily molded. For this reason they are annealed again after shaping. A cable-crimp connection is therefore a connection of the same material but of different degrees of hardness. Electrical currents, electrolysis and corrosion are eliminated.

2.2.3.3
PE-Sleeves

It is always sensible to use sleeves if cables have to be anchored trans-osseously without causing damage. They are made of high-density polyethylene. With a central diameter of 5 mm they create a pressure gradient from cable to bone and prevent any sort of cutting in, thus encouraging strong durable connections.

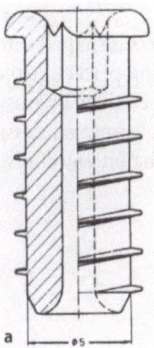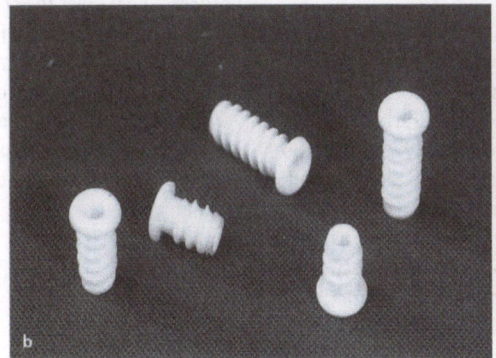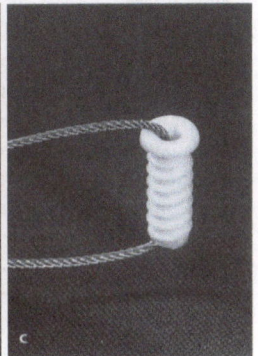

Fig. 19. High density PE-sleeves

The sleeves are 8–18 mm long and are screwed into 3.5 mm bore canals by means of self-tapping threads. Their tops have been fitted with collars which prevent them from penetrating into the bone too deeply and at the same time allow squeezing of the crimp within the free space without losing tension – cf. Fig. 31c and 32. It also has an Allen screw to accommodate the 3.5-mm screwdriver. The central bore is rounded and funnel-shaped both at the top and bottom so that the cable can easily be threaded without sharp kinks. The inner bore has a width of 2.2 mm (Fig. 19).

2.2.3.4
Instruments

To insert and tighten the cables, five tools are necessary:

- One cable tensioner
- One crimp pliers
- One pair cable scissors
- Two awls, straight and curved

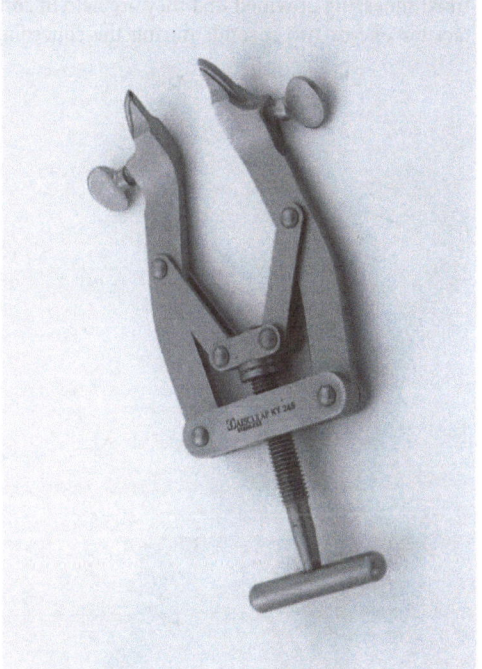

Fig. 20. The cable tensioner

They are carefully crafted with mat, non-reflective surfaces. Their shape reflects their function. The size and strength of the parts transferring force have been calculated, with nothing left to chance. They have been ergonomically designed to ensure a comfortable grip and transfer a feeling of solidity. Working with them conveys a sense of sureness and power.

Cable Tensioner
The cable tension device resembles an extension stirrup. Two movable articulated branches are attached to a crossbar. They can be opened or closed by turning a short T-shaped handle using a double lever construction. They are rounded at the front and have a canal into which the cable is inserted and fastened with a wing nut. To ensure that the crimp pliers can be correctly held between them and used without hindrance, the branches are inclined at 30° at the front. The turning handle is short and can only be gripped with three fingers, thus harnessing the tension force to such an extent that only great strain would break the cable. The cables are tightened by opening the device (Fig. 20).

Crimp Pliers

Crimp pliers have to be relatively large because strong forces are to be produced with their long branches and, by means of the doubly crossed thick claws, transferred to the mouth of the pliers (Fig. 21). With a lever ratio of approximately 1:25, the 200 N hand pressure of the operator is transformed to 5000 N plier pressure. The annealed crimps can be securely squeezed even by women surgeons.

Two force-limiting knobs are fixed between the grips of the pliers. They have a double function and guarantee two things: as excess pressure limiters they protect the anterior lip of the mouth of the pliers from deformation due to being too forcefully pressed together and in addition they guarantee optimal squeezing provided that they are held in contact for one or two seconds during the squeezing process. That gives the crimp enough time to be able to *flow* and arrange itself.

The mouth of the crimp pliers is shaped with geometrical accuracy, thus offering perfect grip of the crimp. It would be crushed when tilted or grasped at an angle. Squeezing would not prove successful; in fact the gripped cable would be bitten off instead – cf. Fig. 40.

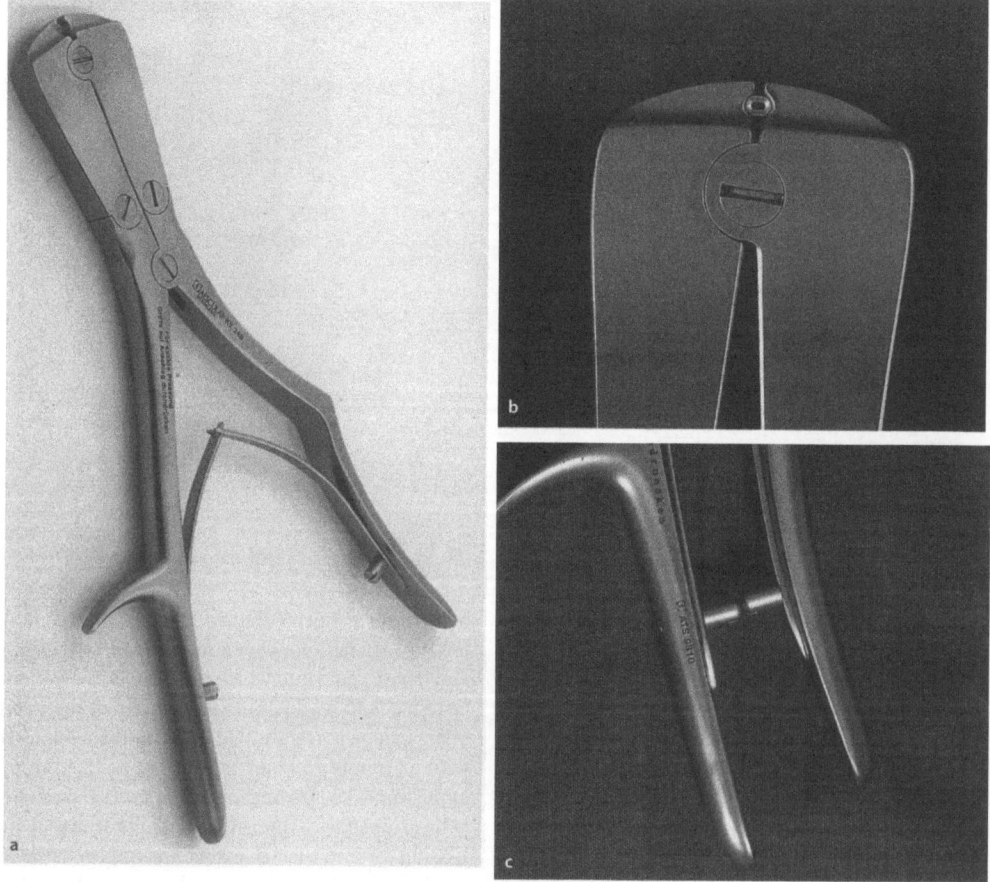

Fig. 21. The crimp pliers: **a** whole size, **b** correct grasping of the crimp, **c** force-limiting knobs during crimping

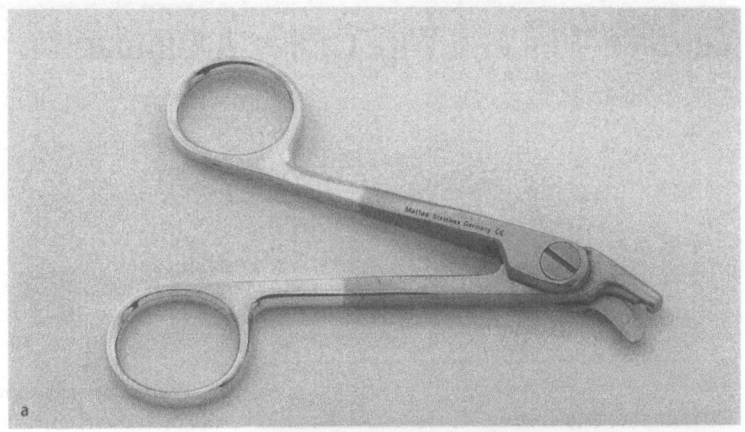

Fig. 22. Cable scissors

Cable Scissors

For a smooth cut of the 49 filaments of the wire cable, special cutters with compact double blade guidance have been constructed. They have two short curved cutting surfaces with crescent-shaped, hardened, sharp cutting notches which grip the cable firmly. On cutting, it is not crushed or twisted, but cleanly cut through as if it were one single strand (Fig. 22).

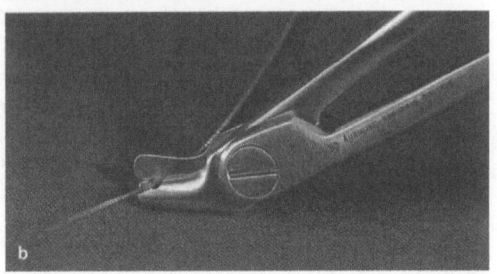

Awls

Awls are required to guide the cables through tissue. At the end they have funnel-shaped, slit, longitudinal hollow bores into which a cable may be guided easily and is fixed by applying finger pressure. One can choose between a curved and a straight awl. They should be gripped only at the compact part with flat pliers (Fig. 23).

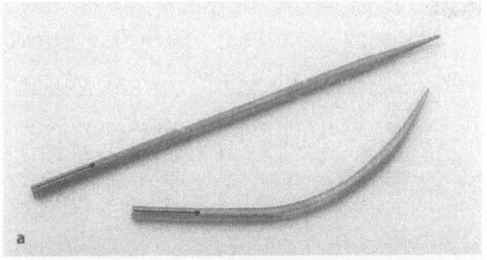

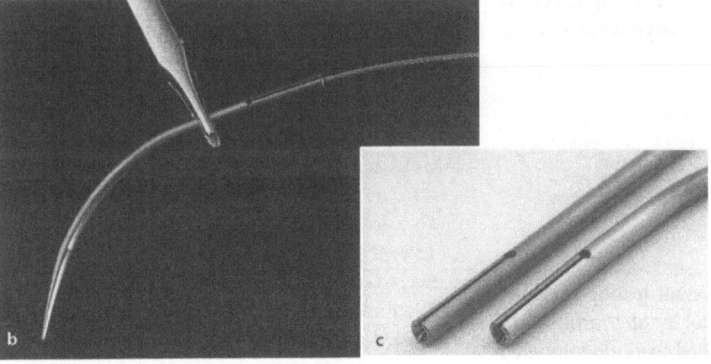

Fig. 23. Two different types of awls and their handling

CHAPTER 3

Cerclage Wire and Wire Cables: A Comparison

3.1
Performance and Testing

All those who are still bound to using cerclage wire, either by regulations, tradition, or simply from force of habit, are well advised to weigh up the results of a comparative mechanical test of wires and cables. Based on experiments it is actually possible to determine various grades of quality. The first attempts were made in 1974 together with K. Bowe from the Institut für Werkstoffkunde at the Ruhr University in Bochum. At that time we tested conventional and bilateral tension bandings on patella and olecranon fractures with tension and pressure experiments and found that this new, until then only theoretically based procedure, was also better in the experimental tear test than other known methods. [198, 202]. However, it could only be achieved with cerclage wire under favorable experimental conditions using smooth model bones. The rigid wire could just be stretched on the low-friction surfaces. These investigations established that stiffer cerclage wire is unsuitable for osteosyntheses and for this reason would have to be substituted for wire cables, which at that stage we used to refer to as wire strands.

Meanwhile the experiments have been updated. We wanted to clarify for practical osteosynthesis reasons:

1. How cables and wires behave as such
2. How they behave in their association with crimps and twists under increasing tension loads
3. When loops and kinks in the cerclage wire begin to straighten

A modern ZWICK 1478 universal testing machine with a linear deformation velocity of 20 mm min^{-1} was used. The results measured were documented automatically in diagram form. Four standard cerclage wires by well-known manufacturers and our wire cables were exposed to tension loads until they tore. All test pieces were 100 mm long and had a fixed diameter of 1 mm.

To characterize the implants the following technical data were established or calculated:

1. The actual diameter of the individual samples before the load and on tearing.
2. The surface and material cross-sectional area before the load and on tearing. With homogenous round wires the cross-sectional area, as a geometrical cross-section, and the material cross-sectional area were the same. Because of the *air in the cable*, its actual cross-sectional area – the space between the 49 individual components – at 58% is clearly smaller than the geometrical cross-sectional area.
   The values of 1 and 2 are allocated to the variables measured under tension load.
3. The tension resistance Rm in Mpa – a technical variable, which allows direct comparison of material because it always relates to a cross-sectional area of 1 mm^2. This variable indicates the level of the tension load at the break (= tear), not taking into consideration the stretch (= lengthening of the sample under tension) occurring up to that point.
4. The tension load R in N at the break of the individual sample. This marks the force which leads to tearing of one of the samples with an individual cross-sectional area – in this case the break load of each individual wire model. This value omits the stretch that also accompanies it.
5. The stretch A in %. This indicates the plastic lengthening of the samples up to the tear. Since we used 100 mm long test pieces, the percentage corresponds to the elongation in millimeters.

We established the values of 3, 4, and 5, because they are quoted as quality features for osteosyntheses [139, 259]. In reality they are *completely unsuitable* for the characterization of practical osteosynthesis compatibility because they also include the stretch. Stretching of osteosynthesis material under tension would mean nothing other than distraction of the fractured pieces.

6. The tension load in N on attaining Rp 0.2 (the so-called 0.2% stretch limit) at which the test piece stretched approximately 0.2% – i.e., only very slightly. This value signals the border between the reversible elastic deformation and the beginning of the irreversible plastic elongation.

▶ **The results of point 6 are the most important and the single relevant reference value as regards the quality of the operation of individual implants, because they describe the level of the possible tension forces which can be applied to each wire or cable in the osteosynthesis where they are effective as interfragmentary compression.**

3.2
Results

The results are represented synoptically as a diagram (Fig. 24) and in Table 1. The different qualities of the samples can be seen at a glance from the different levels of their curves: cables do much better than traditional cerclage wires.

3.2.1
Tensile Strength of Cerclage Wire and Wire Cables

The load-elongation diagram represents a graphical relationship between the load applied in N and the resulting lengthening of the sample. The lengthening attributable to a specific load is made up of one elastic component and one plastic component from the elastic limit Rp 0.2. This elastic limit is a common value in engineering that marks the end of Hooke's line describing the end of the elastic phase. It is distinguished by the fact that the sample springs back to its original length after removal of the load. This is the significant quality feature of every traction-loaded implant. On reaching the elastic limit Rp 0.2 (i.e., an overall stretch of 0.2%) the wire cables and the cerclage wires undergo irreversible plastic deformation. (The initial slight plastic deformation at Rp 0.1 may be neglected.)

The length of Hooke's line shows the elastic force reserve with which an osteosynthesis can be made taut. For the four measured cerclage wires, this aver-

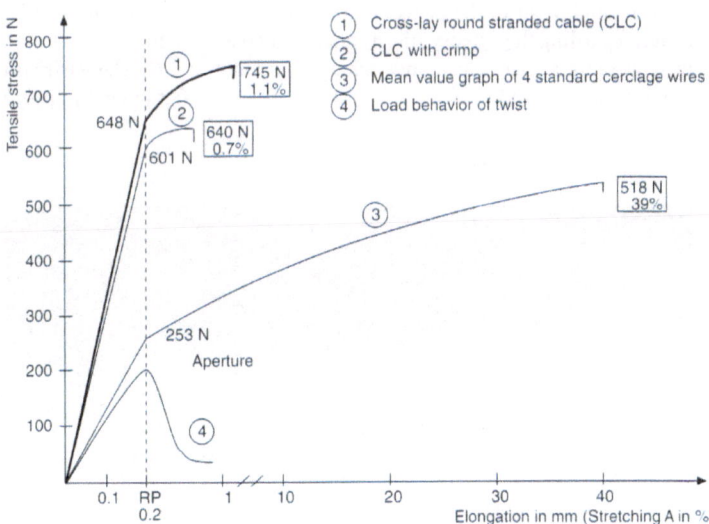

Fig. 24. Load behaviour of wire cables, cable crimp connections, cerclage wires and twists

Table 1. Material ratings of four standard cerclage wires compared with cross-lay cable CLC 04441

	Cerclage wires of 1-mm ∅				Average of A–D	Wire cable of 1-mm ∅ Without crimp	With crimp
	A	B	C	D			
∅ (mm)	0.997	0.990	0.997	0.991	0.989	0.985	0.985
∅ in crack	0.814	0.802	0.808	0.790	0.804	–	–
Difference	0.183	0.188	0.169	0.201	0.185	–	–
QS (mm^2)	0.7807	0.7697	0.7496	0.7713	0.7678	0.4489	0.4489
QS (mm^2) at crack	0.5204	0.5052	0.5127	0.4900	0.5071	–	–
Difference	0.2603	0.2645	0.2369	0.2813	0.2607	–	–
Rm (MPa)	694	656	696	653	675	1660	1425
Rm (N) at crack (Rm × QS)	542	505	522	504	518	745	640
Rm (N) on reaching Rp 0.2	265	243	236	266	253	648	601
A (%) (=mm) (RP 0.2 to crack)	38	39	33	46	39	~1.1	~0.7

∅, diameter; *QS*, cross section; *Rm*, tensile strength; *Rp* 0.2, elastic limit; *A*, stretching.

aged only 253 N, and for our cable 648 N, which corresponds to a theoretical safety factor of 2.6. This results in a different gradient for both Hooke's lines. The value Rp 0.2 is attained late in the cable after a steep increase – in round wires it is reached 2.6 times earlier, which is why its line increases more gently. The elastic limit Rp 0.2 can of course also be seen as the starting point of the arc that follows Hooke's line; it describes the elastic properties.

The length of the arc up to the tear is the directly visible measurement of the stretch – the area of load that from its origin would pull an osteosynthesis and its implant apart. With round wires the arc has a long curve – with cables it is very short. The statement of the tear-tolerance of an implant (i.e., the end point of the curve) is misleading because, regarding the osteosynthesis quality, it falsely represents a load acceptance which could not possibly be achieved.

The outcome of these experiments is that stretching of the wires amounts on average to 39% (39 mm for a 100 mm length of wire), with cables only to about 1.0%. Thus, cables possess excellent quality characteristics.

3.2.2
Tensile Strength of Twists and Cable-Crimp Connections

Is it possible to create tension by twisting? How do wire *connections* hold under tension? These questions are relevant for the judgment of the osteosynthesis compatibility of the test pieces. After all, overall construction is only as stable as its components.

Cerclage wire is twisted with a turning device or flat pliers by applying tension. That is the most fre-

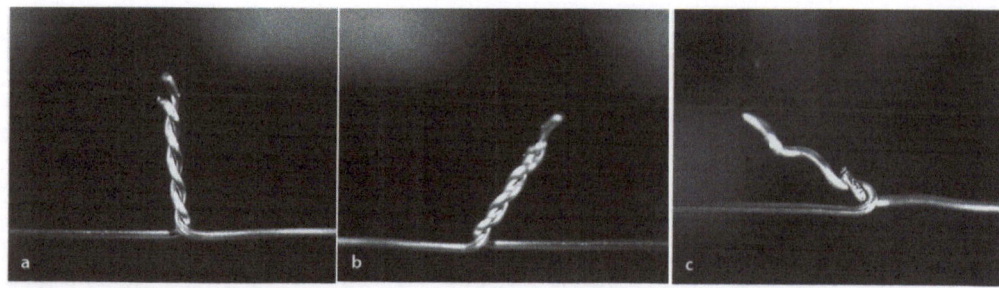

Fig. 25. The loosening of a twist under stress

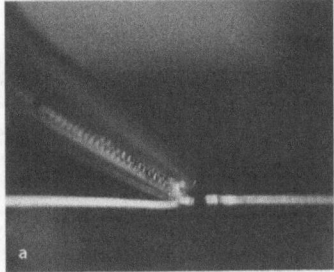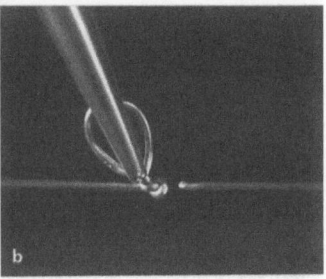

Fig. 26. Breaking of wire in the first coil

quently practised method of fixation, the so-called "twist, wire knot or twist knot" [63, 167, 266, 356, 422].

In a trial, out of two of the wires fastened in the machine, twists with four and eight turns were formed, transversely to the direction of tension. The starting tension amounted to approximately 160 N each time, but decreased on its own in less than 3 s to around 130 N. That happens because of the rebound elasticity of the twists. Unfixed by pliers, the twist bent downwards under tension and opened up; put more precisely, one of the wires unwound itself from the screw-like grip of the other (Fig. 25). Others who carried out the same experiment recorded the same result [135, 145, 422].

In the following trial (Fig. 26), when on reaching a tension of 130 N we turned twists and loops even further using flat pliers in order to initiate more tension, we were unsuccessful. Instead, the first coil broke very quickly (at approximately 250 N), an experience which is not rare when operating [96, 139, 356, 423]. The reason is the cold deformation of the wire through tension and bending on twisting, which makes it brittle and causes it to break. It can be recognized from the mat appearance of the surface in the first coil. Even an additional loop, which under the introduction of higher compressions is put on the opposite side of the wire [136, 284, 323, 339], makes little difference – most of the force is lost in the deformation of the wire.

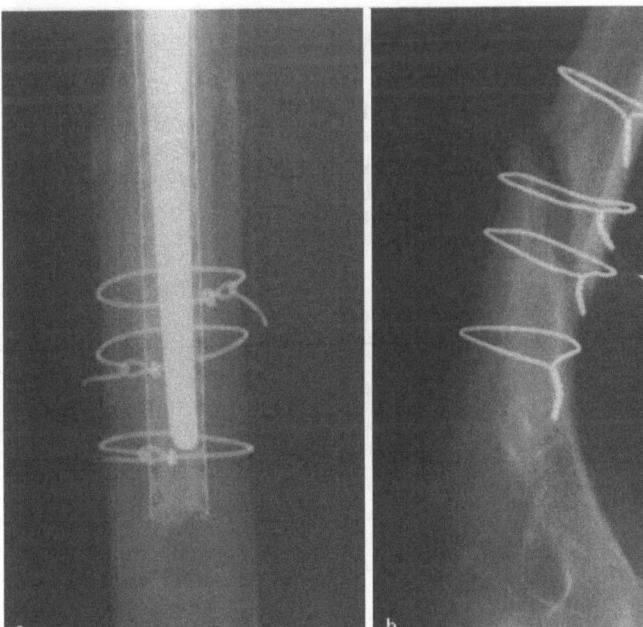

Fig. 27a–f. Clinical examples of relaxed wire loops and turned back and erected twists are frequently found on X-rays. In these cases there is a threat of skin perforation (**e, f**)

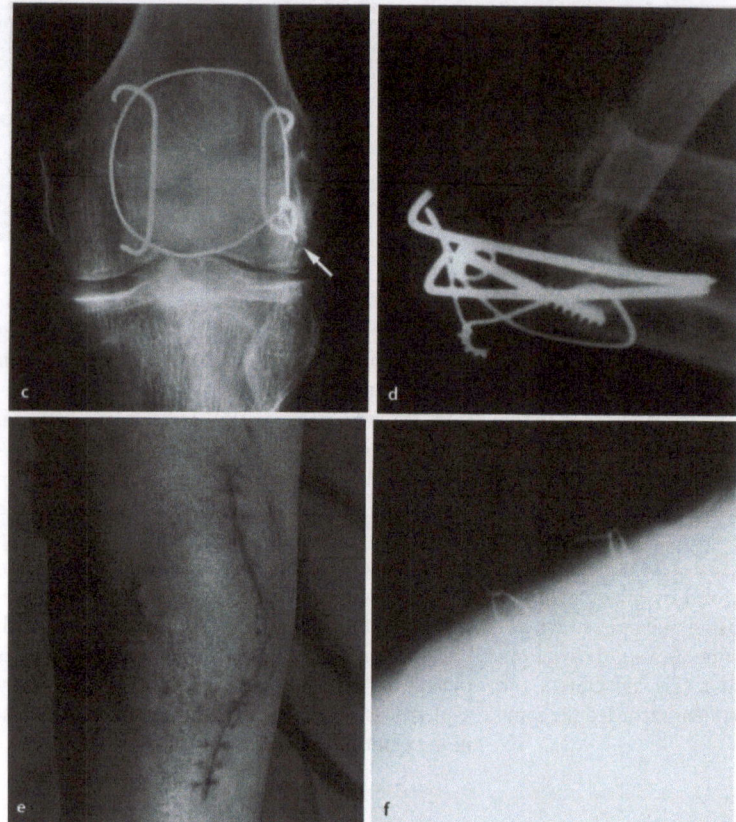

Fig. 27c–f

The stability of a loop knot bent over a pre-fabricated loop has proved even less successful. "Bending and/or cutting the twisted end causes marked loss in wire tension" say Rooks et al. [326] and others [167, 422]; under strain the bent wire end quickly gives way (Fig. 27).

▶ With twist and loop knots no more than an adaptation can be attained intraoperatively, resulting in inadequate bone stabilization [29, 135, 145, 167, 183, 196, 220, 258, 317, 423]. As experience shows, it is high time we replaced wire. As early as 1924, F. König [182] blamed inadequate wire fixation for poor results. In the same year, Steinmann [365], inventor of the Steinmann pin, complained that "often decent anatomical healing fails to come about because the principle of muscle mechanics was disregarded by the operators."

In 1988 Shaw and Daubert [356] gave up, having looked into the possibility of the cerclage fixation systems:

"The wire is prone to break when tightening the twist... *Mersilene tape* appears to be a reasonable alternative to 20-gauge stainless steel wire in terms of fixation capability and ultimate strength." For Franke et al. [95] too, wire osteosyntheses are only adapted because, "...through the torsion of the wire ends tension does not come about because the wire is stressed beyond the yield point and breaks at the first twist."

The cable crimp connections always resisted a tension level of over 600 N. They could therefore be fully subjected to the force of the machine. Their short stretch was not optically communicated; they ripped without warning, always right next to the

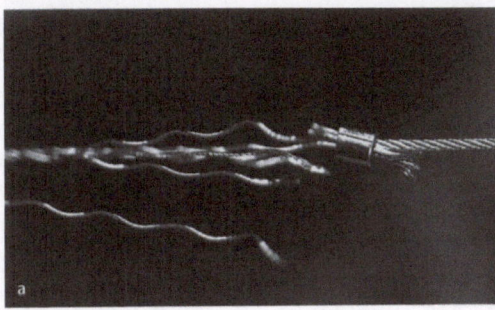

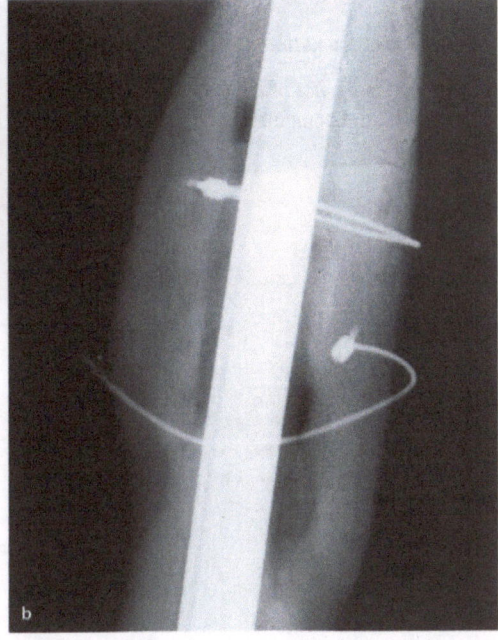

Fig. 28. Tearing of the cable next to the crimper due to the notch-effect

crimp to be precise. The so-called notch-effect is responsible for this. Under a load the crimp aligns in accordance with the resulting forces, leading to slight tilting. Thus a pivot develops in both rims, on which the cable could tear (Fig. 28). In order to minimize this effect, the internal ends of the crimp are funnel-shaped – cf. Fig 18.

To summarize:
A maximum of 130 N can be introduced to twists and loops; with further turns they quickly break.
Over 600 N can be introduced to cable-crimp connections; that corresponds to an improvement factor of 4.6 for the cable.

3.2.3
Tensile Strength of Bent Cerclage Wire

According to Franke et al. [95], "in order to produce effective pre-tension, the wire must neither become bent nor twisted during tightening." But as any X-ray will show, cerclage wire cannot be placed between two points without deviation; it is much too stiff. Therefore a kink can only pass on the force of tension as long as it persists. The force sufficient to stretch it therefore results in the immediate drop of initially attainable pre-tension and finally leads to a loosening of the osteosynthesis [300]. Reproducible results were not attainable in this part of the trial, as the kinks already lengthened with very small tensions. Even if the elongation is only minimal and is hardly or not at all detectable radiologically, this may be a fundamental explanation for the uniting of the fragments, as a rule without tension, in other words merely an *adaptation*, the inherent contradiction of wire *tension banding*.

To summarize:
A kink in the course of the wire straightens under minimal tension. Initial pre-tension will be immediately dispersed.

3.2.4
Evaluation of the Results

From all three parts of the trial the following operation-specific statements can be deduced.

3.2.4.1
Cerclage Wire

1. Cerclage wires can, if at all, only be given very little pre-tension. They elongate early and reciprocally to their rigidity up to approximately 46% of their original length. Their elastic tear-resistance up to the elastic limit Rp 0.2 is not very high, having an average of 250 N. The advantage of better handling of soft wires is negated through low elastic force reserves, whilst stiffer wire can be neither properly laid nor correctly stretched, and so its higher load capacity cannot be utilized [259]. Huberty [139] is opposed to it because of the "powerful tendency to recoil and an associated decrease in tension, and so ultimately the final compression forces are no higher in hard wires than in soft ones."
2. Twists and loops are not particularly resistant to tensions at 130 N; on exceeding this they break without warning at the first coil.
3. Kinks, the unavoidable attribute of any wire osteosynthesis, straighten out under the slightest muscle tension.
   In accordance with these general remarks, with wire tension banding on bony models and cadaveric bones, no or only slight interfragmentary compression was measured [95, 96, 135, 198, 356] and it was recognized that "*none* of the tension banding techniques investigated guarantee active exercise stability" so Brill [29], and that "*none* of the customary clinical tension and fixation procedures for monofilamentous osteosynthesis wire produce permanent tautness" so von Issendorff [145].

3.2.4.2
Wire Cables

1. Owing to their suppleness, cables are to be stretched kink-free – and thus efficiently – between two anchorage points.
2. Cables can be pre-tensioned almost to their tear limit without lengthening plastically. They have a very favorable elastic recoil force.
3. Cable-crimp connections are loadable up to at least 600 N.

From these trials and from textbooks, some general findings may be gleaned: the mode of connection of two tension materials and the way they may be laid faultlessly determine the level of the possible tautness and the load capacity during post-operative treatment. The mechanical properties of a tension material are best characterized by the elastic limits. Tear thresholds at the end of a lengthy elongation process are misleading. Relevant results for cerclage wire disqualify it as a useful implant.

Wire cables are highly effective, based on five results: the most important is the behavior of the pretensed cable-crimp *connection*. Just as a plate osteosynthesis only produces a firm hold after the application of the last screw, so the taut and non-slip fixed tension banding is the adequate state and should remain unaltered within the physiological reduction for the duration of the follow-up treatment, to allow the fracture to heal without complications.

1. At over 600 N, our *cable-crimp connection* made of implant steel 1.4441 is about five times as strong as a twist. It is stronger than cable connections of Co/Cr steel or titanium which have lower load capacities [348].
2. At approximately 1.0 mm the *elongation* of a cable-crimp connection when tearing is very favorable. It guarantees a beneficial level of elasticity, which is based on the cross-lay principle and is regulated mechanically.
3. Cables can be laid with technical precision and great efficiency between two anchorage points – Kirschner wires, screws, PE-sleeves – and remain permanently taut.
4. At, on average, 648 N the cables tested offer 2.6 times higher loadability than cerclage wires in the crucial elastic range although, at 58%, their material cross-sectional area is

only half as big as that of the round wires – 0.4489 mm^2 as opposed to 0.7678 mm^2. Here titanium cables also do badly. They are around 50% less loadable than implant steel cables of the same strength [348]. These disadvantages and undoubtedly higher price are arguments against titanium cables.

5. Another important criterion for the material's quality is fatigue-resistance, that is the number of cyclical tension loads up to the break. It is also substantially higher for V4 A cables than for cerclage wires [104].

3.2.5
References in the Literature

In 1990 v. Issendorff [145], after investigations into tension and fixation of osteosynthesis wires on the patella, came to conclusions that coincide with ours:

1. "Irrespective of the form of tension and fixation of the monofilamentous osteosynthesis wires used in tension banding osteosynthesis, at the end of the maneuver the wire is no longer subject to any traction force. Reality therefore does not match the theoretical observation that tension band wire, in the form of static tautness, balances the dynamic muscle force during movement."
2. "Labitzke's procedure...is indeed the only one of all those tested that still showed a tension at the end of the tension and fixation manoeuvres."
3. "We have been successfully using the Labitzke wire cable for many years for patella tension banding."

Kluger et al. [173] described the differences between cerclage wire and wire cables: "It is precisely this plastic deformability that characterizes every monofilamentous connective wire. Because the customary twist transforms the applied force into the deformation of the wire in the twist to the greatest possible extent, the range of application of the stabilizing tension is limited. That is why as early as 1978 Labitzke introduced the wire cable named after him, which offers *superior values* as regards effective fragment traction forces and also tear resistance and in particular fatigue resistance" – cf. also [439]. However, for reasons not related to the method, this material was not used as widely as anticipated. Over 10 years later polyfile cable was also discovered in America and England to be suitable cerclage material and, due to the producers' activities – without any mention of the first person to describe it – the method once more gained greater interest in Germany and abroad.

▶ **To summarize:**
Based on the results of the experiments and literature it can be safely concluded that cross lay round-stranded cables have proved to be an outstanding material in osteosyntheses subjected to muscular tension – the key words are tension bandings. It may also be deduced that cerclage wire is a means unsuited for osteosyntheses, a temporary measure used for several decades, incapable of transmitting tension forces to the fracture in a controlled manner or withstanding muscular forces during post-operative treatment.

CHAPTER 4

Wire Cables in Everyday Hospital Life

4.1
Introduction

I first experienced wire cables with Schmit-Neuerburg in Essen. During the two decades of their application they have proved to be of such versatility that they have become generally accepted and are in daily use. Wire cables have been of great help in many awkward situations: for example, when an osteosynthesis needs to be given additional support, when a prosthesis has ruptured the femur shaft or when the trochanter has broken off, or in osteosyntheses, where they show better results than ordinary implants. Looking at these types of complications, it may well be said that cerclage wire has proved quite adequate. The stability of a cable osteosynthesis is, however, incomparably higher and allows earlier weight-bearing. When using cables frequently one soon becomes extremely confident; there is a sense of security instead of "apprehension, because even the slightest movement could indeed lead to displacement of the fragments" Winkelbauer already wrote in 1925 [423].

The range of indications for the use of wire cables has meanwhile expanded considerably. Many a procedure that uses other implants has been superseded because cables are more effective. Cable tension banding in fractures of the ankle, the trochanter, the tuberculum majus, or the epicondyli humeri is more effective than conventional wire techniques or a screw. Used together with Kirschner wires and screws, occasionally in conjunction with polyethylene sleeves inserted intra-osseously, the degree of stability or limited movement achieved is such that totally new application methods have been developed, where the rigid cerclage wire could never have proved successful. As examples, take the compression of the tibial head osteotomy for axis straightening [214], cable arthrodesis on the upper ankle joint

and in Pirogoff amputation [211, 215], sleeve-cable tensioning in cases of Malgaigne pelvic rupture [210], Weigand's temporary cruciate ligament protection with a cable [414], and bone transfer across large areas for filling in defects by means of cable tensioning using a fixator [11, 331] (Fig. 29).

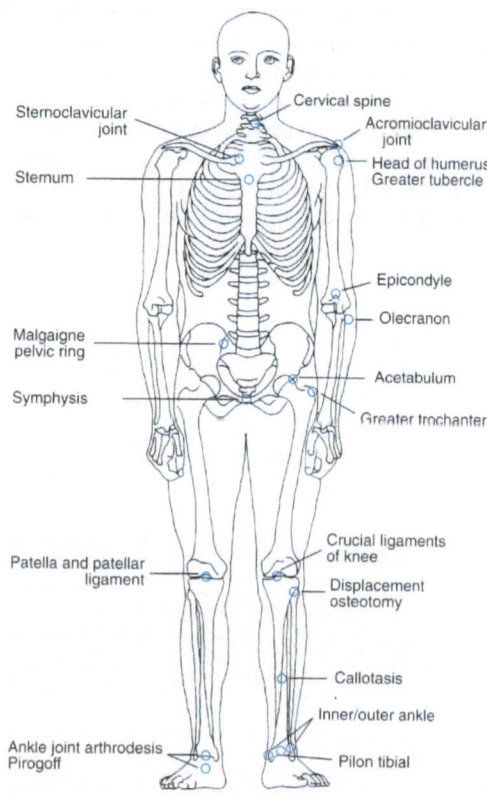

Fig. 29. Application possibilities for wire cables

▶ From 1.3.1982 until 31.12.1995, in the *Surgical Clinic of the University of Witten-Herdecke* at the Evangelisches Krankenhaus Schwerte, wire cables were used in more than 1200 cases with the most divergent indications. That may not seem to be a great number when looking at the time frame, but it is considerable enough to make an unambiguous statement. With approximately 35% of our operative spectrum being accident and restorative surgery, cables are increasingly used; on average 90–100 times per annum. (At the time of printing we surveyed over 1600 cases).

4.2
Technical Instructions for Operations

The following instructions for operations are given according to Blauth's easily applied outlines which he prepared for the journal "Operative Orthopädie und Traumatologie." The technical part of an osteosynthesis, which forms the basis of every actual operation with cables, is described first. It encompasses ever-recurring steps of putting in place, anchoring, tightening, squeezing, and cutting the cable: operative procedures are thus standardized.

There are always *two prerequisites* to be fulfilled conscientiously, namely the *secure anchorage* and the *safe fixation* of taut cables in a crimp.

4.2.1
Tension Band Principle

It is never permissible in tension banding for a cable to be anchored securely to tendon insertions without additional foundation anchorage [36, 339, 434]. Neither a tendon nor cancellous bone, nor the low strain resistance of a bore canal can counteract the force of a cable, neither initially nor permanently. In such a high-tensioned construction cables simply must be secured with Kirschner wires or screws in order to provide tension. These aids are indispensable for tension banding – according to the technical definition: the introduction of force through pretensioning [220]. Weber himself already stipulated this, regarding the olecranon, in his inauguration paper [408] (Fig. 30).

- Position and drill 2 Kirschner wires (1) and (e.g., on the olecranon) also a foundation screw (2).
- Slip on the end loop of a ready-made 15 cm long cable (3) over the free end of a medullary Kirschner wire, cut the tendon longitudinally over the Kirschner wire directly on the bone so that the loop can be guided onto the upper surface of the bone, without interposing any soft tissue, and can be laid there.
- Put the free end of the cable into an awl and guide it *under* the tendon tissue directly towards the bone.
- The process is repeated with a second ready-made cable at the other end of the Kirschner wire (at the patella) or (in other tension bandings) at the foundation screw, which Brunner and Weber [33] also recommended. The screw is *first* passed through the loop and then inserted into the bone.

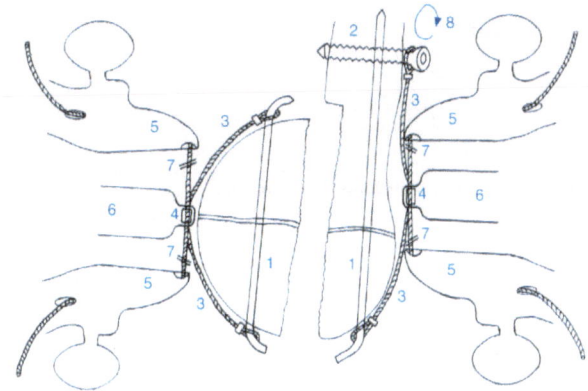

Fig. 30. Technical operating instructions for quasi-axial tension bandings, on the *left*, the patella, on the *right*, the olecranon. The individual steps are shown in numerical sequence, as used in the actual operations

4.2.2
Cerclage

In a peri-osseous cerclage a cable is securely anchored without further measures or aids, avoiding interposition of soft tissue. The pressure resistant cortical bone withstands the tension (Fig. 31).

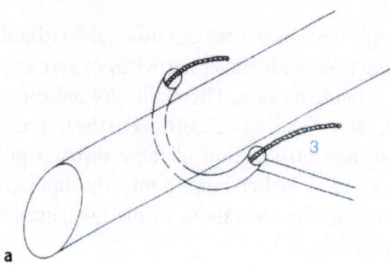

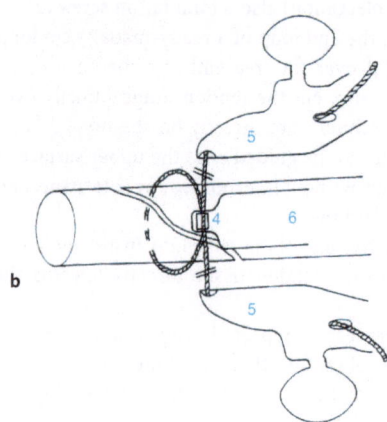

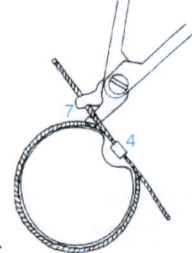

Fig. 31. Operating instructions for cerclages

- Using a hollow Dechamps (or a large Overholt or a curved renal peduncle clamp) passed directly around the long bone, a cable of suitable length (3) cut from the roll is threaded through. Withdraw the guiding apparatus.

- With a narrow chisel or Luer pliers, a small cortical hollow – a free space – is made where the crimp is to lie. This is done because the anterior lip of the crimp pliers is 1 mm thick, the crimp has no contact with bone during the squeezing process. After removal of the pliers the crimp falls down onto the cortical bone. When this happens the circumference of the cable relative to the circumference of the bone is too large and the cerclage too loose. The pre-tensioning attained is consequently reduced or is completely lost (Fig. 32).

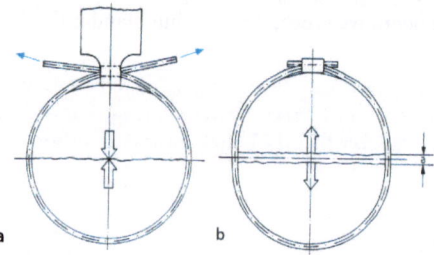

Fig. 32. Effect of crimping directly on the bone surface: loss of tension

4.2.3
Sleeve-Cable Combinations

The third method of providing foundation anchorage [206] is by using self-tapping PE-sleeves (Fig. 33):

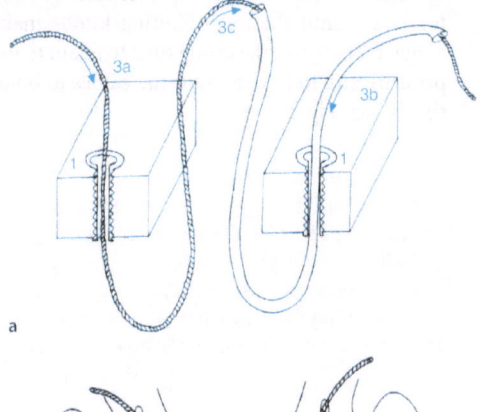

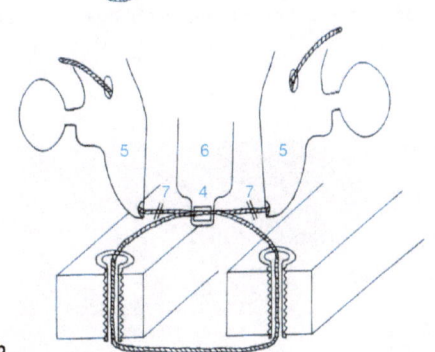

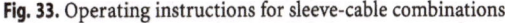

a

b

Fig. 33. Operating instructions for sleeve-cable combinations

- Using the small Allen key, two self-tapping sleeves (1) are screwed into the two bone canals drilled out with the 3.5-mm drill.
- A cable (3a) is then passed through one of the sleeves from above and a cable-carrying tube (3b) is passed, also from above, through the other. A piece of a large lumen venous catheter cut diagonally is suitable for this purpose.
- Now the cable appearing at the far end of the sleeve is threaded at a comfortable distance in front of the site into the far end of the carrying tube (3c) and pulled back together with the carrying tube through the opposite sleeve. (A sharpened Strauss cannula serves the same purpose but is not quite as practical.)

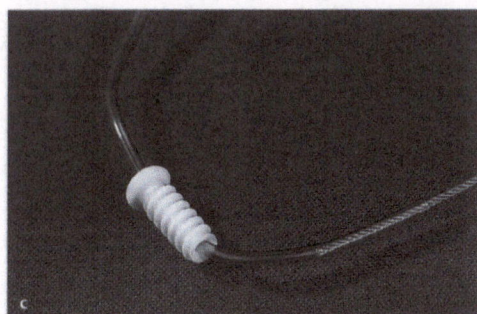

4.2.4
Stretching and Crimping

In the examples in Figs. 30, 31, and 33, two cable ends lie free. They have to be further dealt with (Fig. 34):

- A crimp (4) is slipped over one of the two cable ends and then the other end is passed through it running in the opposite direction. This is best performed with the crimp held between forefinger and thumb.
- Both cable ends are secured in the channels of the cable tensioner (5) by tightening the wing nuts.
- By pulling the easily-opened tensioner away from the bone, space can be made for positioning the crimp pliers (6). Their jaws are slid from one side over the crimp and the latter is gripped in the correct position. It must not jut out at the side – cf. Fig. 40. Gentle plier pressure prevents the clasped crimp from slipping. The assistant holds it in a suitable position over the concave upper surface of the bone or above the excavated hollow.

- Now the surgeon slowly turns the T-handle of the cable tensioner to the right until it becomes stiff and the Kirschner wires bow.
- After tightening the cable the assistant presses the handles of the crimper together continuously for 1–2 s until the force-limiting knobs make contact. That gives the crimp time to adapt to the pressure and to flow, and for the cables to bond firmly – cf. Fig. 21.

> The pressure being applied on turning the tensioner and the sideways deflection of the Kirschner wires to which the cables are attached are indicators of increasing cable tension. Deflection should amount to about 10–15°. Further tightening does not increase interfragmentary compression, but merely bends the wires further.

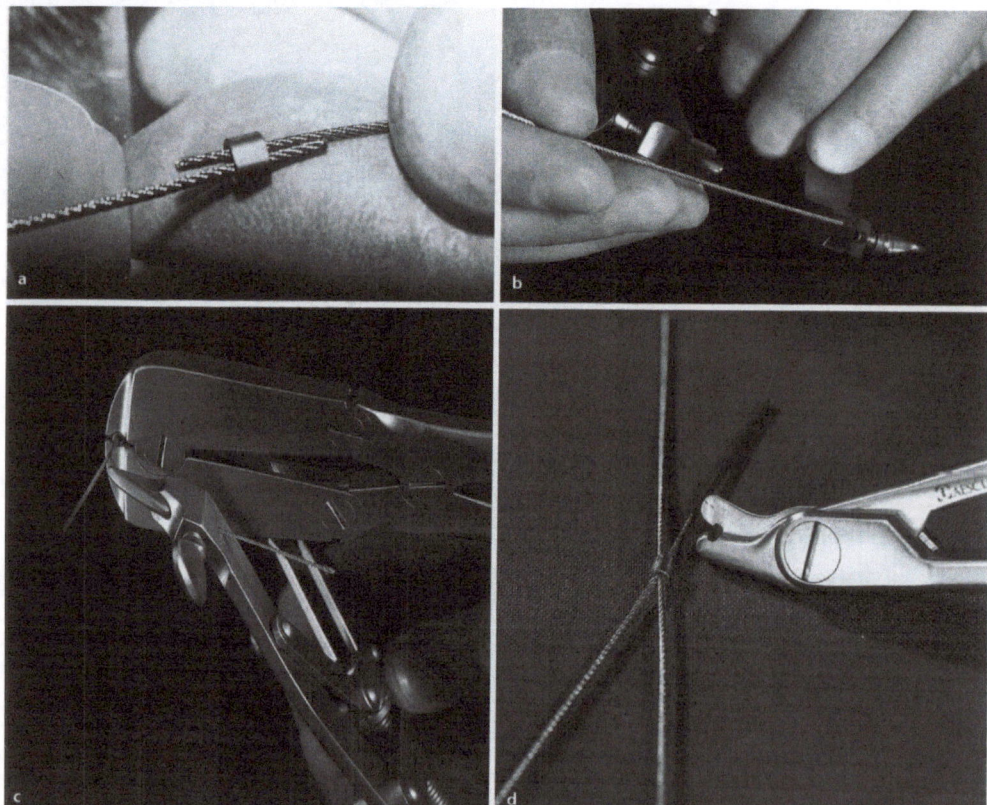

Fig. 34. Additional operating instructions

4.2.5
The Final Steps

- Now the tensioner is loosened a little and pulled away from the bone so that the cable scissors (7) can come into action directly next to the crimp.
- The Kirschner wires are shortened, bent away from the cables (so that the latter cannot slip), and finished off. Pointed telephone pliers may be an advantage here or Zimmer's curved forceps.
- Finally the foundation screw (8) is tightened. The loop sliding up onto the semi-spherical screw head has the effect of producing additional tension due to lengthening of the pathway (Fig. 35).

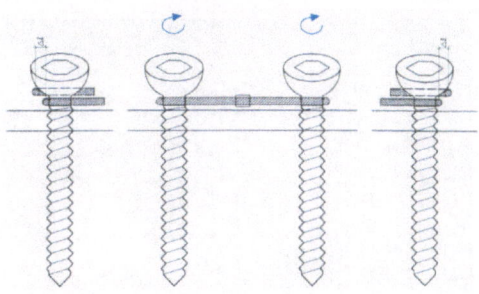

Fig. 35. Effect of final screwing: additional tension

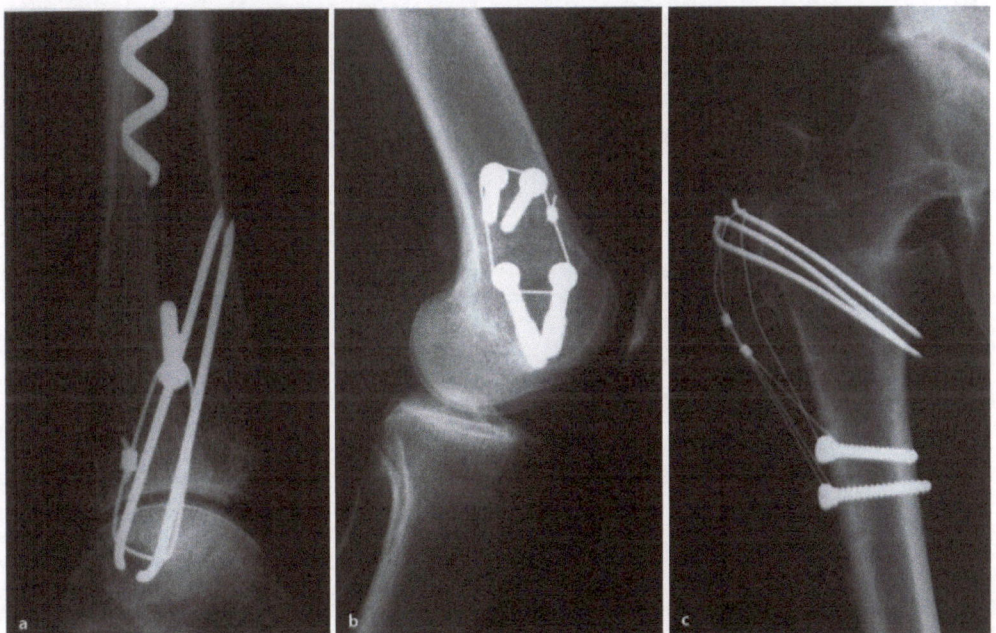

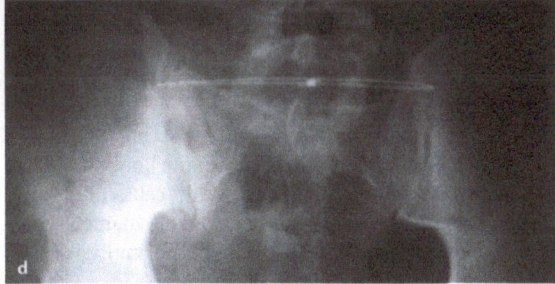

Fig. 36. The high technical standard of cable osteosyntheses can be demonstrated with X-ray pictures. **a** Ancle fracture (above the end of an Endo-Helix, stabilizing a shaft fracture). **b** Supracondylar corrective osteotomy. **c** Secondary distalisation of the greater trochanter after incomplete corrective osteotomy (note the bent K-wires). **d** Sleeve-cable banding of the ileo-sacral joints in a Malgaigne injury

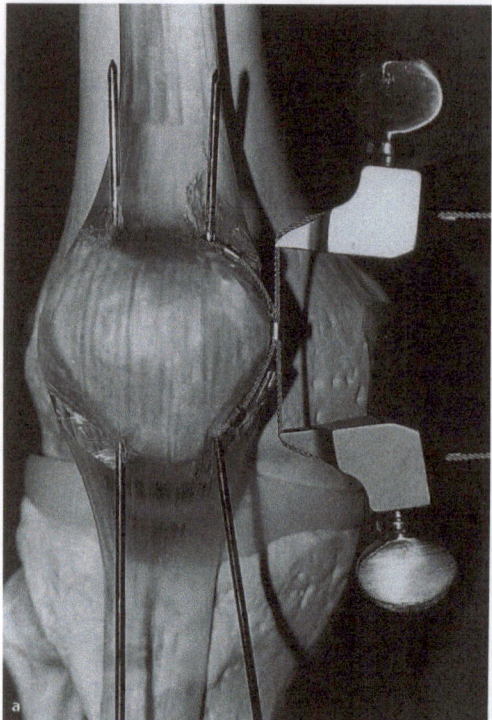

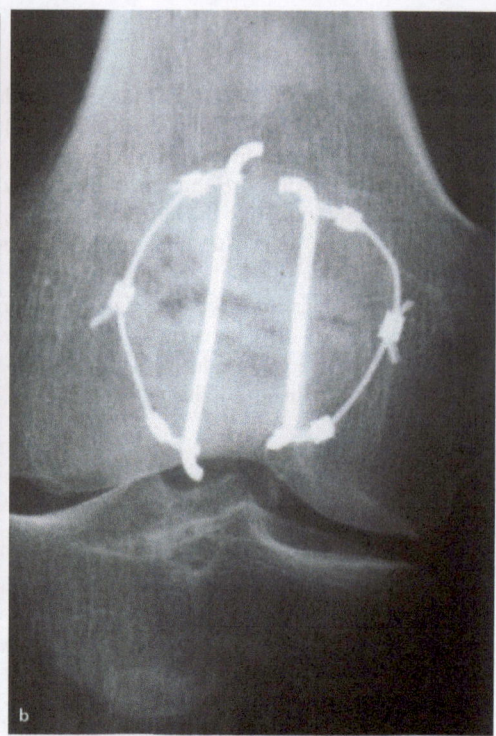

4.2.6
Errors and Risks

> Note: Basic prerequisites for the lasting stability of a cable osteosynthesis are secure cable anchorage and sound cable bonding which does not allow slipping.
> Tension banding means tension on the banded, i.e., anchored traction device!

- Wire cables must only be tightened on the surface of bones and must not cross tendons and soft tissue. The longitudinal incision of a tendon above Kirschner wires is indispensable for this.

Correctly and wrongly positioned cable loops are shown in Fig. 37.

- A loop attached at a distance from the bone surface results, on applying tension to the cable, only in bowing of the Kirschner wires and not in interfragmentary compression; the osteosynthesis works loose.

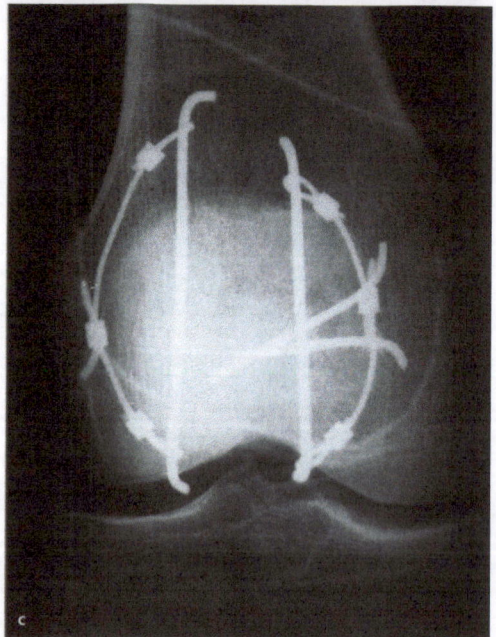

Fig. 37. Bent K-wire as indication for high interfragmentary compression (**a, b**; non-union). Insufficient anchorage of cables may lead to distraction (**c**)

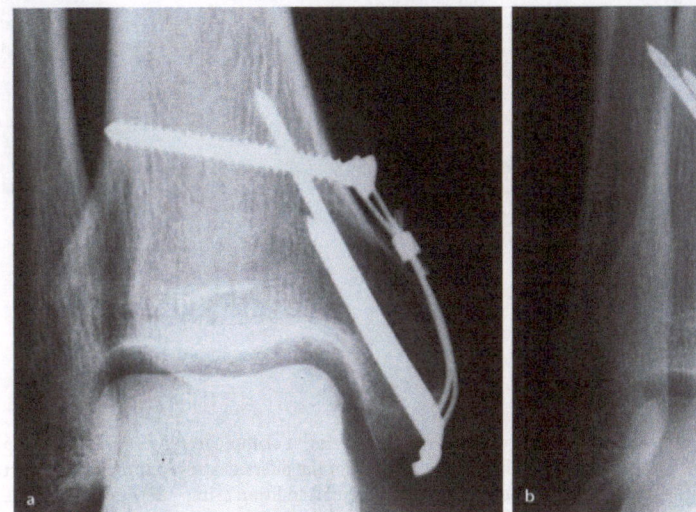
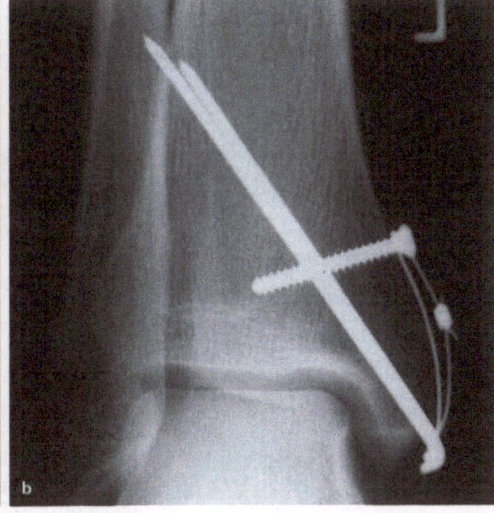

Fig. 38. A screw tightens particularly effectively if it is placed in the direction of strain; note the bent Kirschner wires. Screwed in convergently with the direction of tension, it leads – upon tightening – to a decrease in tension because the distance between the fixation points will reduce

- Squeezing without contact being made between the force-limiting knobs is insufficient because only partial pressure is produced at the jaws of the pliers – cf. Fig. 21.
- The crimp must not project from one side of the jaws of the pliers because it would then only be squeezed partially.
- The crimp must be correctly fitted into the jaws so that it can be safely squeezed. Clasped at an an-

gle, squeezing would not be successful. Apart from that the cable, wrongly held, would be crushed and the anterior lip of the pliers destroyed (Fig. 40).

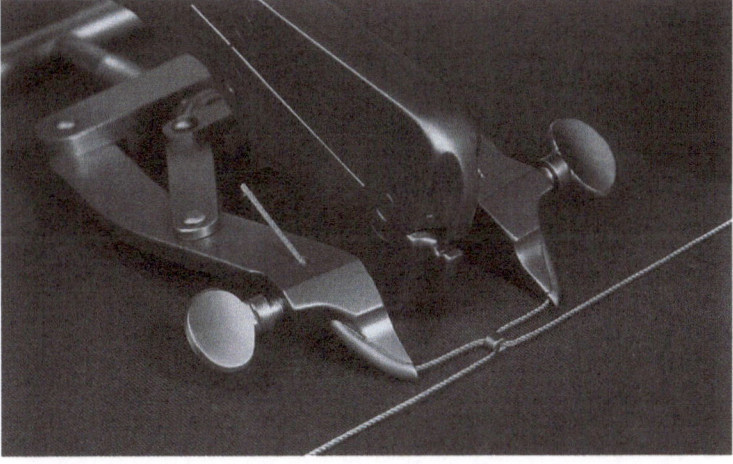

Fig. 39. If both cable ends were passed through the crimp from one side it could not be tightened and squeezed adequately – besides, the crimp would stand on end. Cables slip in the tensioner if the wing nuts are not screwed up tightly enough; full cable tension would not be reached

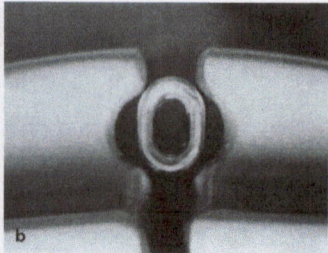
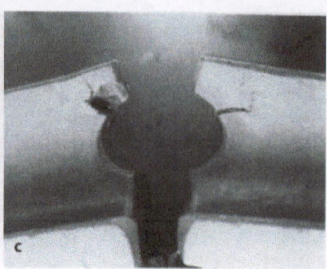
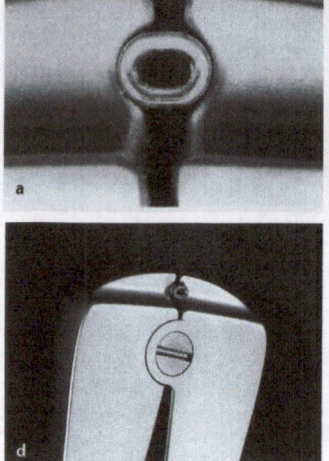

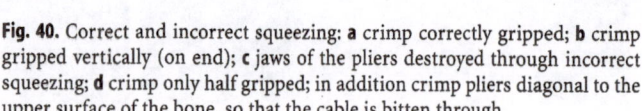

Fig. 40. Correct and incorrect squeezing: **a** crimp correctly gripped; **b** crimp gripped vertically (on end); **c** jaws of the pliers destroyed through incorrect squeezing; **d** crimp only half gripped; in addition crimp pliers diagonal to the upper surface of the bone, so that the cable is bitten through

- Squeezing without a free space on the outer side of a bone concavity or hollow leads to loss of tension after the pliers are removed – cf. Fig. 32.
- If the crimp pliers are not held at a 90° angle (in both planes) but diagonal to the upper surface of the bone, they can crush the cable. In addition, tension would only be partially produced because the cable would be lifted off the bone.

- Not tightening up the foundation screw at the end will result in loss of tension – cf. Fig. 35.
- Do not cut off any projecting cable until the cable tension device has been released and pulled away a little from the bone. This protects the tension banding cable and makes it possible for the cable scissors to make a clean cut (Fig. 41).

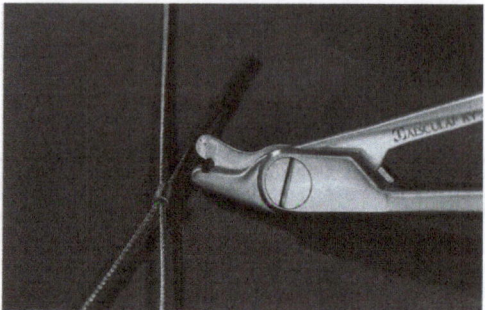

Fig. 41. Correct cut only in the cuting notches

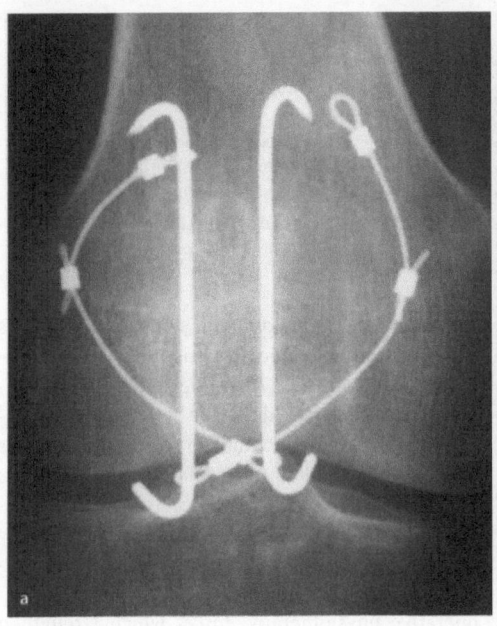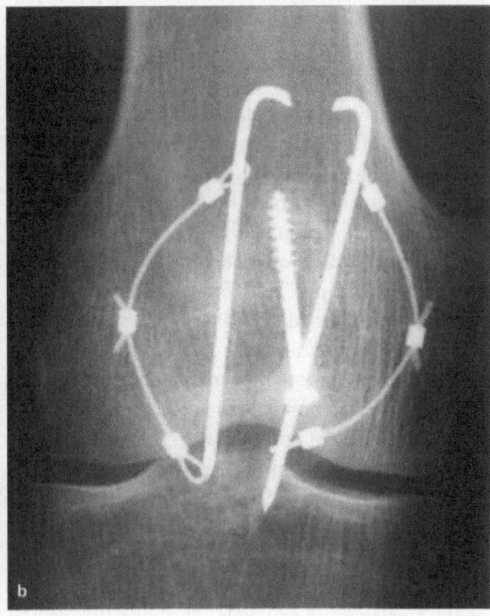

Fig. 42. Cable loops can easily slip down the Kirschner wires when the latter are bent towards them or are not bent at all – then they move

4.3
The Mechanics of Bone Healing

Electrical potentials stimulate the osteoblasts [7, 8, 78]. They develop as a consequence of changing pressure and pulling forces, to which the skeleton is permanently exposed together with many other forces and to which it adapts. Wolff's law of transformation states that only a specifically determined *physiological* force level maintains a balance between construction and destruction of bone [428]. An amount lacking or a certain excess will cause atrophy, whereas a little give within a natural margin has a stimulating effect and leads to hypertrophy. Interpreted mechanically the development of the skeleton of a species can be understood as the result of its adaptation to external forces or, more precisely, to the sum of individual resulting forces. Clear examples of this are the structure and posture of the human spinal column which, during the course of the palaeontology of Homo sapiens, has become erect due to the rotation of the pelvis from the horizontal to the vertical [27, 89, 256, 367, 415], the shaping of the femurs with the formation of a

specific CCD-angle [293, 367], and of an inclination of 9°, which is their frontal "neutral position" [204].

In the case of a fracture external forces shape the callus. With a little too much movement hypertrophic stimulated callus is formed, usually with a gap which remains visible for a long period between the "elephant feet." A large degree of surplus movement results in non-union. Callus develops normally if these forces are restricted to a stimulating level, for example by a plaster cast or non-rigid osteosyntheses.

Primary bone healing [421] differs from natural restitution because movement between the fragments, held together by pressure, is completely excluded; there is no chance for callus formation. This healing of fractures, generated artificially, using rigid implants therefore needs much longer before weight-bearing is allowed; premature metal removal causes re-fracturing. However, this form of osteosynthesis is often necessary, for example in order not to endanger the reconstructed anatomy after joint fracture during post-operative treatment, and for fractures that are subject to particular distraction because of high muscular strain. For such types of fracture, interfragmentary compression is essential, but not for dia-metaphysis breaks.

A primary direct bone union also develops from cartilage-bone transplants which are removed with precision using hollow diamond reamers and inserted ,pressfit' fashion into suitably reamed bony layers [77, 102] – undoubtedly a form of osteosynthesis for the near future.

Weller [418] formulated the school of thought that pressure within a break could be generated in two different ways. "With interfragmentary compression one distinguishes between static interfragmentary compression, i.e., applied once and maintained as long as possible, and dynamic interfragmentary compression, which is constantly renewed through movement and muscle action as well as an additional strengthening effect. *Static* interfragmentary compression can be achieved very simply with the so-called tension or compression screw. *Dynamic* interfragmentary pressure is created with the help of what is known in the technological world as the *tension band principle*. Applying this principle, strain and bending forces are neutralized and converted into pressure forces" [418].

▶ In my opinion this distinction between static and dynamic compression entails a serious misunderstanding, due to the incorrect application of the rules of mechanics to operating techniques. Structural engineers produce stability through *static* processes, by *permanent* introduction at a level of forces which oppose the expected ones and exceed them. Compression cannot be achieved by means of movement within a system which is geared to strength. Movement always means instability and the danger of destruction.

Instead of separating dynamic and static processes it would be more correct to distinguish *flexible* osteosyntheses from *rigid* ones. Flexible interfragmentary compression could then be understood as stabilization introduced through movement in phases and rising and falling as an *addition* to the *static fundamental strength* that is produced by the osteosynthesis. Just as a bridge is given extra rigidity by the traffic load passing over it, in the same way external forces can be put to use by well-directed postoperative physiotherapy; forces which strengthen the primary static stability base of an osteosynthesis. This is valid for plate osteosynthesis as well as for tension banding.

This subject, which is fundamental to the understanding of tension banding, will be dealt with in detail next.

4.4
Biomechanic of Tension Band Principle

In technical constructions very high forces are regularly compensated for by the generation of opposing forces which exceed the expected forces with a safety factor and are permanently effective. Tension banding follows the same principle. It was transferred by Pauwels to surgical medicine and forms its own osteosynthesis category which occupies an akknowledged place in the treatment of bone fractures. Tension banding is best carried out with wire cables which have to be firmly secured in order to be able to produce pre-tensioning and, as a consequence, interfragmentary compression.

4.4.1
Tension Banding as a Technical and Osteosynthecic Principle

The concept of tension banding is associated with Weber. Based on only a minimum of groundwork [118, 294], he drew up a functional procedure that (despite all the disadvantages) improved the results of olecranon and patella fractures and stimulated biomechanical thinking.

My interest in tension banding was triggered off by a non-union of an olecranon fracture which had been operated on in accordance with the acknowledged technique. In the analysis of this and similar cases, disadvantages of tension banding which became evident were increased by the lack of osteosynthesis material. Experiments based on newly acquired knowledge led to *bilateral* tension banding in 1974. Four years later the wire cables described here were first used on living patients [195, 203, 205].

Weber's tension banding on the patella and the olecranon is one of the most impressive examples. It is "viewed as a simple procedure in the surgical treatment of bone fractures, the biomechanical principle of which is easy to grasp." This widespread opinion is not accepted unreservedly by Roesgen and Koch [323], because "the frequency with which mistakes of the most varying types are made are obvious proof that this cannot be so."

Tension bandings demand much higher pre-tensioning than cerclages because they have to counterbalance high muscle forces. The effects of the quadriceps in the case of a patellar fracture would be null and void if the fragments had not been firmly pressed together by means of a tensioning device. Reconstructing a patella with such stability that it can immediately carry out its function correctly without external splinting therefore means giving it such a strong hold by pre-tensioning the osteosynthesis that muscular tension forces influential during the therapeutic exercises are compensated without further ado.

The theory of the tension band has been recognized and understood since Pauwels and Weber. Ekke [81] considered it "the best and neatest principle in functional surgery." The validity of the theory was declared to be beyond doubt by the following claim: on the traction side of a bone fracture tension should be generated with wire, which is transformed into pressure by bending. It is alleged that this should be caused *dynamically*, i.e., through additional movement, and not statically, because that is the very characteristic and significance of tension banding [41, 42, 266, 416, 417, 435]. For this reason it would be necessary for the fragments on the posterior side (i.e., near the joint) to gape [264, 408]. Pauwels was done an injustice with this theory of transformation because he had actually applied it quite differently, using the example of balancing the body *weight* – a *static* force therefore – over the supporting leg, not in fact to the kinetic function but to the "extremely important *static* function of the musculature" [294]. Pauwels expressly called the tension band *compression* osteosynthesis [297]. Obviously that was misunderstood. For tension banding Weller [417] always demanded "functional treatment according to dynamic interfragmentary compression," i.e., movement. We agree with Ecke [81]: "things should be reconsidered".

From a technical point of view, tension banding is the neutralization of forces by the pre-tensioning of special elements of the construction. Its theory stems from concrete engineering. Concrete, a mixture of sand and cement, has practically no tensile strength so that under bending strain severe fissures tend to appear at a very early stage. Everyone has probably already noticed that during the construction of a house the ceiling of a storey is first formed with a steel grid and then concrete is poured over it into a mold. The tensile strength of the steel is enough to absorb safely the comparatively slight bending strain of a floor. Taking particular precautions that are met by using so-called pre-stressed concrete, the bending load-bearing capacity increases considerably without having to fear dangerous cracks. The carriageway of a bridge, highly stressed due to traffic load, requires more than a loosely laid steel net. Here, additional tension banding, i.e., pre-*tensioning and anchorage* of the steel reinforcement, is necessary. An excerpt from the fundamentals of concrete engineering by Dr. Ing. Troche, a civil engineer, may provide further insight:

"The fundamental idea behind pre-stressed concrete is to introduce into the weight-bearing supporting structure additional strains which are directed to counteract those produced by the load. They should be of such a size, that dangerous strains do not occur in the concrete. Pre-tensioning force is applied *statically* to the weight-bearing supporting structure to such an effect, according to position and direction, that it coincides with the resulting force of the inner strains arising from the load" [387].

Pre-tensioning can be produced using the following methods. "In the Freyssinet system the existing strain reinforcement is tightened up by means of a special ‚tension bed'. It is then *anchored* at the ends after hardening of the concrete with the help of special anchors against the concrete. The pre-tensioning force is then removed. The *strain reinforcement has to be of such an extent* that it creates *at least equally large pressure strains in any position* in the concrete as the largest strains that will later appear from the load.

In Finsterwalder's pre-stressed concrete construction the dead weight of one concrete beam with central articulation induces *pressure forces within the entire structure by means of a firmly anchored and strained tension cable*", so again Troche.

The most important part of this theory of pre-stressed concrete is that even from the start such high pressure forces develop in the whole structure through pre-tensioning forces, transferred to firmly anchored strain-resistant elements, that all tension forces which might occur later are neutralized by these forces only – once again according to Troche. The medical profession has continually misinterpreted this part or rather ignored it. In their own definition of tension banding pretensile forces are only required to press together parts of the area, mostly the extensor side, and compression of the whole fracture zone should only arise through additional movements in the operated limb itself and not just as a result of the implant. That is a *fundamental mistake*: tension banding in a technical and therefore medical sense means *achieving permanent pressure in the whole cross-sectional area by pre-tensioning – i.e., statically – and by no other means.*

▶ **The tension band is a *static* principle, a *static* osteosynthesis!**

In this respect it does not differ in any way from other pressure osteosyntheses, such as screwing and plating; they, too, are static principles. But whilst screws, like clamps, press together a fracture *rigidly*, the original tension banding (as realized in bilateral cable tension banding) allows *elastic* alterations in strain, *although without any movement within the fracture*. This stimulates osteoblasts and encourages biological bone healing. If clinically tangible progress is to be attained with tension bandins, these conditions must be accepted and *interfragmentary movements have to be replaced by elastic compression.*

In structural analysis the connection of a strain-resistant element with a pressure-resistant element is referred to as *composite building*. Its characteristic feature is a high degree of strength with minimal material expenditure. Knese [174] and Otto [289] have shown that human bones also correspond to multidimensional composite building, which makes them particularly stable: collagen fibers are the strain-resistant element, calcium apatite as a solid absorbs pressure. These two construction elements form the *basic stability* of the skeleton. They are opposed by external tension banding systems. These are formed by muscles, fasciae, and ligaments which adapt themselves in the development of their forces partly actively and partly passively to external influences, and thus neutralize static pressures, flexion, and dynamic forces which develop due to body weight and kinetic energy during movement. Every fracture annuls the many different components of these *two* tension-banding systems in the bones and in soft tissue of the corresponding sector of movement, or reverses them [204]. A point most vividly illustrated by Pauwels is his comparison of the femur – musculus et tractus ileotibialis unit with a crane: the body weight pushes the broken neck of the femur downwards and both musculature and tractus pull the femur shaft, which now has no resistance, upwards [292]. It results in a pathological varus deformity. The external rotators, predominant as far as forces are concerned, turn the leg outwards, hence the well-known ad hoc diagnosis of fractures of the femur near the hip.

▶ In the living world, a functional element of the highest efficiency is added to basic stability: tissue fluid *additionally* raises resistance to pressure and flexion forces – a type of water cushion effect. It increases the pressure load capacity of the bone framework considerably compared with the substance which is resistant to pressure. This "hydroelastic component", Labitzke 1979 [204], paraphrased by the architect and structural engineer Otto [287, 289] with the not altogether well-chosen term "pneu" (a system of outer covering, filling, and internal tension) and in 1984 called the "hydraulic system" as an element of construction by Draenert et al. [76, 78] – is *the most fundamental principle of stability in nature*. It determines the firmness of a blade of corn, whose length is almost infinitely longer than the minimal width of its cross-section and it increases the load-bearing capacity of a human vertebral disc under the stress of weight-lifting; it helps to keep total endoprostheses firmly implanted and it raises the resistance of cancellous bone (like that of the patella for instance) to the cutting in of thin pre-tensioned wire cables. It is not, as Pauwels [294] thought, tension banding that is the first principle of construction in nature, but the hydroelastic system! The "pneu," a term coined by biologists and architects in Stuttgart in 1973 [288] is, according to Otto, "*the* construction system and construction element of *living* nature," which determines the active part of all natural and many technical building plans (Fig. 43).

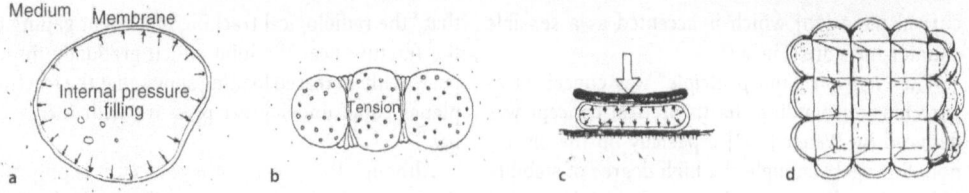

Fig. 43. So-called "pneus", a *living* construction which forces balanced distributes to all directions and by that reduces (from [287])

The non-existence of this hydroelastic stability grafted to basic stability in the case of cadaveric bones falsifies every in vitro experiment, which will be considered in detail later – see page 64.

Where treatment is concerned, the only procedure that can show optimal results is the one that endeavors to replace effectively *both* tension band systems, the inner and the outer. This works most successfully with an osteosynthesis. It has the capacity to imitate the collagen fibers in the bone ripped by the fracture until they heal and to raise quickly reduced hydrostatic pressure within the bone, as well as being able to neutralize the external forces on the fracture that gradually become effective through exercise and partial weight-bearing, provided that the implant is strong enough and has been correctly placed from a mechanical point of view.

In principle, six treatment categories are available for the healing of a fracture and therefore for the restoration of the natural tension banding systems: conventional, medullary cavity stabilisation, plate osteosynthesis, tension banding, the external fixator, and the Kirschner wire pin. The last two procedures are not relevant for the understanding of tension banding.

In conventional treatment forces are neutralized from outside using immobilizing support bandages, extension of the limb, or, particularly on the upper limbs, by including gravity as a functional counterforce to the muscles.

Medullary cavity stabilization in the form of the medullary nail is, mechanically speaking, the optimal osteosynthesis because the nail lies along the axis of the bone. Thus it blocks influential forces on the fracture from the inside and allows additional compression during recovery due to body weight and acceleration. Albeit mechanically sound, in addition to the trauma, the biologically important endosteal vascular system is damaged by the ream-

ing out of the medullary cavity, required for its implantation, or rather by the relatively large mass of a compact nail, quite apart from the embolic consequences of the increase in pressure. The flexible EndoHelix [213, 216] avoids these disadvantages as it is inserted atraumatically – cf. Fig. 106.

In contrast to the medullary nail the *plate* lies eccentrically outside the neutral axis directly on the cortex of the bone. For this reason it is not in a position to exclusively absorb the forces of movement; unfortunately it also generates forces. The visible gaping of the opposite cortical layer is thus a cause of plate breakage and non-union. It occurs, in particular, with high pre-tensioning using a dynamic compression plate. This is avoided with the hollow

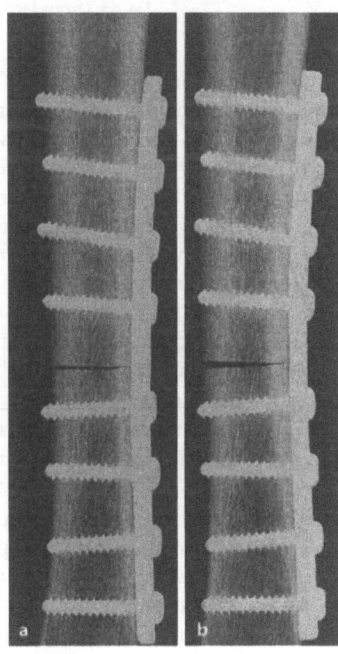

Fig. 44. Gaping opposite cortical layer at 700 N and 1400 N plate tensioning (from [109])

curved plate [70] which is accepted as a sensible counter-measure (Fig. 44).

The *"tension band principle"* was conceived as wire tension banding. Its theoretical concept was deduced by Weber [408] especially on the olecranon. Strangely enough, the high degree of stability to be attained by a plate is not called for in tension banding. Analogous biomechanical findings concerning plate osteosynthesis [70] are deliberately *not* transferred to tension banding: here "dynamic strength" should be adequate – mechanically a contradiction in itself [220].

On the condition that an ulna together with the olecranon would correspond to a horizontal beam loaded at three points, Weber proposed the positioning of the tension band wire on the traction side (Fig. 45).

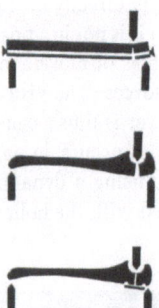

Fig. 45. (from [408])

However, because these conditions do not apply to the bone – it would be as if one wanted to expose it permanently to *isometric* strain (which is neither possible nor desirable) – this location as a means of traction cannot be practical because in the region of the fracture it generates forces whose strength and direction are reversed with the change from resting to exercise and in so doing "disturbance in the fracture region" [41] is produced. In 1963 Pauwels [295] wrote that the counterforce for the muscles is "the weight of the lower arm, possibly plus a load." Povel et al. [305] pointed out a discrepancy, namely that the investigations and calculations carried out by Fick [89] and Pauwels were always based "on a considerable, if not even *maximal* loading of the lower arm," but that correctly understood post-operative treatment "consists of so-called non-weight-bearing exercises where the weight of the lower arm alone represents maximal loading."

Wire banding on the eccentric extensor side brought forth a firmly established principle and a general credo. It was judged by Weber as a good sign

that "the radiological tracking of a slight gaping of the fracture near the joint which gradually disappears with increased loading shows that the fracture planes come under great pressure with increased use."

Although this statement is correct, it is only half the truth. The complete compression of the fracture crevice through movement requires *unconditionally* that the operated ulna is actually strained *isometrically* at three points. However, that would demand permanent triceps activity against the fixed lower arm. Because of the misunderstood analogy with Finsterwalder's articulated concrete beam – fixed at both ends and pressed together statically by a taut and firmly fixed strain element and which, as a result of its weight-conditioned quasi-isometric sagging in fact puts its contact surfaces under pressure, comparable with interfragmentary compression – the two most important fundamental principles from *pre-stressed* concrete construction are not being applied to osseous tension banding, namely:

1. That pre-tensioning should be introduced in such a way that "it coincides *everywhere* according to position and direction with the resultant of the internal traction forces from loading"
2. That it should be so large that "dangerous strain…can no longer occur *at any point*" [387]

This basically means that, instead of compressing, in each procedure, the *whole* fracture with pre-tensioning, in order to be quite sure of eliminating "dangerous breaks" (Troche) or rather a "slight gape" (Weber), – note the interpretation! – Weber's tension banding presses together only a fraction of the crevice, namely that part which lies directly under the tension band wire; the far larger part is *pulled apart* (like the opposite cortex of a long bone using the plate). Here stability is not fully utilized! Instead of *immediately producing pressure over the whole fracture gap during the operation by means of focused traction in the wire* its supporters demand the application of additional external force through *movement* so that the fracture is at least temporarily compressed. Naturally this entails an increased risk factor for the stability of the osteosynthesis. Structural engineers apply strain *from the very beginning* with a resultant force the size and direction of which guarantee that the *whole cross-sectional area* remains permanently compressed *even under traction loading*.

If a force is not exerted in the axis, or more precisely in the *core cross-section*, a defined central part of the surfaces of the whole cross-section, but outside of this region, a gap develops on the opposite side, which technicians call a gaping crack or split. Here it is obviously a question of a region *without any compression, which is all the larger the more eccentrically the force acts*. The width of the gaping crack cannot be a measure of the strength of the tension banding but only a measure of its eccentricity [196, 199]. The more the cerclage is tightened and the further outside the bone axis it is positioned, the more widely the break is *bound* to gape on the opposite side, and the *smaller* is the region actually compressed. This accords exactly with plate osteosynthesis (Fig. 46).

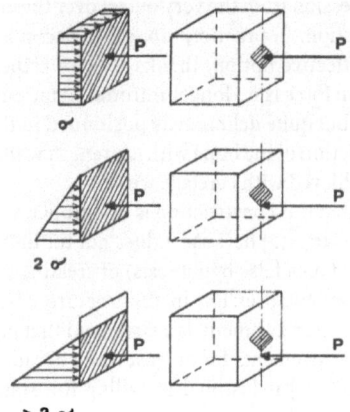

Fig. 46. Effects of different exerting of forces of the same strength

No comment describes the general misunderstanding of this fundamental mechanical principle more vividly than the following by Huberty [139]: "Tension banding fixed eccentrically to the bone axis causes a turning moment in the region of a fracture or osteotomy away from the wire, and thus the development of an additional interfragmentary pressure force (Pauwels, Danis, Weber et al.)." This dorsally directed turning moment naturally does not produce any additional interfragmentary compression, but a gaping crack devoid of pressure. This statement also acts as an example of inaccurate quoting, because none of the authors listed has ever maintained anything of the kind.

Ecke [81], too, was undecided about the developing forces: "Pure flexion forces are indispensable prerequisites for using tension band osteosynthesis without rotatory moments because the rotation would quickly destroy the stability." The objection to this is that flexion without a turning moment is mechanically impossible.

Wondrak [431] confuses cause with effect: "Unfortunately tension banding has a weak point which lies in the relative instability of the bore wires in the medullary cavity." In order to restrict their movement, anchoring them in the opposite cortical layer is recommended [86, 153] or using non-sliding pins with thread or loops [224, 432]. Kirschner wires do not however loosen upon their own accord, but only if they are not made fast by a taut tension band wire. "Symptomatic metal prominence was particularly common after AO tension-band wiring, occurring in 80% of olecranon fractures" [272].

The eccentricity of tension banding is essentially determined by the *diagonal positioning of the wire* – the resultant R in Fig. 47. With a shortened distance between Kirschner wire and the bore canal, it and its unwelcome consequences are increased [196, 327], which becomes blatantly obvious when using thin Kirschner wires – cf. Fig. 81.

A gaping crack, extended incongruent joint surfaces, and steps – these purely mechanically induced disadvantages represent the *at-rest-condition* of conventional tension banding, the *unstrained* situation, for they are caused solely by wire pre-tensioning – if

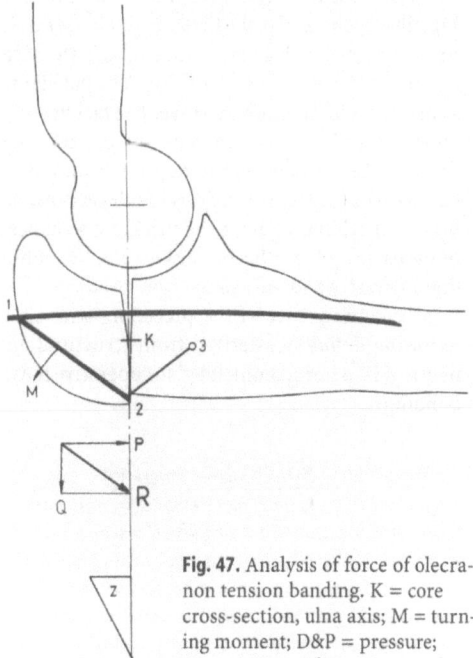

Fig. 47. Analysis of force of olecranon tension banding. K = core cross-section, ulna axis; M = turning moment; D&P = pressure; Q = transverse force; R = resultant; Z = traction

such tension can be produced at all with cerclage wire. Only *isometric* loading – extensor strain with fixation of the limb or lifting against gravity – produces a situation similar to that achieved with Finsterwalder's prestressed concrete, the beam loaded at three points.

However, who wants to take the risk of secondary dislocation through isometric post-operative treatment? As long as external aid is required for an osteosynthesis in order to achieve interfragmentary compression of the *whole* fracture zone, disturbance is *bound* to impair its stability and as a consequence result in loosening, distraction, and destruction. Ritter [317] correctly assessed conventional tension banding: "It is certainly not a completely functionally stable osteosynthesis." The stability that can be attained is not always felt to be satisfactory as is increasingly seen in text books. This will be discussed in more detail for individual fractures.

The consideration of the above-mentioned disadvantages inevitably leads to the observation that the eccentric tension band, speaking purely from the point of view of construction technology, is *not* in a position to restore durable joint anatomy – particularly not if one should manage to pre-tension it powerfully. The tension band using cerclage wire, generally only slightly stretched or positioned in a modified way, does not necessarily have to lead to cracking, tilting, and a step, particularly not if the extremity is protected with a plaster cast or, as in the case of the olecranon, does not bear strain. The patellar tension band is much more sensitive. The fact that many tension bandings heal fairly well anatomically paradoxically lies in their *lack of tension*. If moved only passively or held with a support bandage, cancellous bone can rebuild without the principle weaknesses of the osteosynthesis becoming evident. Non-unions develop rarely and only in the worst cases.

As a consequence of the preceding analysis the following *definition*, derived from structural engineering, is to be recommended for operative tension bandings:

▶ Tension banding is a *static* principle. Using optimized arrangements devised by engineering, and pre-tensioning of an effective traction device, the *whole* fracture zone should be statically and permanently compressed with such firmness – without additional external forces – that it cannot be distracted by developing muscle traction during post-operative treatment.

Currently, wire cables are an effective means of traction – compression of the whole fracture surface has its analogy in the hollow curved plate. Forces should be used that can be *introduced primarily through biomechanically safeguarded procedures and a suitable implant*, and which do not require external energy from weight or movement in order to put the fracture under pressure. A possible solution for patella and olecranon fractures – until now the only one put down in writing – lies in bilateral cable tension banding in which the means of traction is not on the extensor side, but is stretched over both sides of the bone [195, 203, 220]. It optimizes the principle of tension banding from the theoretical basis via a static introduction of force whose resultant produces compression from the very outset over the entire cross-section. In practice, too, it has become a viable and effective option, thanks to wire cables. Cable traction force is no longer introduced far outside the axis but quite deliberately positioned in the core cross-section of the bone with a strength which cannot be achieved with cerclage wire.

To assert that this construction is not proper tension banding [40, 330] because it does not fulfill the precept (based on a false hypothesis) of creating interfragmentary compression in the fracture crack through dynamic movement, is a statement that has prevented improvements for at least three decades. Schmelzeisen [343] is justified in calling it a static pressure osteosynthesis.

From a historical point of view as well as from their anatomical and functional significance, treatment of patella and olecranon fractures (as well as fracture of the trochanter major, the tuberculum majus, and the medial malleolus, prime examples of avulsion fractures) can be described as classical tension band. All these fractures are characterized by rough dislocation of the fractured pieces and functional failure. An osteosynthesis of these bones must not only neutralize muscle forces – it must also not be voluminous because the small anatomical dimensions of the fracture pieces do not allow for large implants. Consequently these fractures were the first to have been systematically sutured with wire and, since Weber, to have been banded with wire [119, 130, 162, 177, 238, 239, 377, 388, 402, 408]. They are dealt with in the following sections.

4.5
Patella Fracture

Topographical anatomy shows the patella as a bone which fits into the quadriceps in order to improve its effect. The bulk of the tendon fibres stretches, according to Kästner [162], towards the anterior surface of the patella "like the strings of a violin over the bridge" where they form the galea tendinea, that goes distally into the patellar ligament. This is indeed useful, for, with this position and inclusion in the musculature, the physiological significance of the kneecap lies in its lengthening the virtual lever for the quadriceps, which with its help requires less force for the same turning moment than without it. That reduces the pressures acting over the whole knee joint, in *all* compartments, not only the retropatellar area [12, 100, 113, 159, 245, 246]. The overall interrelation of all the joint compartments is also reflected correspondingly in the proportional increase in femoro-tibial arthroses after poor treatment of patella fractures [84, 262]. However, in strong flexion the length of its lever becomes irrelevant, for the patella then embeds itself deep into the channel between the condyles. Now its inward pressure even decreases because of the "pivot effect of the quadriceps tendon" [112]. These conditions make the dispute whether or not the kneecap is a sesamoid bone irrelevant: it acts as such, but is a separately developed center of ossification which only later developed contact with the quadriceps tendon. It is not the mechanical product of friction of the quadriceps tendon on the articular surface of the femur or an olecranon-like process of the tibia [12]. It is "a very important part of the knee joint" [100] and "not an excess of nature" [162]. The traction, pressure, and flexion loading caused by its function determines its design. In 1902 Joachimsthal [151] was the first to cut sections of it and interpret them. Traction trabeculae run slightly anteriorly longitudinally convex, with pressure trabeculae perpendicular to them.

Next to the main extensor apparatus, extensively formed from the rectus femoris, the restraint mechanisms of the reserve extensors lie parapatellar to the right and left, predominantly formed from distal fibers of the vastus tibialis and fibularis, the fascia lata, and parts of the joint capsule. If this remained intact, the lower leg can still be raised with reduced strength – similar to the foot using the plantaris muscle in the case of a ruptured Achilles tendon – without the fractured pieces of the patella inevitably being pulled apart. Only if the lateral extensor apparatus is also torn, which forms a functional unit with the quadriceps and patella, will the fragments be pulled apart by the quadriceps. For this reason the treatment of a patella fracture cannot be separated from the repair of the extensor apparatus. Thiem (1905) [377] and Schultze (1924) [353] set great store by this. If the lateral restraint mechanism of the extensors was able to achieve so much stability merely by suturing that the patella remained adjusted and the lower leg could be freely raised, then its osteosynthesis would be optional. That, however, is pure theory because the principal force of the quadriceps is transmitted via the rectus femoris via the kneecap *directly* to the tibial tuberosity and onto the cartilage forming the articular surface. That is why the anatomical reconstruction of the joint surfaces of the patella is the most important restorative measure in fractured and torn extensor apparatus. On X-ray diagnosis of patellar fractures, however, one always has to bear in mind that with few exceptions this is the visible expression of the tearing of more or less large parts of the whole extensor apparatus. Seen as the comprehensive joint injury which it is, a patellar fracture is no simple break. It consistently requires qualified treatment and is not a suitable practice osteosynthesis for beginners [84, 157, 205, 317, 323].

Max Schede [341] confirmed this in 1877 with the following episode: "As is well known, it is extremely difficult to achieve bony union of the fragments in transverse fractures of the patella so that at times the possibility of doing so has been denied. Malgaigne relates that Pibrac offered a prize of 100 Louis d'or to the person who could show him a kneecap completely mended with bony callus."

By now the prize would have been won a thousand times over. The bony reconstruction of cancellous material is no longer the main problem, yet "numerous failures and rather mediocre results of operative treatment indicate that the patellar fracture which appears so simple is not without its problems," according to Holz et al. [133] as late as 1990. The anatomy attainable or attained through surgery and the joint function resulting from it, which should be permanently painfree, are still to be seen as challenges. An improvement can only be achieved through biomechanics and implants in an optimized osteosynthesis technique, because in the long term the operation alone, its principle, its standard, and its practical feasibility decide the *post-operative*, *not post-traumatic* fate of the patient.

As early as the turn of the century "patellar fractures made up 1.4% of the total number of bone fractures presented," indicated Kästner [162] in Leipzig in 1924. That has remained so to this day [277, 324, 340, 416]. However, where once men between 30 and 50 were mainly injured through accidents at work, in fact three times more than women, nowadays with a decreasing dominance of the male sex, a first peak arises as early as 18–30 years of age [97, 252] as a result of speed traumas.

A distinction has always been made between *direct* and *indirect* breaks. The first, formerly called fracturae verae or shock fractures, occur as a result of impact and are now called *dash-board-injuries*. According to the course of the fracture line they are divided into transverse, longitudinal, oblique, star, multiple fragment, and comminuted fractures [36, 43, 133, 162, 434]. Kneecap fractures occurring indirectly due to a reflex-triggered impulsive muscle contraction which usually leads to *polar avulsions* are rare and obviously presuppose weakened bone as found in the elderly or dialysis patients as a result of secondary hyperparathyroidism [36]. Kästner cited Desault who had known a man who, due to pain during a lithotomy without anaesthesia, "in the truest sense of the word acquired a tear fracture." In 1880, Hamilton had even assessed 107 out of 127 patellar fractures as tear fractures [302] – in comparison with today an indication of change in accident type. He is also said to have disputed the possibility of bony healing. This statement, which was already no longer tenable eight years later, underlines the rapid advance in operative procedures and their success.

4.5.1
Historical Procedures

"The numerous publications on the treatment of fractures of the kneecap, which we find in surgical literature, show how this injury, which brings with it such heavy functional disturbances, has always caught the interest of a large number of surgeons." This was how Pletzer [302] summarized the matter in 1888 and it still holds true today.

"An enumeration of all forms of treatment would be almost impossible. In 1880, Lossen had already mentioned around 25 forms and this number has probably multiplied six-fold since then if all forms and varieties are included. After all, Berger, Paris, was recently able to list 90 appliances designed for bringing the fractured pieces of the kneecap together and holding them there, a figure that shows that

obviously none of these devices achieve perfection. For the patella, suturing offers the only guarantee for complete anatomical healing" explained Carl Thiem [377], Cottbus, the co-founder of the "Monatsschrift für Unfallheilkunde" (monthly journal on traumatology), in 1905 at the German Surgical Congress in Berlin. He conducted a discussion during which he firmly established: "All patellar fractures with extensor paralysis or considerable extensor weaknesses and those with gaping fracture pieces are to be treated by open suturing."

In this nothing has changed today, and operation of a joint fracture is a therapy of choice. Looking at therapy and prognosis Bühren et al. [36] proposed a pragmatic classification that is orientated towards the degree of dislocation and morphological damage:

1. Non-displaced fractures without cartilage damage
2. With cartilage damage
3. Displaced fractures without cartilage damage
4. With cartilage damage.

This division goes beyond earlier differentiations. With the desire for immediate functional exercise treatment, even intraligamentary breaks without steps are operated on if a larger diastasis exists. Such injuries should at least be arthroscoped in order to discover the extent of damage and to be able to initiate therapeutic measures immediately. Böhler, whose mastery of conventional treatment is well known (after aspiration of the hemarthrosis), treated over 60% of cases with plaster casts (quoted from [36]) as late as 1961, the rest by merely suturing the extensor apparatus. For a joint fracture this procedure has proved to be inadequate, a fact known for some time. Böhler [20] did not think much of cerclage wires, which he only used in exceptions "because a thin wire cannot hold the load of the body in simple movement."

The technique of operative treatment of patella fracture has changed many times. It consists of three overlapping chronological phases, in which the procedure was relatively uniform at any one time:

1. That of closed epi- and subcutaneous adjustment
2. That of open bone suturing around or through the patella
3. The era of tension banding.

Old literature – a very first compilation from the years 1867–1883 of 38 operated cases is found in work by Wahl [402] – provides a large number of authors and modifications that were used only once or on very few cases and have remained without influence on innovative developments (survey in [12, 26, 119, 130, 162, 252, 283, 400]).

During the pre-antiseptic era up to around 1890 one tried to adjust the fragments without opening the joint by means of percutaneously executed thick silk or catgut sutures. These were removed again after the plaster cast had set in order to keep the extremely high risk of joint infection as low as possible.

Leaving the historically unverified bone sutures aside the following chronology can be derived.

4.5.1.1
Closed Adjustment

▶ In 1868, Richard v. Volkmann (Volkmann's triangle, Volkmann's contracture), who worked in Halle from 1867 to 1889, in 1872 co-founder of the Deutsche Gesellschaft für Chirurgie (German Society of Surgery) and "one of the most outstanding surgeons of the nineteenth century" [165], appears to have been the first in the age of antisepsis to have operated on the patellar fracture. "In two cases I pulled a simple thread loop through the quadriceps tendon and patellar ligament and knotted both loops together on the patella. Then a tightly fitting plaster bandage was applied, a hole the size of a four-groschen piece was cut into it, the threads were cut and pulled out." From 1880 he apparently used silver wire and only removed it after fixation of the break [398]. Kocher [177] warned at the time: "Antisepsis still has great advances to make before the operative treatment of the patellar fracture – opening wide the knee-joint – can be generally indicated."

▶ In 1906 Schäfer [337] reported of Oskar Witzel, Düsseldorf (Witzel gastrostomy) that he had "used for many years a method of patellar suturing, which is recommended as much for its harmlessness and simplicity as for the result achieved with it and enjoyed the approval of every specialist."

Witzel, as the diagram shows, had used the same technique as v. Volkmann with silver wire. Ideas often develop simultaneously (Fig. 48).

▶ In 1889, M. Robson [320] from Leeds stuck a long steel needle with a glass head, a "woman's shawl pin," right next to the edge of the patella transversely through the quadriceps tendon and the patellar ligament and tied it epicutaneously for three weeks with

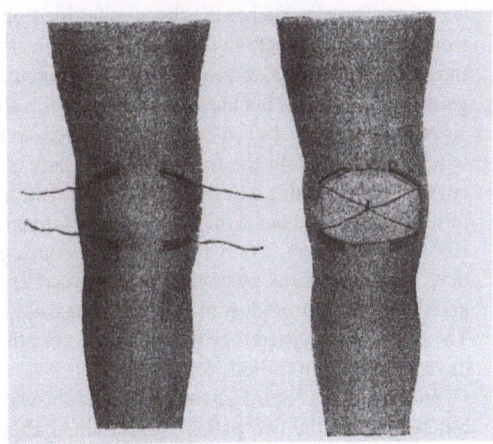

Fig. 48. Witzel's and v. Volkmann's "tendon suture" (from [337])

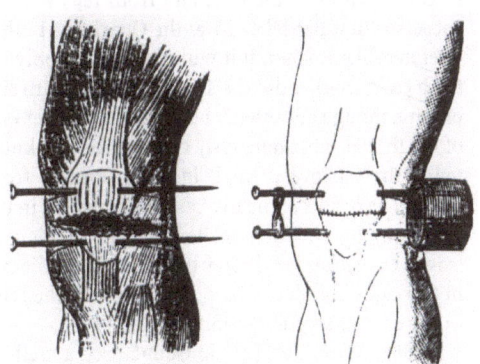

Fig. 49. Anderson's procedure (from [4])

a figure-of-eight thread. In 1892 William Anderson [4] from London used a similar procedure but he fixed the needles for three weeks with a cork on the one side and a wire twist on the other (Fig. 49).

Both procedures are not dissimilar to a frame fixator; one could even establish a loose theoretical relationship to the bilateral tension band.

Whilst the sutures described so far were positioned anteriorly, the ones in the following variants are placed around the patella in a sagittal plane, for the first time also with wire. Pulling rigid foreign bodies transversely through the articular surfaces of a joint is incomprehensible to us today. This is explained by the fear of infection, due to which one endeavored in all circumstances to leave the joint closed, and indicates that movement was prevented by means of a plaster cast.

▶ In 1880, Theodor Kocher (Kocher's collar incision), working from 1872–1917 in Bern and at that time the most important Swiss surgeon and the most famous goitre surgeon [165], his life's work earning him the Nobel prize in 1909, pulled "a strong, doubled silver wire through beneath the fragments by means of a curved needle, passing it in at the lower edge of the inferior fragment and out at the upper edge of the superior fragment. Because only the needle punctures go deep down, asepsis is guaranteed with all certainty and therefore the procedure may find universal usage. The threads are twisted together on Krüll gauze that has been soaked in carbolic solution."

Kocher did not record when he removed the wire, but "neither of the two patients complained about the threads pulled through the joint" [177].

▶ Bernhard Riedel ("Riedel's goitre"), working from 1888 until 1911 in Jena, and Franz König, who worked in Göttingen for some time and from 1895 was the successor of v. Bardeleben's at the Charité in Berlin, operated like Kocher, but with catgut and only on fresh cases. Barker did the same as Kocher with silk or wire, though admittedly he passed the upper end of the thread subcutaneously downwards and knotted it there above a small incision (quoted from [119]). The results of the five cases operated on in the same way by W. Körte in Berlin were, as his colleague Oehlecker [283] reported in 1905, "mediocre; in two cases the silver wire pulling through the joint cavity caused severe discomfort" and broke.

▶ In 1886, Anton Ceci [46] in Genoa used a method which already belonged to real bone suturing, because he passed the wire (still using a subcutaneous

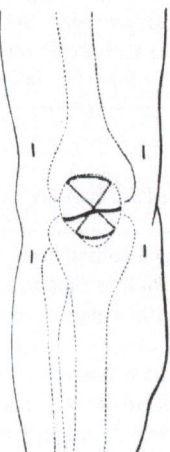

Fig. 50. Ceci's technique (from [46])

technique) through the patella. Holding both fragments together externally and using a homemade bone awl, a "cylindrical steel rod, which on one end was shaped like a raspatory, but with an eye," he drilled through them twice diagonally and connected them with a silver thread. Its ends were "twisted together and then pushed into the substance of the bone using strong tweezers" (Fig. 50).

4.5.1.2
Open Bone Suture

▶ Around 1870, Lord Joseph Lister, working from 1859 till 1895 in Glasgow, then later in London, the father of the antiseptic era [237], developed and standardized the first real intra-osseous bone suture, using it on different bones. He is therefore also the founder of the basic concept of osteosynthesis, the systematic bone suture. In 1873 he performed it for the first time on the olecranon. His friend H. Cameron, to whom he had described his project meticulously, preceded him on the patella by several months, because he had had the first patient.

Lister [239] describes his first patellar wire suture in 1877 as follows: "On October 26th, I accordingly proceeded to operate, making a vertical incision, about two inches in length over the patella, exposing the fragments, which were then one inch apart. My inability to bring down the upper fragment into contact with the lower became explained when the parts were exposed; for there were found between the fragments extremely firm coagula, with fibrous tissue, fascial and periosteal, mingled with them, constituting so firm a mass as to make it quite impossible for the two fragments to be brought into contact. The clots having been completely cleared away from between the fragments and from the interior of the joint, I applied a common bradawl in the middle line of the patella, drilling each fragment obliquely so as to bring out the drill upon the broken surface a little distance from the cartilage. Pretty stout silver wire was then passed through the drilled openings, and the fragments thus strung upon it were pushed firmly home, and so brought accurately into apposition. The ends of the wire were now twisted together, and the wound was closed with sutures and a small drain inserted. The wounds healed without any suppuration. At the end of eight weeks, the wire was removed by an incision through the cicatrix. This, I believe, is the first instance of a recent case of fracture of the patella being treated by wire-suture antiseptically applied" (Fig. 51).

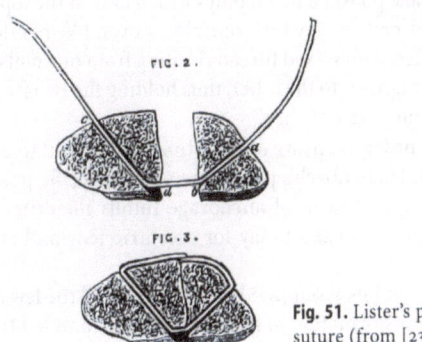

Fig. 51. Lister's patella suture (from [239])

▶ Even before 1900, Johannes v. Mikulicz-Radecki (Mikulicz clips, first oesophago-bronchoscopy) working from 1890–1905 in Breslau, and Sauerbruch's mentor, had strengthened Lister's suture in the middle of the patella with two wire sutures placed next to each other [130]. F. König from the *Charite* in Berlin used the same technique in open fractures [73].

▶ Dating back to Paul Berger in 1892 [14], working in Paris, and called *cerclage* by him, is a procedure still occasionally used, which Eduard Rehn [90] described in 1958 as follows: "After clearing the patellar wound a Krupp wire is pulled through the quadri-

ceps tendon in the frontal plane and then through the patellar ligament using a large needle; the fracture pieces are fitted exactly together and finally the ends of the threads are tied" (Fig. 52).

▶ Quenu modified Berger's technique slightly by taking hold of the largest fragment trans-osseously in a hemicerclage. From 1903 he bored through both fragments and thus performed a Payr suture at approximately 90° to the horizontal. According to Hoffmann [130], even these procedures seem to have had precursors: "So far as I know, this form of suturing was taught much earlier in Austria."

▶ Around 1900 a procedure was attributed to Erwin Payr (Payr Incision), a general surgeon specializing in bones and joints, and working, after Greifswald and Königsberg, as Trendelenburg's successor from 1911 until 1936 in Leipzig. For decades this procedure enjoyed the same popularity as Berger's cerclage. "The great disadvantage of a lack of stability," wrote Hoffmann, "is met to some extent by a kind of wiring, which Professor Payr has already been using for years. Through two approximately parallel bore holes, which perforate the patella superiorly on both sides of the quadriceps tendon and inferiorly on both sides of the ligamentum patellae proprium, a strong silver or better still aluminum-bronze wire is passed to form a square with rounded corners, which is fastened as is most convenient superiorly or

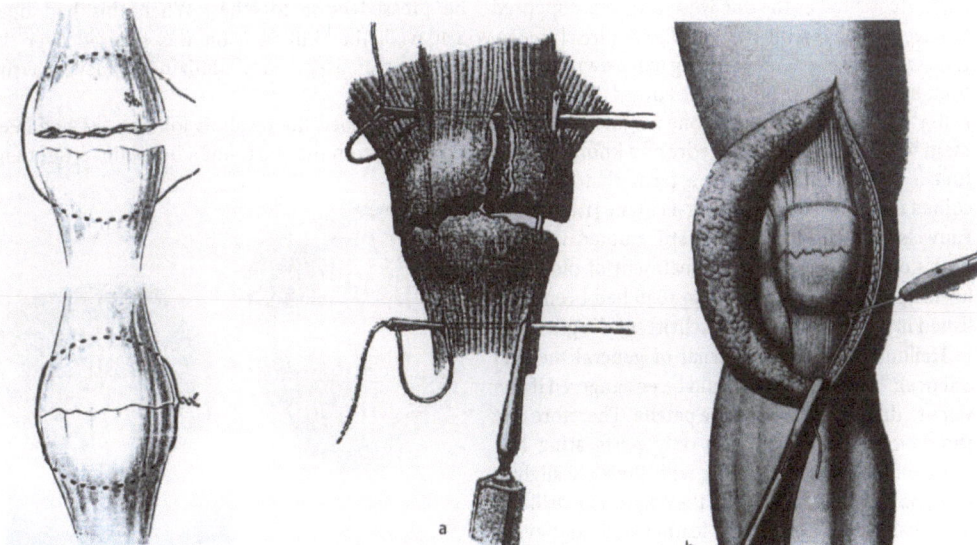

Fig. 52. Berger's cerclage (from [90])

Fig. 53. Payr's method (from [171])

inferiorly, laterally or medially close to the edge of the quadriceps or the ligament and sunk into the soft tissue. The placing of the suture is not as simple as in the customary patellar suture, yet it is by no means difficult" (Fig. 53).

Both procedures – the cerclage as well as the Payr method – were only superseded by Weber's tension banding, as old textbooks verify [32, 90, 171, 182, 264, 344].

For decades almost all authors have placed great emphasis on removing coagulations, periosteum, and fascia interposed between the fragments. Thus a diastasis and callus inhibiting influence which are attributed to them might be avoided. Where it was no longer possible to bridge diastasis in old cases, the tibial tuberosity should, as Ernst von Bergmann had recommended even before the turn of the century, be chiseled off diagonally up to the joint (quoted from [119]) to relieve the strain of the suture. As it was always very difficult to hold the adjusted patella securely together, E. Rehn regarded as useful every procedure that fulfilled the requirement "to make the union of the fragments really close fitting, independent of whether the suture included the kneecap itself or only the lateral extensor apparatus."

4.5.1.3
Tension Banding

▶ The very first tension banding in the functional sense seems to have been used by Johann Dieffenbach. He is cited as the one who in 1846 is supposed to have carried out the first patellar sutures [90, 139, 171, 252, 264, 338, 402]. According to his own description, however, it was not a bone suture as known by Lister – perforation of both bone fragments, adjustment by means of pulling on wire and knotting – but first a "suture functionnel," a term that was first coined 112 years later by Hachez-Leblanc [118], one of Pauwels' pupils. Pletzer [302] still quoted Dieffenbach's original work on the treatment of old, nonhealed patellar fractures that in 1846 had been published in Campari's "Wochenschrift für die gesammte Heilkunde" (Weekly journal of general medical science): "The knee joint would be endangered if one were to drill right through the patella. Therefore one should content oneself with only perforating two thirds of the latter's thickness with the knee slightly bent, only 1/4 of an inch from the edges. The drill has to be half the thickness of a feather quill and every edge of the break, if it is in the middle of the patella, is drilled twice and plugs knocked in the bores. One

can take polished metal plugs which have at the top a round nail head, which one closes over, like harelip needles, with waxed threads leading from one nail of one fragment to the other, thus holding the two fracture surfaces together."

In order to ensure an infection-free wound treatment, Dieffenbach's procedure with a specific positioning and form of anchorage fulfills the criteria that are still valid today for eccentric tension banding.

▶ Even Julius Wolff [428], who formulated the law of the transformation of bone and in 1890 founded the first orthopedic clinic at the *Charité* in Berlin, performed a form of tension banding – without knowing of the principle formulated later by Pauwels – in the same manner as Dieffenbach had half a century previously: "I had prepared four horseshoe-shaped double nails of approximately 1 cm in width and of similar height. The nails were sharpened well so that they could easily be driven into the pre-drilled holes in the bone. Every horseshoe was provided at its blunt end, that is on the curve connecting the two nails of the horseshoe, with two holes next to each other at a distance of 5 mm, through which strong silver wire could be pulled... After I had satisfied myself that the double nails hammered into the drilled holes were completely firmly in place, the wires connecting the lateral nails and equally the medial nails were pulled firmly together until the two pairs of nails opposite each other were pulled close and at the same time caused the fragments to be pressed close together. When this had been achieved, the skin incision was sutured over the nails and an aseptic immobilizing bandage was applied."

He described the result as follows: "As had been expected from the start, not a bony, but a tight and

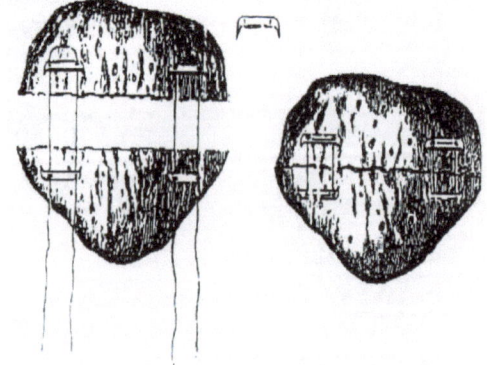

Fig. 54. Wolff's "tension banding" (from [427])

strong ligamentous union had developed, such that functionally it is tantamount to a bony one" (Fig. 54)

Hachez-Leblanc [118] was in 1958 the first to emphasize the generation of increased resistance against the traction of the quadriceps by positioning the cerclage "en avant" and by improving stability – the first *consciously* applied biomechanics.

The new age began in 1963 with Bernhard Weber [408]. Pursuing further Pauwels' and Hachez-Leblanc's observations, he made biomechanical theories concerning treatment strategies for bones under constant muscle traction. For the patella it seemed sensible to him to absorb the pull of the quadriceps tendon *by extensor-side positioning and pre-tensing* of the cerclage wire. With this, two fundamental principles were introduced into operative procedure, which clearly make it far better than simple adjustment by means of bone suturing or cerclage.

Although the rigidity of traditional cerclage wire is contrary to the intra-operative realization of his eccentric tension banding concept, which makes the introduction of pre-tensioning almost impossible [29, 95, 104, 135, 145, 220, 356], its procedure has for many remained until today the method of choice. However there was never complete unity in carrying out Weber's tension banding. At the second Reisensburg Workshop [41] in 1974 in a vehemently led discussion about cerclage "guided around tendon insertions, this procedure was considered to be sufficient, additional Kirschner wires only being indicated where shearing forces have to be controlled in corresponding orientation of the fracture surfaces." If one were to use Kirschner wires in general on the patella, then the tension band wire should "only be fastened on one side, as otherwise too strong a tilting moment arises on the wires, which leads to a dorsal gaping of the fracture." If this, "at least in individual cases, is detectable radiologically," then it would surely speak for "the good clinical experience of this procedure, that the fracture is not subject to changing loads." Apart from none of this information having been biomechanically verified, clinical experience cannot be quoted as scientific proof; at most it can only substantiate it. What doubts prevailed are made clear in the choice of words used in the summary of the meeting. It was stated that: "... a whole series of objections raised on principal as well as those

gained from practical experience are opposed to the wire sling fixed cranially and caudally next to the bone in the banding apparatus. This theoretically captivating method from the biomechanical point of view should therefore be combined with other compression, or at least safe adjustment techniques, because exercise stability is only rarely achieved, as numerous failures or moderate results show."

Attempts to achieve more stability were therefore prematurely made through operative variations per se. The first to put the disadvantages of Weber's tension banding down to its eccentricity were Wenzl and Krüger [419] in 1971. To them the gaping crevice near the joint no longer seemed advantageous – they merely saw it as a pressure-free gap. They tried to prevent it by laying a second wire in the form of a cerclage *near to the joint* like a ring around the kneecap, which should absorb the strain on extension. At the time Ritter [317] considered this method to be the best ever. It is still recommended today in observed instances of defective stability [36, 42, 324]. In 1977 our own observations [202] confirmed the findings of these authors and led to bilateral tension banding for patella fracture too.

Since this workshop, hardly anything has changed in interpretation. To date the principle of tension band is defined worldwide as being *dynamic*: through movement traction is to be transformed into pressure [416]. This principle – which was, however, opposed by "objections of principle" [36] – leads to the conclusion that it is worthy of criticism. It can definitely not be applied to the technical assumption of *static* stability; it is unstable. It is for this reason that since Lister "many osteosynthesis procedures have been developed and described without one being spoken of today as a unanimously recommended and accepted method" [36]. As an example, the simple tension band is to be used without Kirschner wires. According to Ziegler and Regazzoni [434] as late as 1991, these should "not be used routinely, but only where shearing forces are to be expected." The "modified tension band" fastened to Kirschner wires [13, 42, 277, 300] is regarded as an extended procedure.

The operative procedures can best be judged on their results. The results of the first decades are merely of historical interest; they cannot really be taken into account, because thinking at that time to a large extent was directed towards avoiding infection and not towards technical details. A considerable achievement lay in promoting the indications for operation. In 1905 in Berlin these were already laid down for most patellar fractures and had generally been acknowledged, because non-surgical intervention was "not suitable in cases with diastasis and tearing of the extensor apparatus." Kästner [162], who supported Thiem with this statement, gave the following summary:

Thirty-five surgeons achieved bony healing in 87.3% of 292 patellar fractures operated on in various ways, as compared with just 19.4% after conven-

tional action – a considerable result and an indication of the potency of cancellous bone. But almost always flexion difficulties and other unsatisfactory, not specified, results were listed, 72 poor results out of 182 (= 40%) and 22 poor results out of 49 (= 45%) in the subgroups – whatever that may have meant.

The frequency of wire breakage is also to be seen as an indication of poor osteosynthesis quality. v. Brunn [31] found 11 out of 12 silver wires broken into several pieces and, when they had strayed into the joint, associated with clear functional disturbance. Why does wire in most cases break in so many places? he wondered and replied: "The essen-

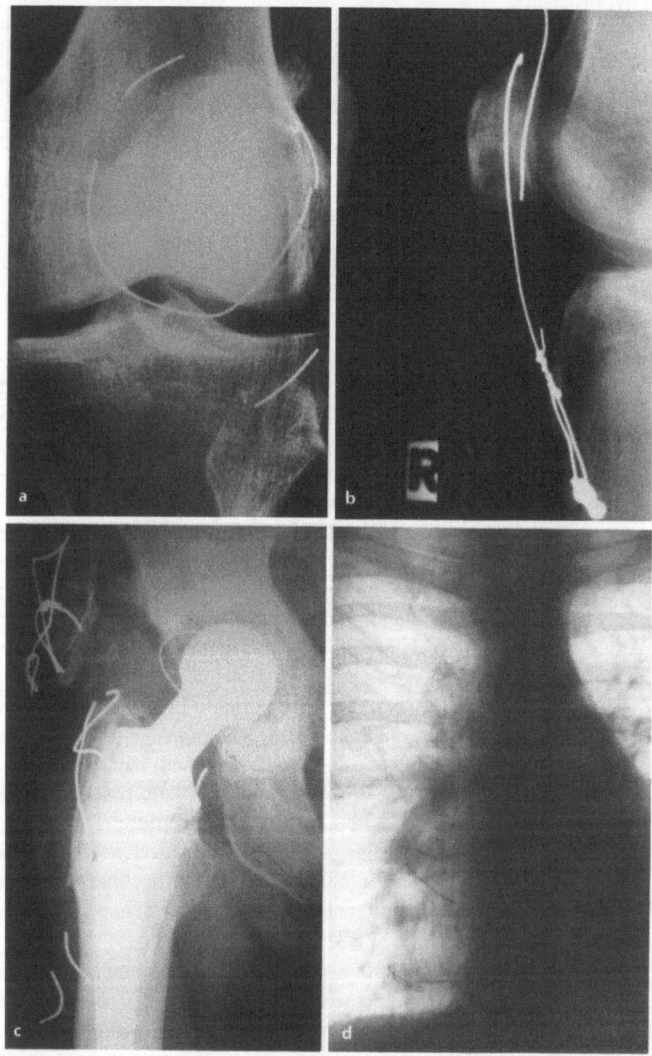

Fig. 55. Cerclage wire breaks everywhere as a consequence of its rigidity

tial element seems to be disintegration, that is, flexion which exceeds the elasticity of the wire... This is proved by the cases where, despite bony healing of the fragments, breakage of the wire occurred." A correct explanation.

Wire breakage in all areas where it is indicated, not just in the patella, may have been a reason for silver wires being superseded by the stronger aluminum-bronze wires [388], of which ostensibly only every third one breaks. Even today it is a well known [16, 333, 390] albeit usually silently ignored fact (Fig. 55).

▶ Weber's wire tension banding with Kirschner wires should be a benchmark for comparison with the *bilateral cable tension banding*, which we view as an optimal and contemporary patellar osteosynthesis.

The number of publications dealing with wire tension banding, especially concerning the treatment and results of patellar and olecranon fractures, is staggering. Consequently the selection must remain subjective; adequate space however is given to the supporters of the conventional technique. Their results have never been satisfactory in any respect. After initial optimism over the more favorable results achieved in comparison with bone suturing and cerclage, critics soon emerged, including Weber [29, 133, 185, 356, 419].
▶ The best success rates of simple and extended patella-wire tension banding were seen in the last ten years with 61–78% [97, 178, 277, 324, 434]. Hung et al. [142] find 72% satisfied patients, but state that "objectively 81.3% had an excellent or good result." The prevailing opinion is that they could have been even better. Surgical error [157, 323, 324] and a lack of post-operative treatment [277] or "damage to the cartilage due to the trauma, which could not be repaired even by such an ideal repositioning and stabilization technique," were named as reasons for unsatisfactory results [97]. Only Holz et al. [133] blame complications on the failure of tension bandings – as a single opinion a somewhat weak clinical confirmation of identical experimental findings.

Clear statements cannot always be drawn from a study. Often the results are obtained from the entire non-homogenous operative spectrum [324, 364], or partial statements in a publication are difficult to reconcile. The two following highly contradictory sequences come from *one* study by Jaskulka et al. [148]: "In our follow-up group the tension band osteosyntheses were by and large affected with a failure quota

of at least 13%, whilst an ideal result was only attained in 43%" and " Tension band osteosyntheses clearly lie ahead of wire cerclage with 87% ideal and adequate results compared with the latter's 72%." Apart from the fact that ideal and satisfactory results should not be merged into one figure, these reports could, uncritically cited, be reproduced also with 87% good and 13% poor results. The work is suspect also because of the too highly rated results after cerclage, which really should no longer be considered as a suitable procedure for the patella. In the cadaveric knee on extension, Buzzi et al. [44] measured distractions of 30 mm whilst pulling on the quadriceps tendon!

Immediately after the "modified tension band osteosynthesis using two Kirschner wires bored in parallel to the patellar longitudinal axis" had been stressed as a reliable procedure by Neumann et al. [277], they quoted Rogge [324], who had seen "unsatisfactory results in only 1/4 of cases." He, however, declares "a very good to good result in 77.8% of all screwed longitudinal fractures, all partial and total patellectomies of the knee and simple ventral tension band osteosyntheses" – for quite a number of the most varied procedures therefore and thus inadmissible. His table, nevertheless, shows only 31 very good or good results (= 61%). Rogge however quotes the Reisensburg Workshop of 1974, where it was said to have been "lastingly confirmed" that the "wire tension banding osteosynthesis introduced by the AO in the operative therapy of transverse and also multiple fragment fractures is the method of choice." Anyone who was present or who later reads the discussion and recommendations [329] will confirm that nothing was said in the statement about sustainability.
▶ For more critical members of the medical profession the rate of very good and good results lies only at around 50% or less [133, 148, 234, 340]. Egyed and Kazar [84] in 1977 identified only "tendential, statistically insignificant differences" between cerclage and tension band wiring on the patella, which, considering the low acceptance of cerclage, represents a very critical evaluation of tension banding. In 1978 Moschinski et al. [262] noted that "3/4 of all patients complained about different degrees of subjective pain. Approximately half of the patients showed more severe arthrotic changes in the femorotibial and femoropatella joint; in comminuted fracture cases it was 2/3."

In fact, in 1989 Jaskulka and coworkers' figure of just under 50% of "ideal results" [148] could only be achieved because they put 86% of their patients in a long leg cast for three to six weeks – such little faith had they in the capacities of tension banding, which according to Rogge et al. [324] however "should al-ways be so stable that a complication-free functional post-operative treatment is possible."

Holz et al. [133] recapitulated in 1989 that the "operative treatment of patellar fractures is affected by a relatively high rate of complications in the post-operative stage." As such they named pain, movement deficiency, morphological changes, widening of the contours of the patella, and 40% arthrosis as early as one to five years post-operatively.

In 1989 Peterson et al. [301] noted, after the most stable tension banding anchored with Kirschner wires in 37 operations, 9 secondary dislocations and displacements of more than 3 mm (27%) – an unambiguous indication of deficient interfragmentary compression. From this it can be further concluded that *all* cases were only adjusted, because he did not evaluate gap formations less than 3 mm which indeed likewise signal loss of pressure.

▶William Anderson's remark which he made in front of the London Association of Surgeons in 1892, is still relevant: "Gentlemen – there are few fractures that give more trouble both to the patient and to the surgeon than those of the patella" [4].

> ▶ The fact that conventional tension bandings exclude better results per se lies in:
> 1. Their principle of eccentricity
> 2. The deficient quality of cerclage wire, which is not a means of traction
> 3. Pure procedural shortcomings, for example the renunciation of stabilising K-wires.

The exact analysis of wire tension banding on the patella will confirm the correctness of these statements.

4.5.2
Weber's Patella Tension Band and its Biomechanical Analysis

The tension band for the patella is quite simply *the* osteosynthesis procedure. In order to be able to judge it, the effects of the interaction of different forces on the intact patella have to be known as well as the forces that prevail in a fracture stabilized using a tension band. The analysis is – as our own investigations from 1977 show [202] – not simple, but absolutely necessary, if one wants to know the influ-

ence of tension banding on the fracture gap and determine the quality of the osteosynthesis.

1. Determination of the external and movement-dependent forces on the *intact* patella
The total force Q of the quadriceps through the kneecap is broken up into the components Q_1 (quadriceps tendon) and Q_2 (ligamentum patellae). Since a muscle can only exert tension, the patella is exposed with *every* movement, that is with every extension *and* flexion, to constant tensile stress. Owing to the angled radiation of the quadriceps tendon and the patellar ligament as well as depending on the starting position and velocity of the movement (acceleration), partial forces Q_{1y} and Q_{2y} develop, which in a fracture surface would give rise to a shearing effect with a tendency towards step formation. $Y1$ is the length of the lever, over which moments of flexion are generated, P is the inward pressure of the kneecap in the femoro-patellar articular surface (Fig. 56).

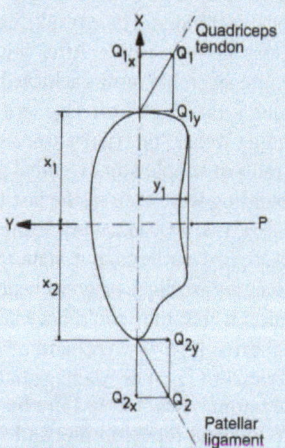

Fig. 56. Analysis of the forces on the intact patella which affect the kneecap via the quadriceps tendon and the patellar ligament as Q_1 and Q_2

Because the tendon fibers predominantly radiate on the extensor side into the kneecap, the result of all forces produces a different tension pattern in the intact cross-section of the patella: it is exposed to higher strain on the extensor side than on the juxta-articular dorsum. The turning moment which arises generates pressure near the joint only when flexion occurs (Fig. 57).

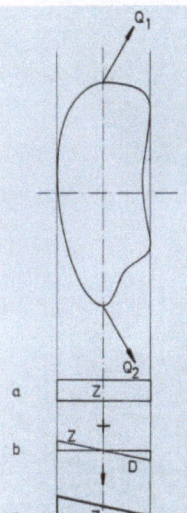

Fig. 57. Strains in the cross-section of the patella. Traction strains within the patella result from the muscle tractions Q_1 and Q_2 on flexion as well as on extension. Z = strain; D = pressure: **a** axial traction strain; **b** moment effect as a result of angled force application; **c** summation of the strains as total tension force in the cross-section of the patella on extension of the joint

2. Determination of the forces which the eccentric tension band produces *at rest* **in the patella fracture gap (Fig 58)**

The forces produced through pre-tensioning can be divided into axial pressure forces D and a turning moment as a result of the cerclage wire which lies eccentrically and which causes on the extensor side additional pressure and, with increasing wire tension, a proportionally larger juxta-articular gaping region Z, an effect that is also to be observed very clearly in plate osteosynthesis – which is likewise eccentrically applied – and should be suppressed using suitable measures – cf. Fig. 44.

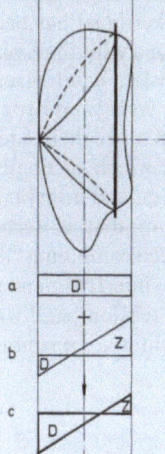

Fig. 58. Resting tension in eccentric patellar tension banding: **a** axial pressure strain; **b** picture of moments caused by the eccentricity of the wire; **c** summation with gaping dorsal fracture region Z

3. Determination of the *movement dependent* **forces that the eccentric tension band causes in the patellar fracture gap (Fig. 59).**

Unravelling the interplay of forces inside the tension banding at rest with those that develop on extension and flexion is complicated. The resulting strains clearly differ from each other. The result of the summation c_2 is in the case of extension a considerable expansion of the gaping crevice Z, which goes together with an increase in the angle of the crevice. Now, the extension position is the one however that is predominantly considered, because walking, even with weight-bearing relieved, occurs with relatively extended knees. Consequently the kneecap treated with conventional tension banding is exposed to traction strains most of the time. Only a small extensor side region of the fracture is affected, and even then only when *in effect* pre-tensioning can be introduced into the wire. Recommendations to begin extension and contraction exercises as soon as possible after the operation and only to load the outstretched knee [40, 266, 416], are to be rejected as particu-

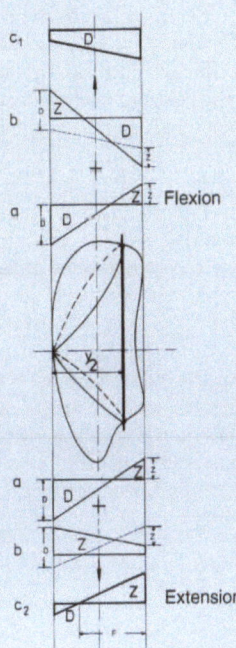

Fig. 59a–d. Interfragmentary movements are harmful, not "dynamic"! In the worst case they lead to distraction
a = inherent resting tension

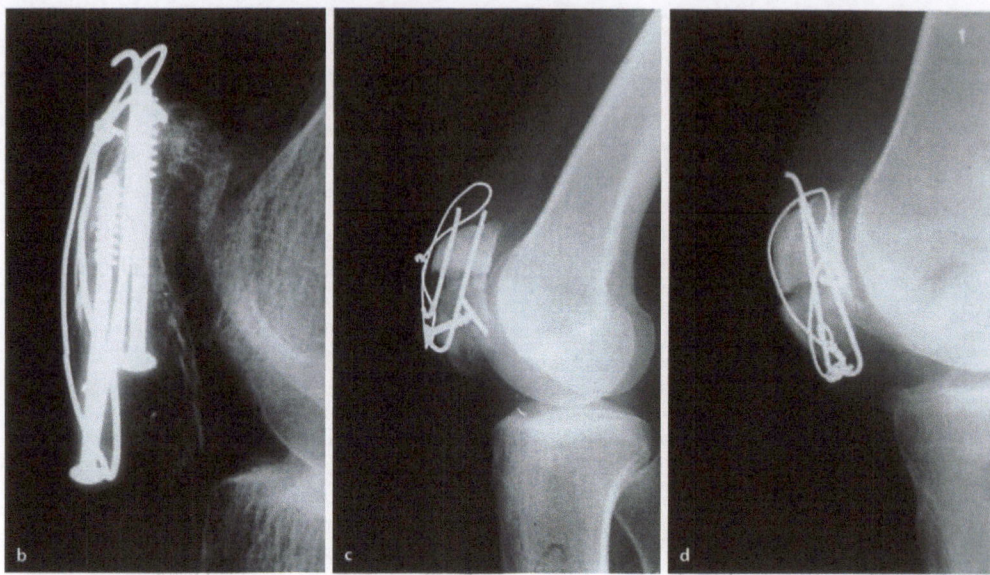

Fig. 59 b, c, d. Clinical demonstration of the biomechanic analysis

larly harmful because it is precisely during these movements that the fragments are powerfully pulled apart from each other.

Merely by flexing, a turning moment can be generated via the long lever Y_2, which gives a certain compression in the summation c_1 in the whole fracture area, *provided that* the tension banding is sufficiently stable. If it is not, the fracture fragments are pulled apart from each other even on flexion. The moments of flexion are intensified too during flexion which can lead to tilting of the kneecap. In stable osteosynthesis pressure can develop indeed *only during the course of* flexion, and not during rest in the flexed position (which gives the illusion of pressing together) because in the rest position muscle traction almost ceases and the basic to-nus generates no mentionable strain. This condition corresponds mechanically to a loose cable on a roll. Hence it follows that rest in the flexed position has no compression effect on the fracture gap.

▶ Where the conviction of having a stable osteosynthesis procedure with wire tension banding on the extensor side comes from remains a riddle given the biomechanical facts as outlined. It also contradicts the concern about adequate sta-bility which contributes to the tendency of wanting to achieve more stability with more wire [36] and of protecting this with generously prescribed plaster casts [148, 324].

In addition to such trials which do not follow a system, variations were also soon published that were supposed to be more stable. Tönnis [382] in 1970 wanted to achieve greater exercise stability using two longitudinal-ventral cerclages fixed to Kirschner wires. Lotke and Ecker [241] has been pursuing the same goal since 1980 with their ventral, longitudinal anterior tension band placed trans-osseously. As mentioned, Wenzl and Krüger [419] were the most consistent with their additional juxta-articular cerclage, which in English circles bears the name Pyrford (quoted from [42]). For Perry et al. [300] none of that is secure enough. Since 1988 they have been combining "the standard fixation technique (interfragmentary cancellous screws or modified tension band wiring)" with a safety wire, as is common for rupture of the patellar ligament.

All of these specific variations are still based on the principles of the eccentric tension band and demonstrate the knowledge of lacking stability.

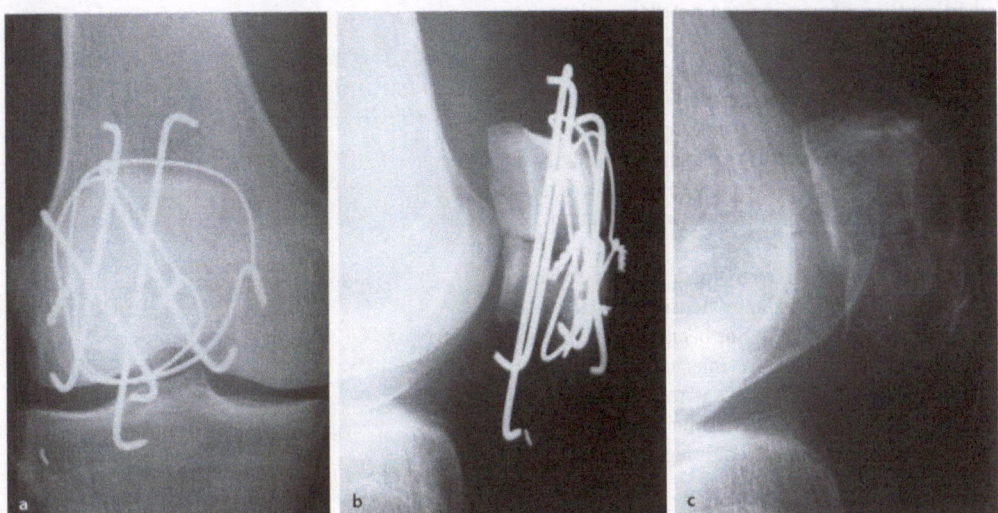

Fig. 60. "A lot helps a lot" – a false concept. Healing with obvious step formation and angulation

Brill and Hopf [29] in 1987, after *trials on the cadaveric kneecap stiffened on the inside with Palacos bone-cement,* even wanted "to replace the currently predominant tension band osteosynthesis with wires by double tension screw osteosynthesis." This hardly practised method will certainly not displace tension banding from the operative repertoire. Even if in vitro results may not be transferred easily to the living system [204, 220, 289], several statements of the authors stand up to critical consideration. They

are, as far as the strength of eccentric wire tension banding is concerned, crushing. The trials have established "that all investigated tension banding techniques guarantee *no* active exercise stability. Moreover *no* tension band effect could be proven experimentally anyway. Therefore it appears that the tension band principle adapted from mechanics using ordinary cerclage wire in patellar fractures is *not* practical!" Brill laid the responsibility for the hardly detectable tension band effect in particular on the

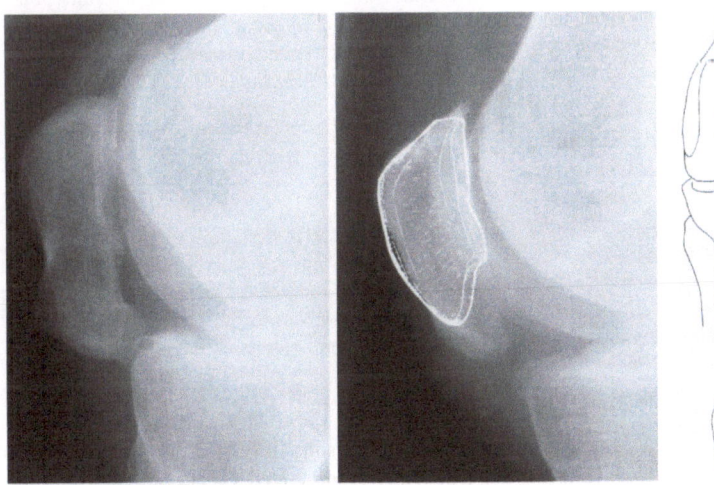

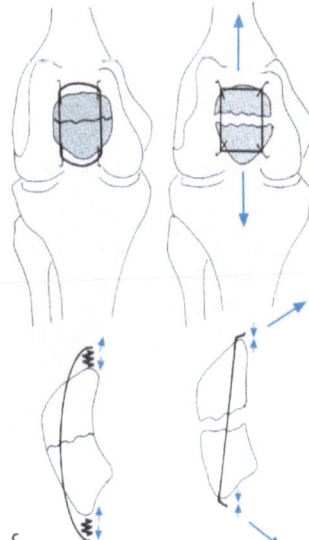

Fig. 61. Typical elongation of the patella, as seen after conventional therapy (**a**) [92] and after wire tension banding (**b**) [83] – the patella of the opposite side was overprinted – and Brill's explanation (**c**) (from [29])

bad nestling of wire on the patellar contours, on yielding soft tissue layers between wire and bone, as well as on the lengthening of kinks and loops – statements, which have to be agreed with (Fig. 61).

(Note, the expression "the principle adapted from mechanics" is incorrect. The mathematically based technical procedure is of course correct; it was transferred into medicine with wrong interpretation).

▶ Why these findings remained without response from researchers is incomprehensible. A stable osteosynthesis has certainly not been sought. As such, and as the benchmark for internal fixation [13, 41, 142, 266, 301, 324, 418], AO wire tension banding continues to be accepted at a time when proof of the quality of medical treatment is legally required.

It was said that the bilateral cable tension band tested by Brill indeed achieved the highest interfragmentary compression forces of all tension bandings, but then the cables cut through the soft tissue and on further tensioning even frontally the kneecap. Such a drawback had never been encountered with wire tension bandings; thus cables were deemed unsuitable for osteosynthesis.

Here, of course, certain points must be made:

1. On mechanical and biological grounds cables must always be passed underneath soft tissue.

2. The Palacos-filled kneecaps were resistant enough to withstand the forces generated by the cerclage wire laid on the extensor side, because they are not high. Gaping occurred and consequently the force sensor placed within the osteotomy could not measure any pressure.

3. When viewed in detail, the cutting into of the patella observed for the lateral cable tension band due to the tensile force of the cables actually proves to be an advantage. It is proof of its superior quality. The explanation of this apparent paradox lies in the "hydroelastic system" [76, 78, 204, 289], that is an exclusive characteristic of living tissue; see page 46. It is the most important mechanism that gives to the *living* skeleton exceedingly good stability which is far above the mechanical strength of the hard bone. It absorbs, in particular, the high kinetic forces that develop on forced movement. On jumping even from a small height the loading on the bone reaches a multiple of the body weight. In spite of this the bone does not break. That is because of two highly efficient synergistic systems working independently of each other. They act as hydroelastic shock absorbers:

1. On the fluid-filled living cells, i.e., on the cell aggregations in high tensile surroundings and collagen fibre nets

2. On the blood vessel system which immediately stops the venous drainage via muscle tonus increased by reflex action without impairing arterial supply.

These two intra- and extra-cellular fluid compartments create spaces, which are not compressible, and therefore distribute pressure in all directions and thus remove the pressure peak. The effect of cell aggregation could be compared with the function of a water-cushion, that of the blood vessel system functioning as a kind of steam-kettle. This is where the distinction between living and dead bone is made. Therefore the results of cadaveric trials *must never* be applied to living structures without further consideration! In death, hydroelastic systems break down, the pressure resistance of bone disappears. This explains why the highly loadable wire cables *had to* cut into the cadaveric kneecaps. In the living, on the other hand, in several hundred osteosyntheses not a single cable has cut in! These findings regarding the mechanical significance of tissue fluids are confirmed by Schröder and Gall's [352] investigations of the biomechanical influence of synovial fluid on joint function: "The cartilage tissue undergoes its smallest strain when its material characteristics equal in fact those of a fluid. Accordingly, its pressure resistance vis-à-vis static loading is produced by intra-cartilaginous hydrostatic fluid pressure."

▶ Correctly interpreted, Brill's experiments show that *all variants of wire tension banding lack pressure and are not resistant to muscle strain, but that the bilateral cable tension banding is a compression principle of great value.*

In 1977, in personal investigations [202] on a subtrochanteric amputated cadaveric leg with transverse osteotomy of the patella we measured the forces existing in the fracture gap after eccentric and after bilateral tension banding during extension and flexion over the quadriceps tendon, using cerclage wire, because at that time cables were not yet available (Fig. 62 and Table 2). Natural conditions could be more closely imitated than in an isolated patella fixed in a machine with implanted anchors. Because above all it was the *distribution* of force within the fracture which was of interest, two piezo-electric pressure sensors were built in juxta-articularly and on the extensor side. The results with eccentric tension banding were very similar to those of Brill: on extension, interfragmentary compression could not be detected anywhere. But in bilateral tension banding, on the other hand, it was possible to induce tensioning three times as great, so that the whole fracture area remained compressed on extension. This correlates with results from traction experi-

ments in an artificial patella. In these, after bilateral tension banding nearly three times higher distraction forces were necessary – 490 N as against 170 N – until a gap was just visible.

Mechanically an osteosynthesis already lacks pressure before a gap can be seen. It is not therefore worth measuring the forces which are necessary to produce a several millimeter wide gap [301], because their stability is not genuine.

In principle it can be stated that:

1. Eccentric tension bandings are unsuitable osteosynthesis procedures, which both at rest and during movement partially pull apart every fracture (of the patella and of other bones).

Table 2. "Isometrically" measured interfragmentary pressure after eccentric and after bilateral wire tension banding on a patella transverse fracture on cadaveric knee

Stress (N) in fracture gap	At Rest		In active horizontal extended position (high quadriceps reflex)		In 90° flexion (low quadriceps reflex)	
	AO-TB	Bilateral TB	AO-TB	Bilateral TB	AO-TB	Bilateral TB
Extensor side	51	80	0	36	4	42
Near joint	0	71	0 No pressure in fracture gap	43	24	48

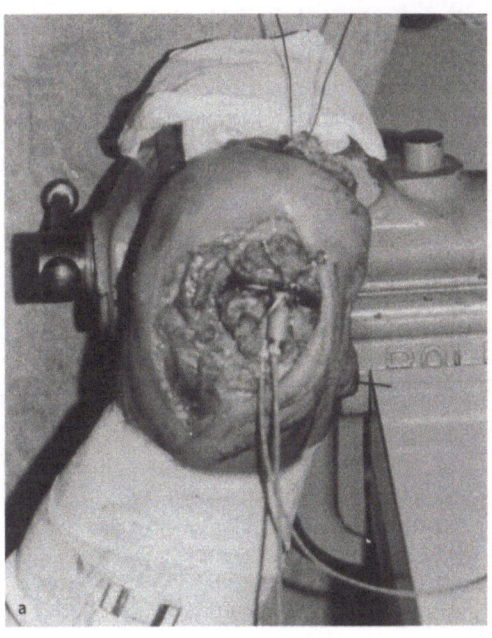
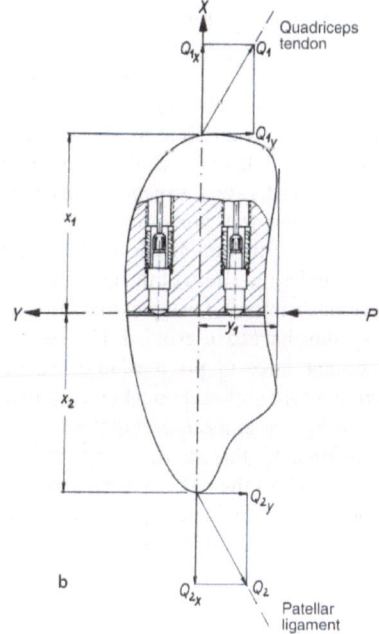

Fig. 62. Measuring interfragmentary pressure on an in-situ patella on a cadaveric leg

Ritter et al. [145] think it is "not justified to continue regarding this principle as the theoretical basis of tension banding." Its results are not optimal. According to Hackenbroch the fractures, which have healed, despite everything, in the cancellous area often with insufficient anatomical precision are a *prearthrotic deformity*.

2. Because of ever-present shearing forces eccentric tension banding tends to lead to the formation of steps and with every movement produces disturbance within the fracture, which can lead to secondary dislocation [146]. This is not a dynamic osteosynthesis, as has been said before, because the forces freed during movement are destructive. Then there is also no stimulus to promote healing.

4.5.3
Bilateral Cable Tension Band and its Biomechanical Analysis

The principle of bilateral tension band was developed in 1974 and immediately applied to the patella [195, 202]. Tension resistant wire cables pull a fracture so firmly together that a "stable pressure osteosynthesis" [29] develops. Additional demands, such as rest in the flexion position and flexion movements or beginning with stretching and straining exercises as early as possible, in order to make the osteosynthesis "strong" as it were, are unnecessary but as a rule are possible without giving problems.

A fundamentally different means of introducing force makes the bilateral technique far superior to its predecessors. Its aim is to generate in every single case interfragmentary pressure over the whole region of the fracture and at a level that guarantees that even under the strain of the quadriceps it does not become distracted. On top of this the forces that lead to gaping have to be avoided. This requires that the resultant force of pre-tensioning should run through the core cross-sectional area or, more precisely, through the anterior part of this area. Technicians understand this to be a surface arranged around the axis of the body – cf. Fig. 46. Thus, the formation of harmful bending moments and shearing forces is excluded; the tendency of the patella to bend during flexion is neutralized. Further advantages lie in securely fixing the foundations of the cables using Kirschner wires and opening the joint bilaterally giving a clear view.

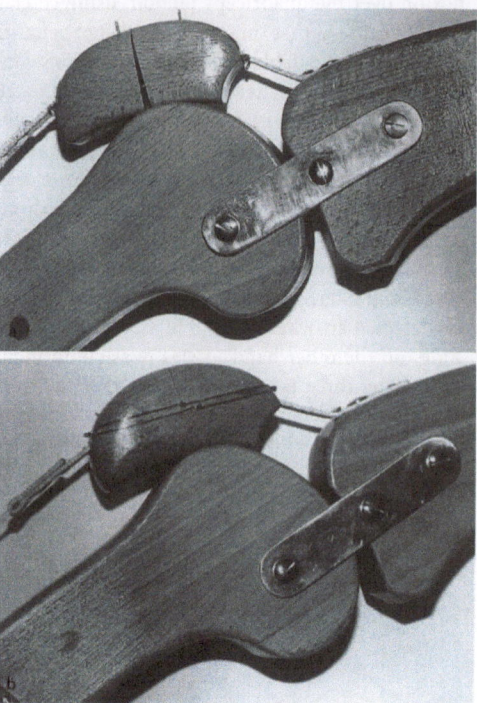

Fig. 63. Difference eccentric – bilateral tension banding

On a wooden scale model loaded at the lower end with 50 N the differences between the two procedures are clearly demonstrated. Following conventional treatment the fracture shifts during active flexion and extension; after bilateral tension banding it remains compressed throughout every phase (Fig. 63).

Principle of Operation

Static interfragmentary compression is produced by means of permanently acting cable tension banding firmly grasping the patella bone laterally and attached to two longitudinal Kirschner wires. It is easy to draw a parallel with the internal fixator. The resultant force of the tension banding runs, as is anatomically necessary and thoroughly beneficial (because the majority of the tendon fibers pass through the anterior area of the patella), through the anterior center of the fracture. Smaller fragments can additionally be held in place with further Kirschner wires and/or screws (Fig. 64).

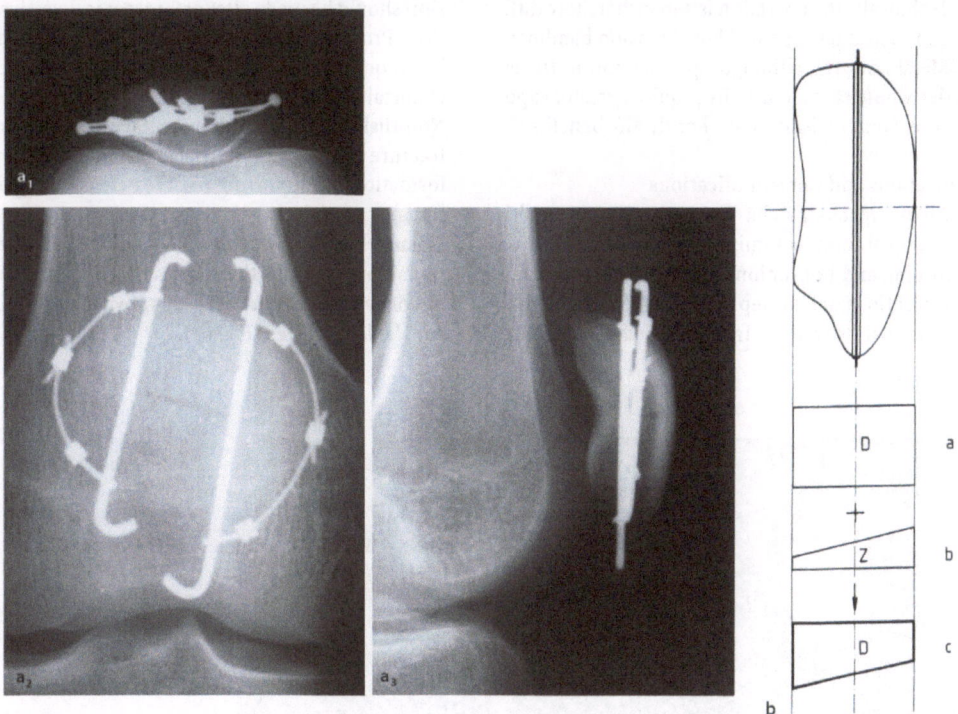

Fig. 64. The principle of operation generates high interfragmentary compression which is not to be completely reduced under movement (c in **b**)

▶ Note the absence of interposition of soft tissue in the problem region of the Kirschner wire-cable loop, as well as the inward bending of the 2-mm wires, the exact lateral position of the tension cable, and the crimp lying directly under the attachment of the joint capsule.

The strain-at-rest of bilateral tension banding is high and evenly distributed provided that the core cross-sectional area has been pin-pointed exactly. The quadriceps tension b is subtracted but leaves sufficient interfragmentary compression c remaining so long as it is exercised with reasonable partial loading in post-operative treatment.

Despite varying opinions [36, 416, 434] it has to be emphasized that Kirschner wires are necessary in every case – cf. Fig. 4. They have to be of adequate size, that is, not less then 2 mm thick, in order to perform their tasks. These consist of:

1. Forming secure anchorages for the means of tension
2. Neutralizing the *ever* present shearing and bending forces

3. Stabilizing fragments through additional pinning

▶ K-wires are in fact an imperative prerequisite in *every type* of tension banding.

Advantages and Disadvantages

✦ There is stability for exercise and partial weight bearing.

✦ Bilateral para-patellar incisions produce a good view over the joint surface of the patella, which can also be assessed visually and by palpation *after* the osteosynthesis.

✦ The joint surface, anatomically firmly fitted together is the most important criterion for the quality of the resulting effect.

✦ Everywhere the cables lie directly on the patella. Soft tissue is not compressed and therefore blood flow is not disrupted. Pre-tensioning or rather interfragmentary compression is not lost.

✦ Treatment with a plaster cast is unnecessary in 2/3 of cases; there is no need to fear secondary dislocation.

– Technically the operation is somewhat more difficult than extensor side "false" tension bandings.

– Metal removal, although optional and in the elderly unnecessary, usually requires greater exposure. Point incisions have hardly any benefits.

Indications and Contraindications

+ All distracted patella fractures, simple, multifragment and comminuted fractures, delayed healing and non-unions as well as corrective interventions due to step formation following conventional operation. In dubious cases the decision should be made after arthroscopic investigation. Proximal and central fractures, in particular, require especially high stability on biomechanical grounds [230] (Fig. 65 und 66).

– Non-dislocated intra-ligamentary transverse fracture without significant lengthening and step formation in supporting reserve extension apparatus.

– Isolated small bony polar avulsions without functional loss [149]. In these cases decision in favor of conventional functional therapy. Four different stable fractures (Fig. 67).

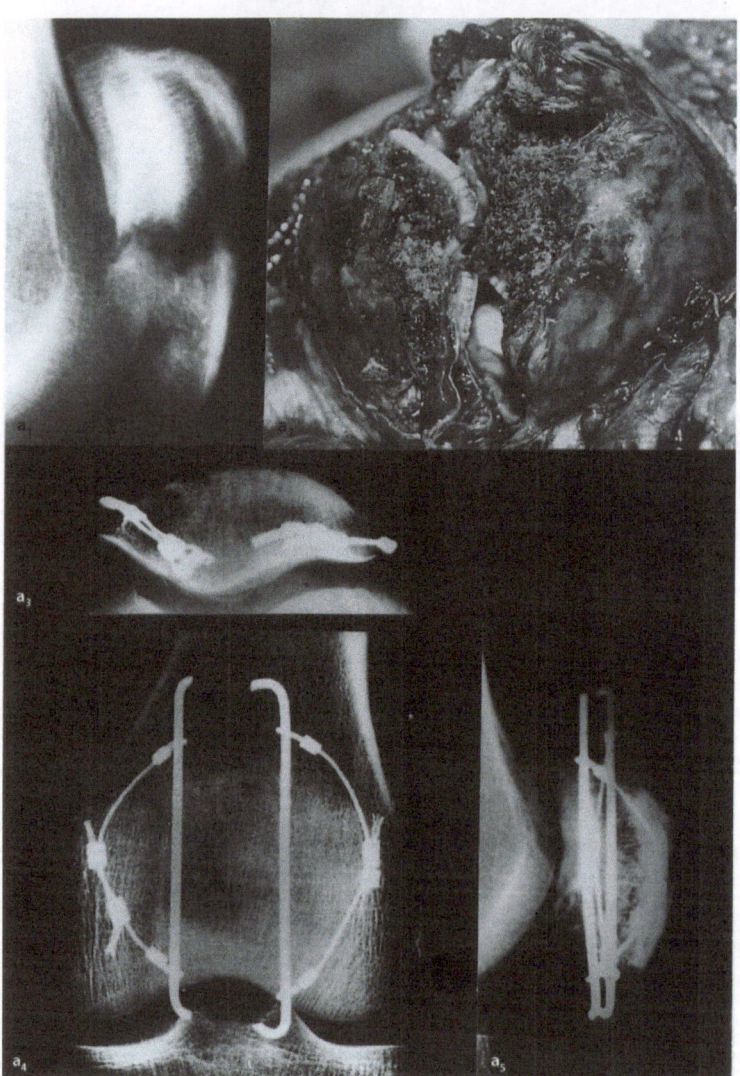

Fig. 65a–c. Indication. Comminuted fracture of the patella. The very first application of a wire cable in traumatology on 7th November 1978: H. T. 50-year-old male; 4 weeks plaster cast. Metal removal in 5/1979; fully functional from 6/1979

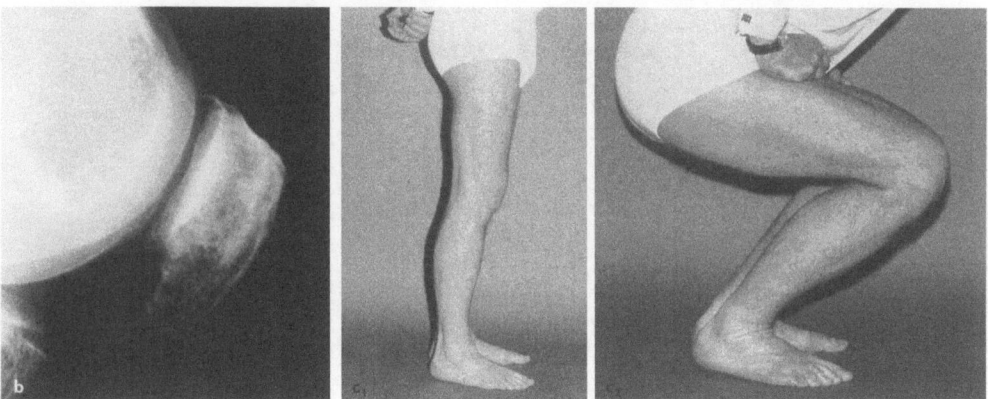

Fig. 65b, c

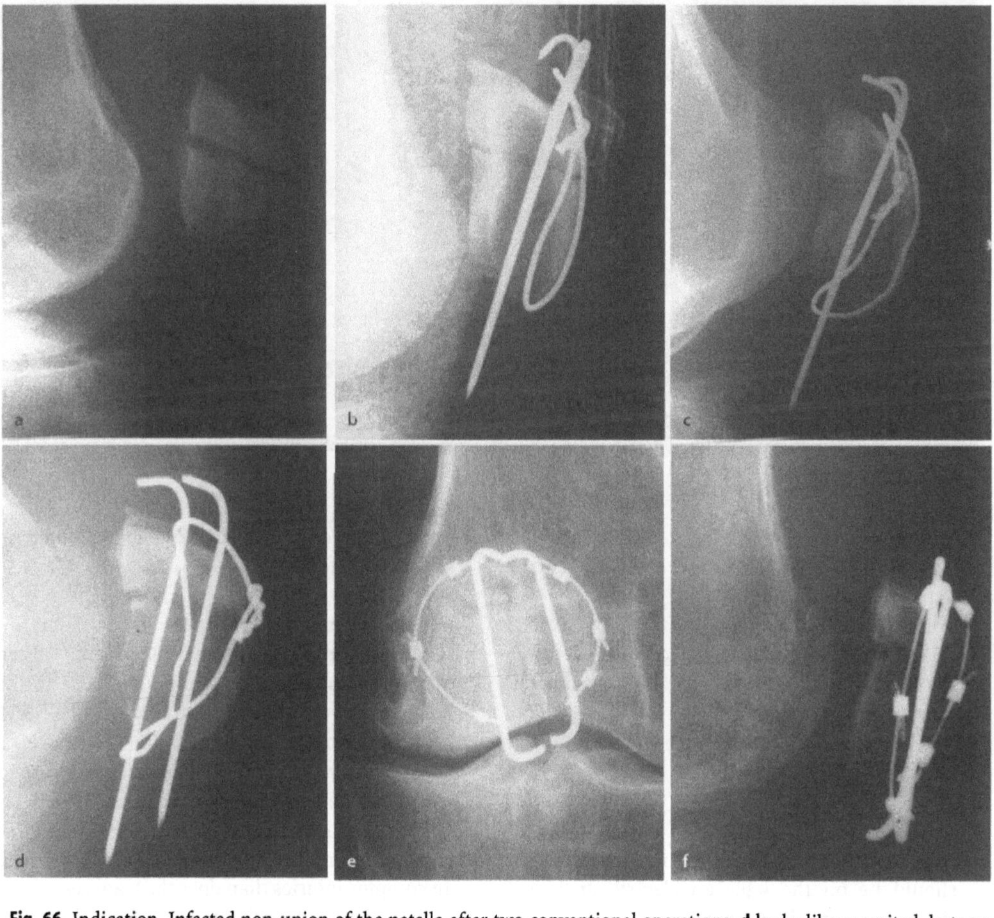

Fig. 66. Indication. Infected non-union of the patella after two conventional operations. **d** looks like re-united, but was not. Healing with flexion deficiency of 20 °

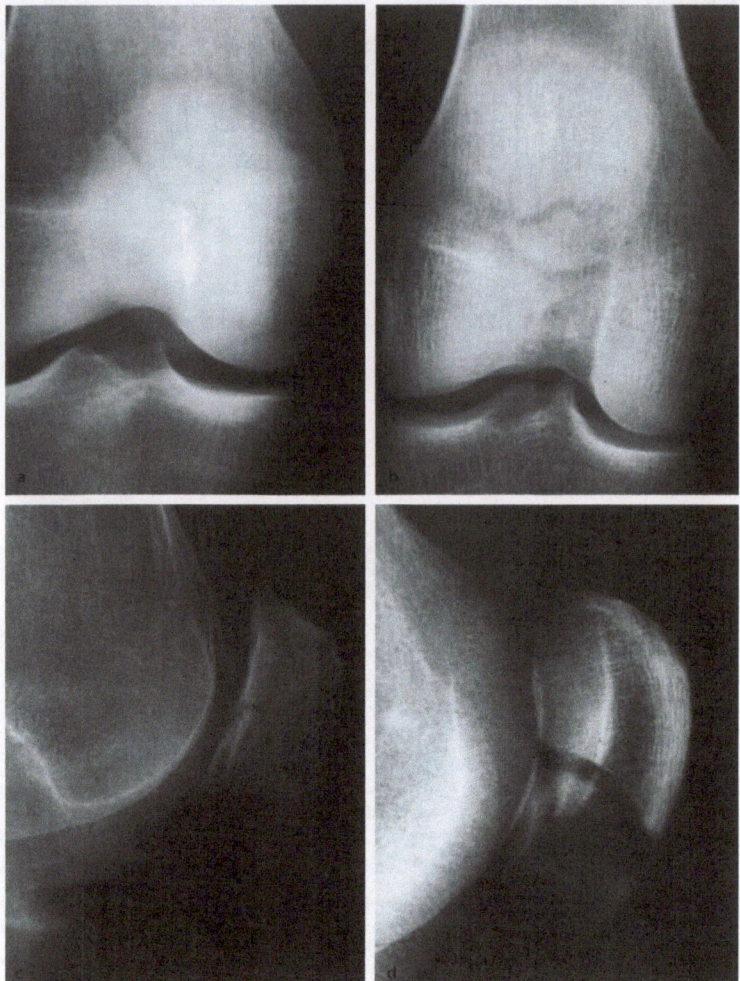

Fig. 67. Conservative treatment in non- or nearly dislocated fractures

Positioning

- Thermal mat, supine position, right and left side supports
- Wash the leg from hip to toes
- Foam rolls under the affected knee. Slight lowering of the opposite leg allows the surgeon freedom of movement
- The lower leg is placed in sterile wrapping to 5 cm below the tibial tuberosity

Instruments

- In addition to the special cable instruments there should be on the table an electric drill, drill sleeves, 2 mm Kirschner wires, side cutters, curved pins, pointed and flat pliers or Zimmer

forceps, as well as two small and large pointed repositioning forceps.

Operation Technique

- The incision is always non-standard. Lister, v. Bergmann, Payr et al. gave preference to the longitudinal incision because it spares the nerve structures more, especially the infrapatellar nerve. Today it is therefore generally performed on the fibula side. The transverse incision dates back to Mikulicz-Radecki [36, 162, 361]. Longitudinal incisions do not expose the joint any better in complex injuries than does the transverse incision, which we have favored for a long time. Performed generously enough, it provides very good access to the torn extensor apparatus, a free view into the joint and is functionally and cosmetically optimal.

After division of the skin and blood-rich subcutaneous tissue the broken kneecap is exposed. Tracing the infrapatellar branch of the saphenous nerve that runs beneath the pes anserinus is not necessary.

- Remove the coagulation and the torn pre-patellar bursa so that the inner joint can be freely inspected.

- Incise the joint capsule in a longitudinal direction approximately 1 cm on the right and on the left next to the patella. The vessels radiating proximally and caudally into the patella are not touched.

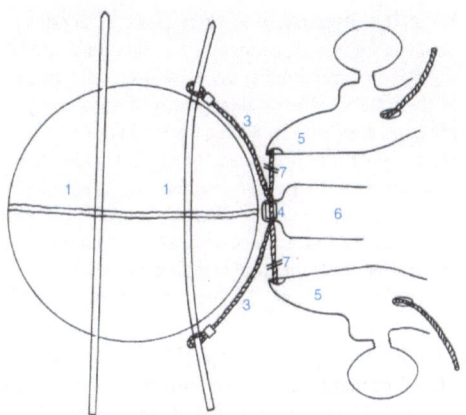

Fig. 68. Operation technique

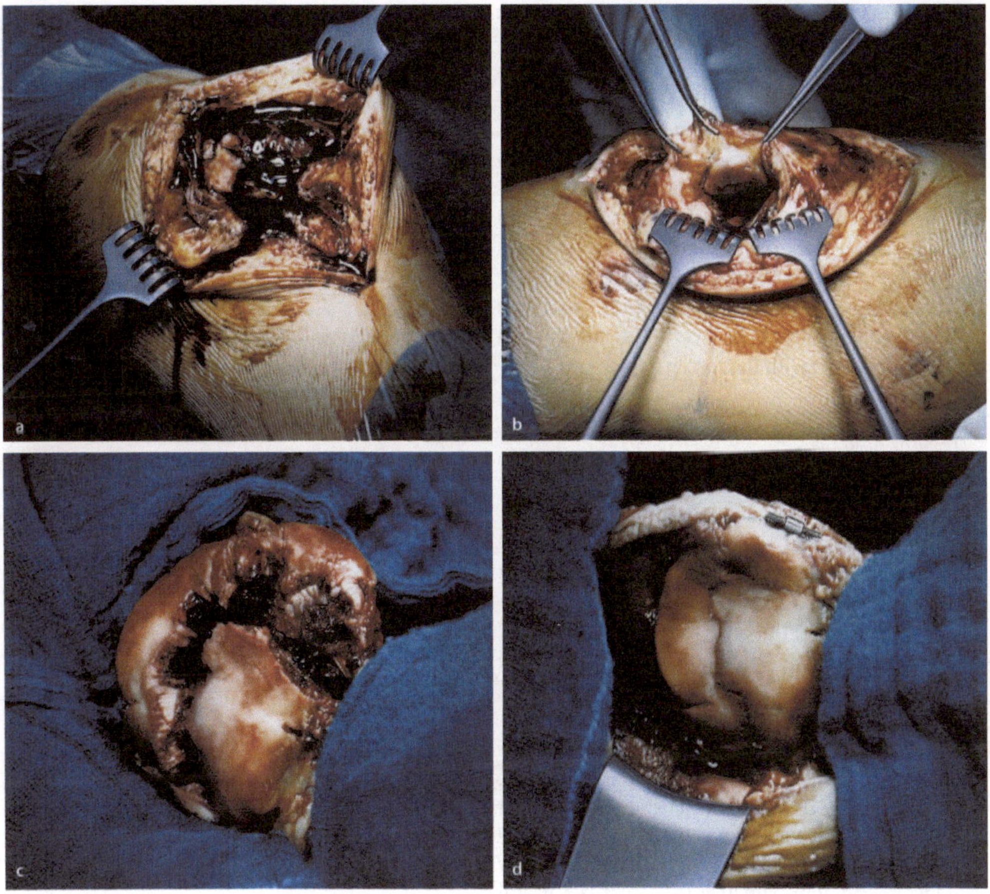

Fig. 69. Site at the start and end of the operation: **a** fracture hematoma; **b** para-patellar longitudinal incision of the capsule; **c** extent of the fracture; **d** patella joint surface after treatment

Note: This preparatory work carries a great advantage, for it permits an exact understanding of the fracture and definite digital and visual control of the results of the re-alignment and the stability of the osteosynthesis. Such a possibility does not exist in positioning a means of tension on the extensor side. In that case repositioning, as is well known, has to be assessed indirectly on the upper surface of the kneecap, because after adjustment of the fragments the joint is no longer visible; it is impossible to test the stability of the joint surface.

The individual operative steps (Figs. 68, 69, and 70):
- Re-alignment takes place with the knee over-extended. The fragments are held together with two large pointed repositioning forceps.
- The ligament and quadriceps tendon are longitudinally incised with the scalpel up to the immediate circumference of the kneecap.
- Two 2-mm Kirschner wires (1) are now screwed in via this incision as parallel as possible distally to proximally, or the reverse, while continual control of the joint surfaces in the slightly flexed knee is maintained.
- Two wire cables (3) are attached by their loops to each Kirschner wire and are threaded as a pair using an awl through the incised soft tissue from above and below directly onto the lateral surfaces of the patella. The bent awl is advantageous for this purpose as it takes the cable ends and allows for safer guidance. If it is very difficult its solid part is gripped with flat forceps.

Note: The lateral surfaces of the kneecap form a small channel together with the capsule attachments which is wide enough to give the cables a firm anchorage and strong hold so that they do not slip into the joint.

- Both free cable ends of the one side are put through a crimp (4) in opposite directions and afterwards fixed in the cable tensioner (5).
- The cable tensioner slightly pulled away from the bone makes room for the crimp pliers (6), the jaws of which must correctly grip the crimp.
- The pliers with the gripped crimp are brought into the desired position and given to the assistant. By turning the handle of the tensioner to the right the surgeon tightens the cables firmly until the ends of the two Kirschner wires above and below have bowed approximately 10°. That is a useful visual indication of sufficiently high cable tension – cf. Fig. 37.

- The crimp pliers are firmly pressed together until the force limiting knobs make contact for 2 s, so that the crimp can shape itself. In doing so it loses its oval form and becomes round and somewhat longer.
- The loosened tensioner is drawn away from the kneecap to make room for the cable scissors (7). Now the excess cable can be cut off in the notch of the scissors, right next to the crimp.
- The opposite side is dealt with in the same way. If they are not in the way the repositioning forceps can be left in place until the final tensioning.

All four Kirschner wires are shortened and first bent *ventrally*, both proximally *and* distally. Immediately afterwards they are turned *medially* so that the cables cannot slip off.
- Finally the posterior surface of the patella is once again digitally and visually assessed. It also has to remain stable during flexion of the lower leg. If it is not the tension banding should be repeated and/or a plaster cast applied.
- The para-patellar longitudinal incisions are closed with Vicryl, strength 2 × 0, after one or two Redon joint drains have been inserted.
- Finally the torn reserve extensor apparatus is sutured. The skin is clipped or closed after separate subcutaneous suturing with the self-adapting Medi-Zip wound closure. – cf. Fig. 94.

Note: Fig. 71 shows the theoretically best position for the Kirschner wires. It is position c which is found through the 45° angle to the horizontal in the center of the patella. At this point the existing pressure force P developing from the resultant R is the same size as the transverse force Q. This has always to be counterbalanced by the 2-mm Kirschner wires. The lateral cushioning of the bone is thick enough to prevent them from possibly pulling out as in b. In a on the other hand interfragmentary compression becomes too small relative to the transverse force.

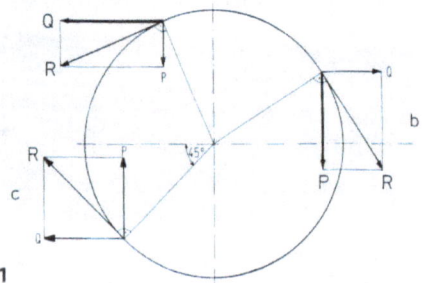

Fig. 71

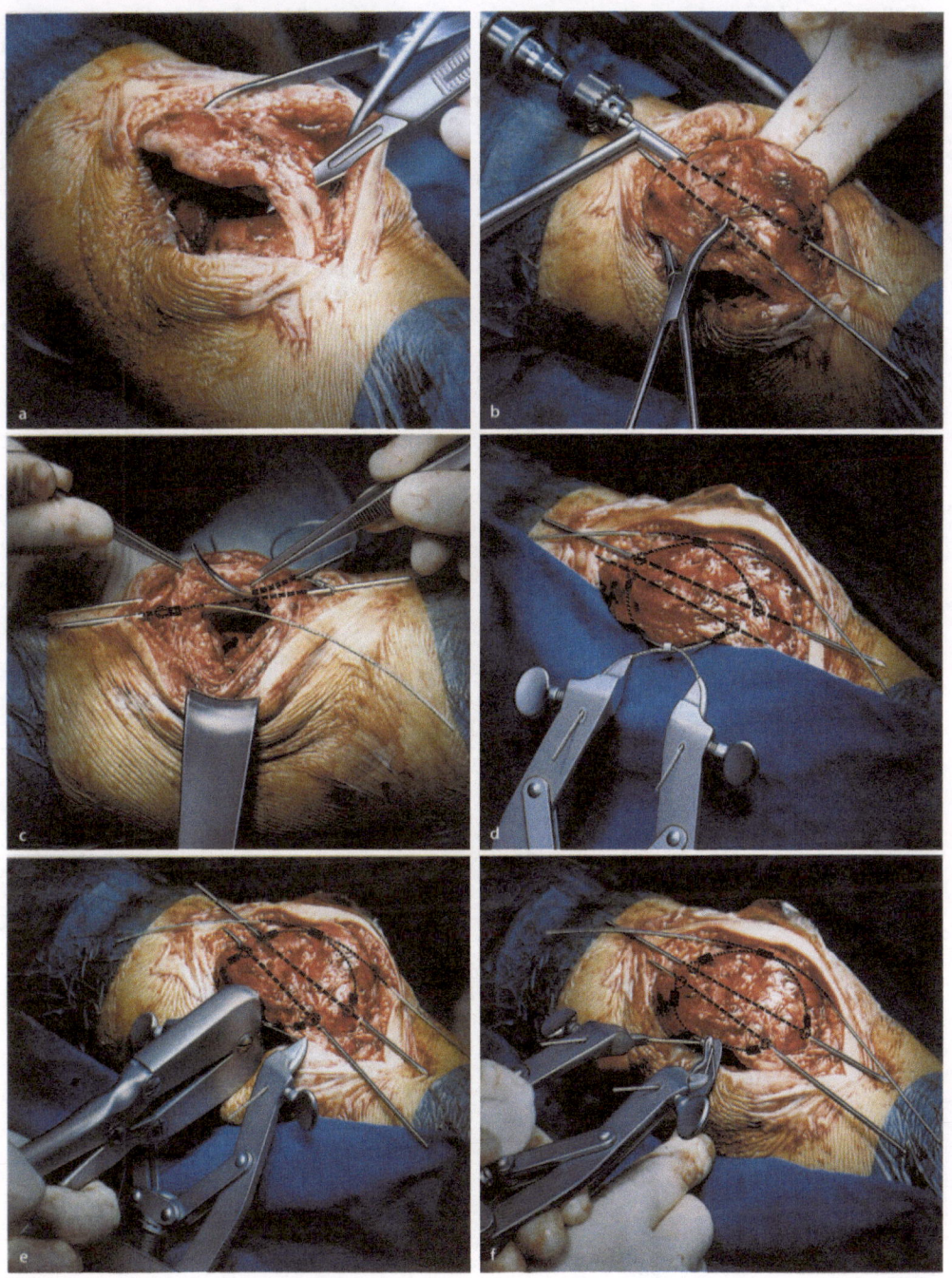

Fig. 70. The individual operative steps. (The operation photographs in Figs. 69 and 70 have been provided by Mr. Leibinger, by kind permission of Aesculap AG Tuttlingen)

Operative Peculiarities and Variations

- Bilateral incisions allow for quality control of the restored joint surfaces of the patella and the stability of the osteosynthesis.
- Before tensioning of the cable the lower leg is overextended by raising the heel. This relieves the strain on the patella.
- With smooth joint surfaces a poorly adjusted fragment on the extensor side does not cause a disadvantage. The Kirschner wires, not bent distally, moved proximally. Therefore four weeks in a plaster cast. Anatomical healing with free function (Fig. 72).
- Multi-fragment and comminuted fractures require smaller fracture pieces to be first joined to each other with Kirschner wires or screws to form, if possible, only two or three main fragments, which allow the application of tension banding. Cartilage-bone fragments are fitted back in; isolated cartilage fragments are removed. A defect is filled in with spare cartilage and is, contrary to a step, tolerable. By crossing the cable over itself at the poles one attains additional partial cerclaging and with it support for comminuted zones. But then the Kirschner wires must be bent *outwards*! This variation is being used more frequently (Fig. 73).
- In distal bony ligament avulsions an additional cable protection of the ligament structures is advantageous – see Chap. 4.14.1.1.

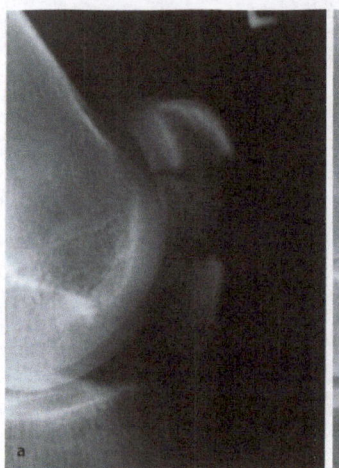 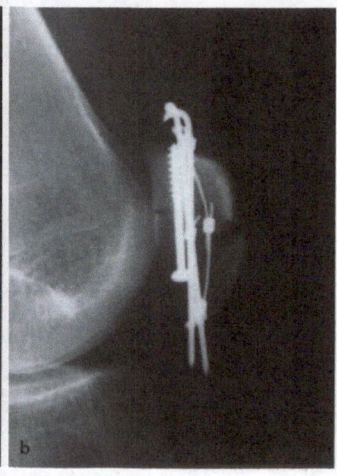 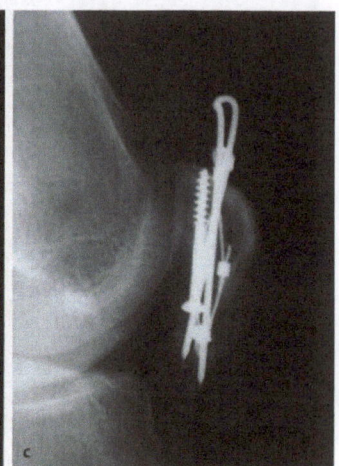

Fig. 72. Expression of a good osteosynthesis is the exactly adjusted cartilage surface, not the extensor side of patella

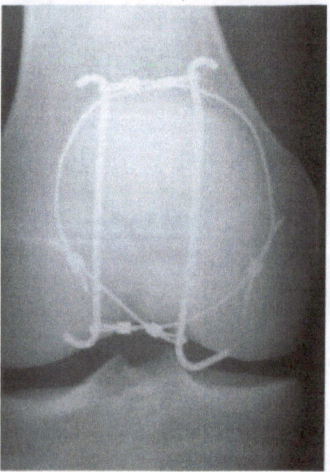

Fig. 73. "Crossed over" cable tension banding (Prof. Contzen, BG-Clinic, Ludwigshafen, 1987)

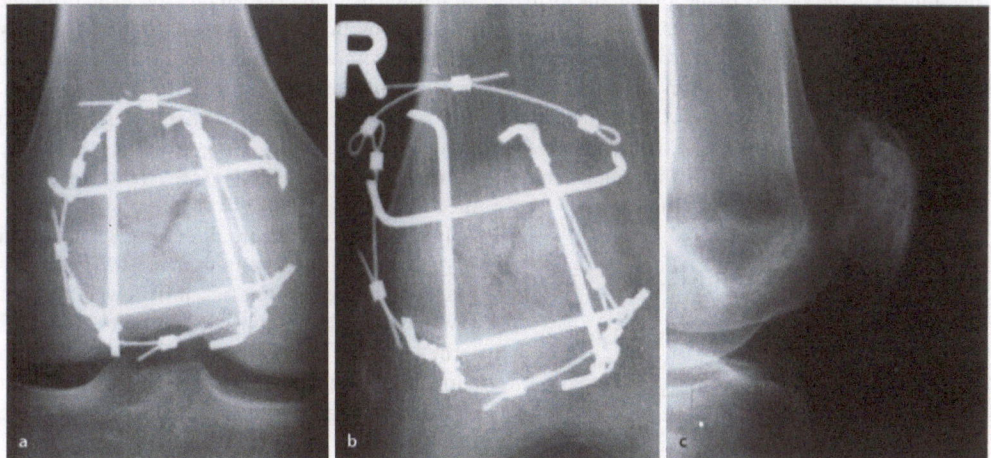

Fig. 74. Excessive demands on the emergency team: **a** atypical treatment of a star fracture. Cables not stretched directly on the bone, Kirschner wires incorrectly bent. No primary plaster; **b** loosening after a few days. To maintain fragment adjustment, application of a thigh cast; **c** healing. After careful functional treatment with movement splints between 0/10/40 degrees from the third week out of plaster good function six months post-operatively

Complications, Mistakes, and Dangers

- A comminuted fracture should not be treated as an emergency during the night, but the next morning at the earliest (Fig. 74). There is no indication for primary patellectomy.

- Inadequate exposure of the injury and half-hearted para-patellar incision prevent the exact re-alignment and lateral positioning of the cables and the post-operative assessment of anatomy and stability of the osteosynthesis.

- If soft tissue is left between the cable loops and the kneecap, loss of pre-tensioning can occur during follow-up treatment. The Kirschner wires must be bent inwards proximally and distally – otherwise they slip out of the cable loops and patella on moving the knee during post-operative treatment; the same is true of laterally bent Kirschner wires – cf. Figs. 37 and 42. Kirschner wires with screw threads are not necessary.

- Carelessly fitted cables can slip into the joint causing cartilage damage and loss of pre-tensioning.

Post-operative Treatment

- It is usually without plaster; any necessary plaster remains split for four weeks so that the knee can be moved out of it passively and exercised on the motor splint between 0 – 10 – 40 °.

- In stable treatment after wound healing the patient may walk around on level ground without basic strain relief because, when standing and when walking, traction forces on the patella are safely absorbed by the cable tension banding. Crutches are necessary because they provide security.

- Horizontal active raising of the extended lower leg in bed without physiotherapeutic support as well as weight-bearing stair climbing and squatting are not advisable within the first six weeks.

Results

Up to the end of 1995, 56 patella fractures were treated with bilateral cable tension banding; 21 cases (36%) were placed in plaster for up to 4 weeks due to complex patterns of injury. The average age was 46 years (17 – 91), with both sexes being equally represented; 49 fractures were closed, 7 open, of which 4 were second and third grade. The cases presented – of which 4 were cases of polytrauma – were 16 transverse, 32 multi-fragment and comminuted fractures, and 8 avulsions of the lower pole. The latter, rated as bony ruptures of the patellar ligament, were additionally secured according to Mc Laughlin's procedure [251] with a cable anchored to two screws on the tuberosity, that went around the patella. The fracture was complicated in six cases by accompanying injuries in the vicinity of the joint in the form of condylar and tibial head fractures. Adequate information could not be gathered from four patients. These ten cases are excluded from the assessment.

The X-ray series and completed outpatient clinic notes of 46 cases were evaluated. Here, both result and function are recorded. A few incomplete notes were filled in after further check-ups.

▶ Bony reconstruction occurred in 43 patellae; a non-union did not develop. In one case the tension band of an inferior polar avulsion loosened with peri-patellar cable protection remaining intact. It was renewed and resulted in healing; 36 out of 46 (78%) were rated as very good (free function, unremarkable X-ray, no pain) and good (extension deficit $\leq 5°$ and/or flexion deficit $\leq 20°$, minimal divergence on the X-ray, hardly any complaints), seven (15%) as satisfactory (extensor deficit $\geq 5°$ and/or flexion deficit $\geq 20°$ and/or arthrotic signs on the X-ray with corresponding complaints), three (7%) as poor. In these cases a deep infection after second or third grade open injuries, which could not be controlled, led to arthrodesis.

Even the comparison with eccentric wire tension banding is proof of the quality of bilateral cable tension banding: 78% very good or good results with clear reduction of pre-arthrotic X-ray signs compare with good AO results which rarely exceed 70% at most, and are generally around or below 50%, and frequently describe deformation of the joint surfaces. The arthrodeses due to infection are not detrimental to the procedure. In two-thirds of all cases the high stability of bilateral cable tension banding makes low-risk early functional post-operative treatment; nevertheless an additive plaster should be arranged if necessary.

▶ New findings often bring about a certain degree of "resistance," as is revealed by a report seeking to prevent a publication relating to biomechanics of tension banding [220]: "No original experimental or clinical results have been presented which show the superiority or proof of the superior functional ability of the principle described by the author. On purely subjective assumptions, Weber's principle of performing patella tension banding with ventrally crossed wires is portrayed as being non-functional. The claim is put forward that it is, supposedly, a rigid wire system. This is naturally not the case in classic tension banding. The lateral cable band principle proposed by the author does not lead necessarily however, contrary to the author's assumption, to fracture compression. On increasing cable tension, one can assume that a force in a transverse direction may develop with increasing buckling of the wire rather than a compression force…" (anonymous for the sake of the author)

In contrast to that, Troidl et al. [389] stated in 1993: "For us a lack of commitment as well as ignorance are the greatest sins (i.e., mistakes) in surgery. One must speak of a ‚mistake' and include in this term a state of affairs where a therapeutic goal in surgery is not achieved or is even perverted – just owing to ignorance or deficient care in conceiving the therapy."

Contemporary Alternatives and Conclusions

Wire tension banding as the suitable method of choice is technically incomplete and unstable because "pressure and shearing forces are not neutralized" [146], and the fragments are distracting easily during post-operative treatment. Benjamin et al. [13] found experimentally that poor results "occurred in two ways: *initially* there was fracture separation secondary to the inherent laxity in wiring techniques. *Further* separation occurred by plastic deformation of the wire." Even in dynamic tests on the cadaveric knee the weaknesses of the modified tension band were visible: on average they only withstood 106 defined movements between 0° and 90° before destruction [300]. Burvant et al. [42] measured gaps of 1 mm or more during loading using different methods in a cadaver knee. The variants described by him as more stable with tension band wire fastened onto cancellous screws can lead to the wire breaking under movements on the sharp thread of the screws.

Variations such as the techniques of Lotke and Ecker [241], Perry et al. [300], and Tönnis [382], or the combination with dorsal ring cerclage according to Wenzl and Krüger [419] and Pyrford (quoted from [42]) or the many individual techniques using increased quantities of materials, which are practised in individual clinics, do not lead to measurable improvements. Lengsfeld et al. [230] emphasise after kinematic computer investigations that fractures within the proximal and central part of the patella need a very high stability of internal fixation which cannot be provided by cerclage wire.

Modified tension banding with PDS-cord and pins used on living sheep has given "in comparison with conventional wire tension banding equivalent results" [435] a statement that shows the poor quality of wire tension banding rather than the value of this possibility.

> ▶ A *warning* against this compromise: anyone who wishes to perform an AO tension banding with a wire cable will cause its biomechanical weaknesses to be particularly enhanced because high pre-tensioning can be attained with cable. *Never on any account is eccentric cable tension banding to be employed!*

Brill and Hopf [29] suggested as an alternative the double screw osteosynthesis with washers which they found particularly stable in cadaveric patellae strengthened with Palacos bone-cement. Cement and washers are unsuitable however for the living; moreover smooth transverse fractures, which can be screwed, are comparatively rare. Cancellous screws are simply not up to the bending forces on the living patella during functional post-operative treatment. Their ability to hold permanently is not guaranteed. Benjamin et al. [13] measured only very slight extraction forces and saw some fractures around the screw threads; this caused them to recommend screws only "in patients with adequate bone stock." Perry and coworkers' [300] osteosynthesis with two cancellous screws only withstood ten (!) movement cycles which had been generated by traction on the quadriceps.

Brill and Hopf's proposal has apparently not been adopted anywhere.

Arthroscopic treatment of the uncomplicated transverse fracture with tension screws [334], the mini-fragmentation plate [371], and the mini-fixator

[110] were occasionally described. It is reported that Liang and Wu [235] in 1987 healed 27 transverse fractures with a form of Malgaigne clip.

Fourati and coworkers' [92] conviction, again expressed in 1987 after analysis of 400 cases, that the best results were obtained by conservative treatment, can indeed be taken as scepticism towards operative methods, not as a plea for a rest in plaster.

The problems of primary patellectomy are discussed to a varying degree. Albeit judged predominantly positively [17, 332], there are correct warnings against it and it is described as the last resort in therapeutic possibilities [91, 163, 363]. Various disadvantages such as a feeling of instability and reduction of the circumference of the quadriceps with up to 50% loss of force make it clear that "no restitutio ad integrum can be expected from patellectomy" [Vogt 397; 164, 231, 407]. A primary patellectomy, recommended usually or fundamentally in multiple fragment and comminuted fractures [36, 68, 247, 277, 290, 324, 416], seems to be an expression of resignation.

> ▶ In conclusion, bilateral cable tension banding is a theoretically and experimentally proven osteosynthesis procedure whose high stability in patella fractures is also documented in clinical results. In two-thirds of cases danger-free early-functional post-operative treatment is possible. The morphological weaknesses of the conventional technique such as lengthening, tilting and step formation, delayed healing, dislocation, and non-unions are not encountered in correct fracture after-care; the number of patellectomies can be greatly reduced.

4.6
Olecranon Fracture

It has become standard surgical practice to describe the olecranon as the proximal part of the ulna which extends over the whole articular surface approximately as far as the coronoid process. This is incorrect, because the olecranon is biomechanically defined exclusively as that part of the ulna that forms the lever for the triceps. As calculations show [196], it is defined from the tip of the olecranon process to a limit which is formed by the axis of flexion running through the capitulum humeri during a 90° flexion of the elbow. Lying distally to this limit the

half of the semi-lunar articular surface, which the ulna has formed for the trochlea of the humerus, can no longer be olecranon because the lever of the flexors begins here. This corresponds to the distance distally from the axis of flexion to the insertion of the biceps (or more precisely, to the common imaginary insertion of all flexors). It is longer than the triceps lever. Consequently, no biomechanical identity can exist for the two joint regions. Extensors and flexors must have opposing actions in the same way as must the forces introduced through an osteosynthesis [86]. Unfortunately accepted fracture schemes do not take these relationships into consideration. They differentiate between transverse,

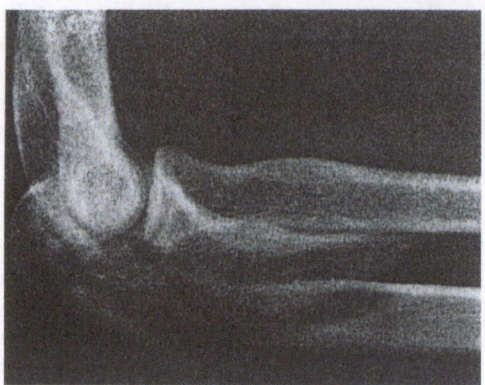

Fig. 75 (from [242])

oblique, and comminuted fractures, taking notice of the position and direction of the fracture [87, 136, 169, 266, 342], and include the intra-articular ulna as far as to the coronoid process as "distal olecranon fractures" [309]. Even the extra-articular ulna shaft, without defining a distal limit is included [72]. A diagram and comment by Lugger and Russe [242] shows this very clearly: "Comminuted fracture of the olecranon with a large volarly dislocated fragment, bearing the coronoid process on the flexor side" (Fig. 75).

This, correctly described, is a combined proximal extra- and intra-articular fracture of the ulna shaft with accompanying olecranon fracture. Lugger plated it. Indeed it could not have been treated with eccentric AO tension band.

Morphologists have classified it more precisely: Rauber-Kopsch [312] too, defined the olecranon only as "that hook-shaped bent bony part of the elbow that surrounds the trochlea of the humerus posteriorly." The limit within the ulna joint surface can be easily recognized by a cartilage lying transversely in the middle of the fossa olecrani [159]. Based on these anatomical demarcations biomechanical findings gained at a later point in time were also corroborated morphologically.

The *definition* of the olecranon supported anatomically and biomechanically reads therefore:

▶ The olecranon as the lever of the triceps is the intra-articular end of the ulna, which lies proximal to the axis of flexion (in a 90° elbow flexion) reaching from the tip of the elbow to the middle of the trochlear notch.

The ulna shaft begins intra-articularly forward of the limit forming the lower arm.

4.6.1
Historical Procedures

As for the patella fracture, similarly a number of different surgical procedures has been practised that can be arranged chronologically. Clearly both types of fracture show biomechanical similarities and can therefore be treated with almost identical methods that only differ from each other in details. These small differences have anatomical but no mechanical causes. Even for the treatment of the fractured olecranon it is a question of neutralizing the strong extensor muscle strain just as much as the bending forces that become stronger and stronger with increasing flexion and which continually threaten to pull apart the repaired region again and displace it – cf. Fig. 78–80.

▶ Lister [239] first carried out his "metallic suture", which for many years has been the treatment method for olecranon fractures, on 28th March 1873: "I made a longitudinal incision, exposing the site of the fracture, and, at the same time, bringing into view the articular surface of the humerus; and, having pared away the fibrous material from the fracture surfaces, I proceeded to drill the fragments, with a view to the application of the suture. I introduced a silver wire in its place and was then able to pass it on through the other drilled opening, and thus the two fragments were brought into apposition. The ends of the wire were twisted together and left projecting at the wound. Healing took place without suppuration or fever, and the wire was removed on May 19th, seven weeks after the operation. The wound made for its extraction soon healed, and the patient returned to Glasgow; and I afterwards had the satisfaction of learning that he was wielding the hammer in an iron shipbuilding yard with his former energy" (Fig. 76).

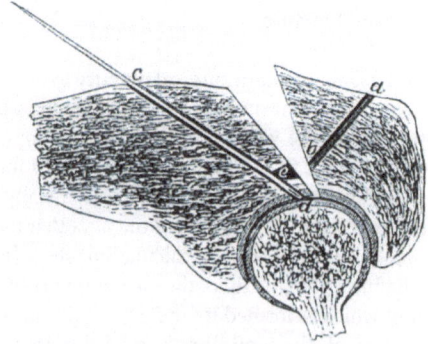

Fig. 76. Lister's technique (from [239])

Around 1900 Lister's wire suture was superseded by Payr's technique [130, 361]. He guided the wire (as in the patella – cf. Fig. 53) in bore canals running longitudinally across the fracture crevice and knotted it dorsally.

Berger in 1902, Böhler in 1929, and Watson-Jones in 1940 made a ring suture, a cerclage, through transverse bore canals, and knotted it crosswise or in an O-shape [87].

In Hachez-Leblanc's functional cerclaging [118], wire loops are stretched between the triceps tendon and a distal bore canal, a precursor better called simple tension banding. It has become obsolete (Fig. 77).

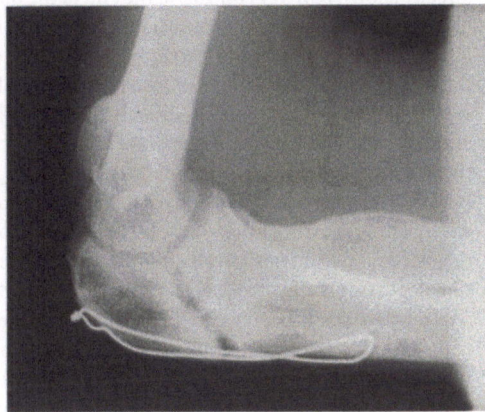

Fig. 77. So-called simple tension banding

In 1978 Scharplatz and Allgöwer [339] had it put on record that in the Basle clinic olecranon tension banding without Kirschner wires was favored for two reasons, which were

"1. owing to post-operative soft tissue problems
2. owing to their preventing the making of fine adjustments".

This concedes that despite osteosynthesis movements are still possible. In 1983 this variant was all but abandoned, comprising only 6% of operations [86].

In addition to this procedure "amongst others were recommended the periosteal suture, the nailing of the fracture with flat-sided or Smith-Peterson nails, the Zuelzer clip, the Maatz feather screw, the U-nail, the use of plates, screwing, the method of wire loops and the treatment of the fracture with Küntscher-nails or Rush pins, the possibility of percutaneous wire fixation with one or several Kirschner wires,

percutaneous threaded pin osteosynthesis (V. Schwier) and the fixation of fragments by means of cancellous screws," according to Bürger and Hennert [38]. In the meantime the use of the plaster cast in the extension position [20] had become obsolete.

From this multiplicity of methods it can be deduced that there was no standard osteosynthesis for the olecranon before that time. Weber's tension banding became the first. As a functional procedure it improved results. In 1957, Eriksson et al. [87] had had to record that out of all possible bone sutures and simple tension bandings, non-unions had occurred in one third (21 out of 64 cases), a rate that has been under 10% since Weber [86, 333], but has occasionally been found to be higher [205, 306]. Its best results are assessed at 80 – 87% [75, 132, 150, 284, 339]; usually very good or good results are situated between 55% and 80% [38, 86, 136, 155, 169]. Not to be outdone are those 97% "good and excellent results in 29 out of 30 cases of isolated fractures which despite minor and functionally insignificant loss of motion in terminal extension" were achieved in Pennsylvania in 1987 [429].

> Weber and Kouwenhoven [185] judged their first very carefully documented cases much more cautiously: although all had osseously healed within a short time, in 8 out of 31 later controls, i.e., in 26%, they found joint steps of approximately 1.5 mm or more, "either already an arthrosis or an incongruency that sooner or later will lead to arthrosis."

Hume and Wiss [141] describe similar experiences: "Tension band wiring resulted only in 37% good clinical and 47% good radiographic results. Post-operative loss of reduction, leading to a significant articular step-off or gap in 53%."

Bony reconstruction is not the main problem – cancellous bone healed well even with early bone sutures [162]. However, unfortunately nowhere near all patients become pain free.

An early critical assessment of results of comminuted fractures in 1972 is to be found in an AO Bulletin [16]. It states: "Out of 13 patients 12 presented restrictions of joint function. Radiologically the causes of the reduction of movement were found to be steps or defects in the joint surfaces, incongruence, dislocation of fragments, pseudarthroses and arthroses." That is why König et al. [184], in 1990, completely rejected tension banding for comminuted fractures – "a sufficient treatment can only be achieved through open re-alignment and plate osteosynthesis." Not everyone is quite as radical, but it has gradually become accepted that non-simple fractures, in particular the distal unstable types C and D, should no longer be treated with AO-tension band [137, 242, 248, 284, 306]. We had already noted this in 1975 [196] because in these pseudo-olecranon fractures, extensor side tension banding increased the bending strains of the forearm flexors.

At a professional meeting of the Berufsgenossenschaft (Employees' Industrial Compensation Society) in 1977 in follow-up investigations for *all* 43 cases, which had been operated on using wire tension banding, "painful movement deficits in extension and flexion directions" of 10 ° in 29 patients (67%), up to 30 ° in 12 (28%), and over 30 ° in 2 patients (5%) were reported [343].

Nothing has changed: in 1994, 24 out of 44 of Jockheck and coworkers' [153] tension bandings – i.e., 55% – showed movement deficits between 20 ° and more than 50 °. Nevertheless their overall assessment was: "With the correct technique tension banding is a safe operation procedure and an exercise-stable osteosynthesis of the fractured olecranon."

> ▶ Irrespective of this optimism, numerous post-operative complications often occur. They are seen as loosening of the osteosynthesis (22% with Povel et al. [306]), soft tissue irritation due to symptomatic metal prominence in 42% with Hume and Wiss [141], 75% with Macko and Szabo [244], and 80% with Murphy et al. [271], as shifting of the joint surfaces and step formation [141, 196, 271] and in the worst cases as distraction and non-unions [60, 205]. In a dissertation [333] in 1981, in 93 wire tension bandings 10.7% showed metal loosening and 8.5% developed non-unions despite an upper arm plaster cast which in principle had to be worn between 4 – 6 weeks.
>
> The collective study of the AO from 1983 [86] therefore concludes: "The results clearly show the limitations of tension banding."

4.6.2
Weber's Olecranon Tension Band and its Biomechanical Analysis

Weber [408], as is well known, had compared the ulna and the olecranon process with the jib of a building crane. Although this analogy does not apply to the elbow during unladen post-operative treatment, the eccentric wire tension band, whose "principle is known well enough from daily life" [343] is regarded as the method of choice.

How blurred understanding of tension banding has become is shown by a quote from 1967 of Bürger and Hennert [38]: "The effect of tension banding is already shown in X-ray controls at the end of the operation. It leads, sometimes associated with a small gaping of the section of the fracture crevice close to the joint, to bending of the Kirschner wires, which were straight when originally inserted. The strain and flexion forces which, post-operatively, are effective further in the fracture region are transformed into pure pressure forces by means of the taut bore wires. These pressure forces increase the stability of the osteosynthesis which even after the use of functional post-operative treatment remains constant, contrary to pure axial osteosynthesis. Therefore, with a simple operation technique a pressure osteosynthesis is achieved which allows functional post-operative treatment to begin a short time after the wound has healed."

In plain English: it is asserted that despite a fracture gap, compression osteosynthesis has been achieved using tension banding. A paradox!

In order to be able to subject AO-tension banding (or rather, the sum of the variations which hide behind it) to tests, first their common denominator must be defined. As in the patella fracture here, too, simple tension banding around the triceps tendon is separated from the modified version, where Kirschner wires, Rush pins, or screws give the cerclage fixation, ensure rotation, and neutralize transverse forces and turning moments [62, 137, 244, 284, 339]. The author's own findings which are quoted here [196, 198, 205, 220] show that *tension banding without foundations is absolutely impossible.* The simple one is even less of a tension band than the modified version; it remains theory, and cannot be seen through to fruition.

As the basic prerequisite for an analysis the external forces acting on a healthy ulna joint during the activity of the triceps muscle *and* the flexors have to be established, the significance of which is neglected by nearly all researchers. It is worth understanding the influence resulting from these forces on the development of bending moments, transverse forces, and strains in the elbow as well as its impairment due to fracture of the olecranon and its osteosynthesis.

For equilibrium in the joint it is an essential condition that the sum of all forces and moments acting on it be zero. Moving *against* gravity in the humeroulnar hinge joint the forearm produces in the joint the total pressure force Rd. Movement against gravity is work. Muscular force and joint pressure are varyingly high in extensor and flexor activity because the levers at the disposal of both muscle groups are not the same length. The forearm can only be extended against gravity if the upper arm is held above the head. In this case electromyographically strong triceps activity (and only very weak activity in the flexors) could be detected, as opposed to high biceps activity (and slightly less in the triceps) during bending of the forearm held normally. Pendulum movements of the forearm during walking show only slight electrical activity in both muscle groups, and can be ignored (Fig. 78).

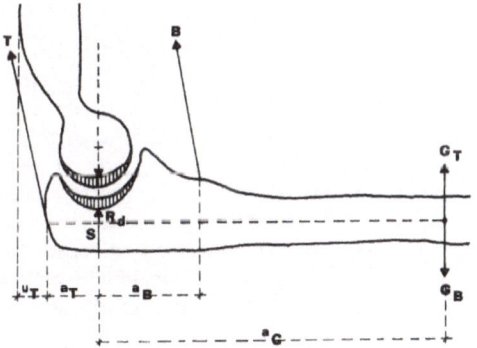

Fig. 78. Levers and equilibrium of forces in the elbow
S = Intersection of the axes of the humerus and the ulna as lines of limitation of the levers uT and aT for the triceps and aB for the biceps
G = Weight of the forearm
uT = Lever of the triceps, which results from the pivoting effect of its tendon reflector on the humerus

Measured in a cadaveric arm, flexion of the elbow requires a force of 96 N and for extension the triceps has to produce 122 N. Therefore joint pressures occur of 78.5–139.5 N respectively. These values were confirmed in 1979 [305].

The relatively small difference of the two muscle forces despite a clearly longer lever for the flexors is explained as a trick of nature: the virtual lever of the triceps extends along the length uT which corresponds to the distance of the projection of its tendon to those dorsally on the furthest protruding point of the humerus up to the tip of the olecranon. One can claim with enough certainty that the functional improvement of the efficiency of the triceps has led to the anatomical angle formation between the shaft and the trochlea of the humerus and thus to the development of this additional lever. Here the same "pivoting effect" takes place, which Goymann and coworkers [112, 113] described in 1974 for the quadriceps tendon after the embedding of the patella in the intercondylar channel of the femur. The inward pressure in the elbow joint (as in the knee) is thus reduced and the force of the triceps is then particularly intensified if stretched out of deep flexion. With increasing extension this effect is lost; it is then also no longer necessary.

Knowing the distribution of pressure and traction strains in the cross-section of the intact ulna – near the joint and away from it – under conditions of isometric loading makes it possible to decide how opposing forces must be introduced through osteosynthesis in order to stabilize a fracture optimally. In reverse, it also allows evaluation of osteosyntheses.

Because a visual representation conveys the facts better than abstract formulae, the force relationships are made clearer by means of diagrams:

Case 1 – Pressure and tension strains on the intact olecranon due to the effect of the triceps (Fig 79)
Loading of the ulna and olecranon due to the contraction of the triceps can only occur if the forearm is stretched against resistance or is held elevated above the head. In that way the weight G is registered upwards. Only in isometric contraction of the triceps against gravity does a turning moment directed dorsally along the whole length of the ulna develop, which has its maximum in the line of intersection S. With the so-called flexion line pulling tensile can be seen to develop on the whole dorsal side of the ulna, i.e., from the olecranon almost to the wrist (the exact limit lies in the center of gravity line of the forearm). They are united with pressure strains of the same extent on the ventral side which likewise have their maximum levels on the line of intersection S.

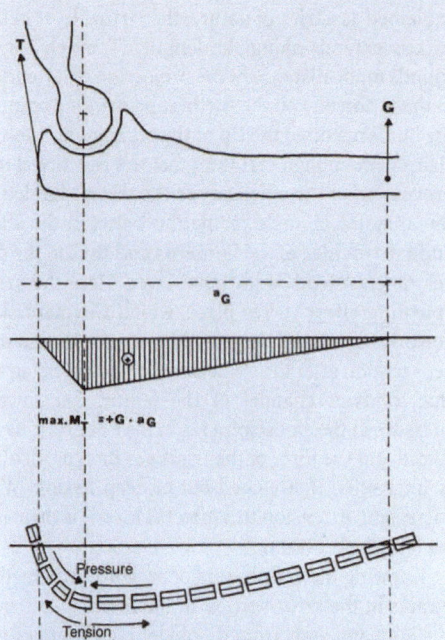

Fig. 79. Case 1 – pressure and tension strains on the intact olecranon due to the effect of the triceps

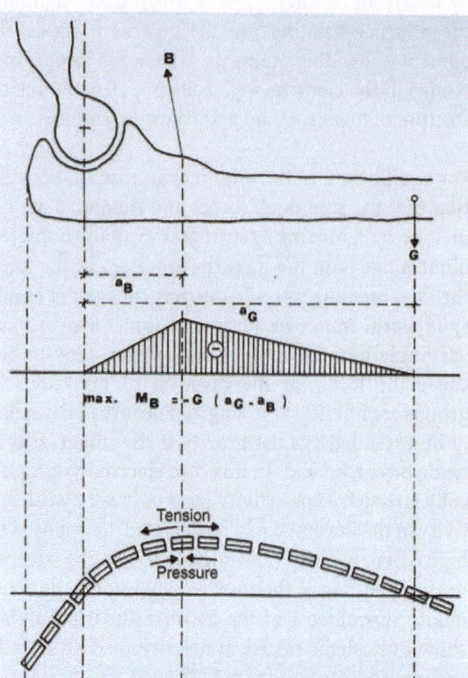

Fig. 80. Case 2 – pressure and tension strains on the intact olecranon due to the effect of the flexor muscles

Case 2 – Pressure and tension strains on the intact olecranon due to the effect of the flexor muscles (Fig. 80)

The diagrammatic representation of planned intersection loading and strain relationships in flexor innovation shows a picture of strain fundamentally different from case 1. An opposing turning moment arises with its maximum over the flexor insertion which, proximally to the line of intersection S, i.e., in the olecranon, is no longer effective at all. It is, compared with that of the triceps, somewhat smaller – understandably so, because the lever of the flexors is longer, which is why its work can remain smaller. From this pressure strains result on the *dorsal* side of the ulna with concomitant traction strains on its *ventral* side – but with the fundamental difference that the olecranon stays completely strain neutral during flexor activity: it exhibits neither pressure nor traction strain, as can be deduced from the flexion line running straight from S. Consequently fractures lying distally to this line should be counted among proximal intra-articular fractures of the ulna shaft. Since anatomical (and biomechanical) demar-

cations are not adhered to in clinical practice, it is to be doubted, cf. [86], that it will gain acceptance. It must be clear, however, that every eccentric tension banding on a so-called distal olecranon fracture *intensifies* the crevice-forming forces developing on flexion in this region. The crevice becomes larger, the danger of dislocation grows; the results of just these C and D type fractures are particularly poor. Consequently conventional wire tension banding is rejected here [86, 137, 242, 284, 306].

Extensor side tension banding theoretically opposes the pull of the triceps, namely when it is introduced isometrically; it is however not in the position of compressing the *whole* fracture. Here, one should refer to the *technical* definition of tension band, which postulates that pre-tensioning forces, applied to securely anchored strain-resistant elements, should generate such high *static* pressure forces in the *whole* element (i.e., over the whole cross-sectional area of the fracture) that all traction forces that might be expected later are neutralized by that alone [387]; see Chap. 4.4. The gaping near the joint, desired for AO tension desired for AO tension banding [38, 266, 408], can only be canceled out during the phase of *isometric* triceps activity and produces short-term simultaneous compression [196, 198]. In the after-care of osteosynthesis however weight-bearing is not advisable because it would lead to destruction. Every *straining* physiotherapeutic exercise is therefore ruled out as a possible form of post-operative treatment for tension bandings as for every other osteosynthesis.

For Weber, radiologically visible gaping of the fracture crevice near the joint is an indication of particularly strong closure of the fracture. Actually this crevice is merely a measure of the eccentricity. Forces being applied from beyond the middle of the cross-section produce traction strains on the opposite edge – cf. Fig. 46 – which lead to the crevice formation. This becomes proportionally larger with increasing eccentricity and pre-tensioning of the tension band wire. The phenomenon is known from plate osteosynthesis – see Fig. 44.

In 1974 in order to learn about the distribution of the forces generated by the tension band in the fracture gap, and in order to recognize how muscle force changes them, interfragmentary pressure forces were measured on an anatomically correctly shaped ulna made of high density polyethylene with two piezoelectric pressure sensors [198]. The electrical

Table 3. "Isometrically" measured interfragmentary pressure after eccentric and after bilateral wire tension banding on a plastic olecranon fracture

AO wire tension banding		With triceps reflex (N)					
Stress (N) in fracture gap	At rest (extended position)	10	20	30	40	50	80
Extensor side	93	78	65	53	42	35	20
Near joint	0	7	15	27	44	58	102
Bilateral wire tension banding							
Extensor side	116	111	100	90	75	65	39
Near joint	98	110	130	140	155	170	215

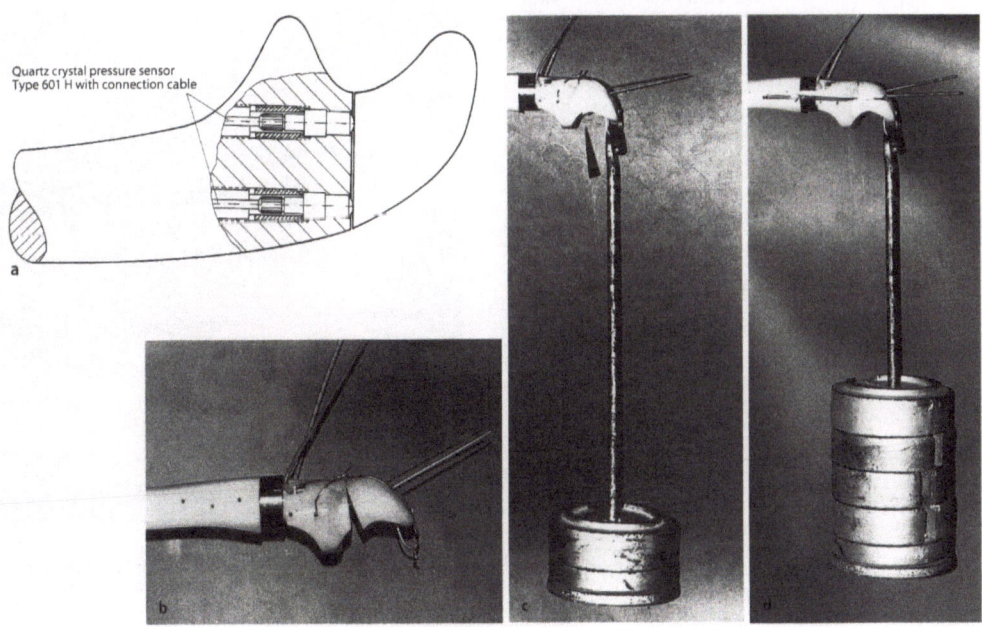

Quartz crystal pressure sensor Type 601 H with connection cable

Fig. 81. Comparison of stability of AO tension banding with bilateral wire tension banding: **a** arrangement of the pressure sensors; **b** the turning moment is particularly clear using thin Kirschner wires (∅ 1.6 mm); **c** step formation due to a transverse force of only 20 N; **d** bilateral wire tension banding: stability despite 50 N strain

charges that were generated by them in proportion to force were converted through amplifiers into voltages and indicated on two analogue measuring instruments. In the fracture region of the olecranon model one of the measuring sensors was introduced ventrally near the joint, the other dorsally on the extensor side. With this positioning it was possible to measure simultaneously the strains produced by the tension bands at rest and during isometric triceps simulation. Some of the characteristic results comparing eccentric with bilateral tension banding can be seen in Table 3 and are illustrated with some photographs of the experiment (Fig. 81).

It can be stated that:

1. *Eccentric* tension banding produces on the extensor side slight pressure and pulls the fracture apart near the joint. A step develops and the joint surfaces become incongruous (Fig 82).
2. Transverse and flexion forces are poorly absorbed.
3. *Isometric* triceps activity reduces pressure on the extensor-side (until distraction occurs) and increases pressure ventrally. Isotonic triceps activity, with the mere function of creating movement, doesn't alter the basic tension of the banding, and the fracture crevice gapes.
4. *Bilateral* tension banding, particularly when wire cables are used, is optimal, as far as production and distribution of pressure, the degree of interfragmentary compression, and the neutralization of transverse forces and bending moments is concerned.

From the experiments it may be concluded that the results of conventional tension bandings for olecranon fractures (and others) cannot exceed a certain level. The more force and the more eccentrically introduced by means of wire tension banding, the greater are its biomechanical disadvantages. This applies particularly to wire cables which are therefore contraindicated for eccentric tension bandings. Anyone who uses them must also decide in favor of static tension banding!

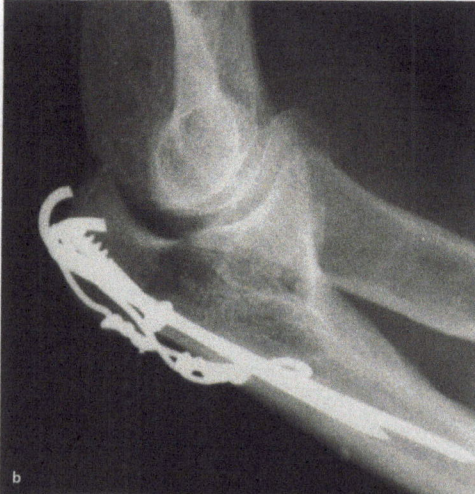

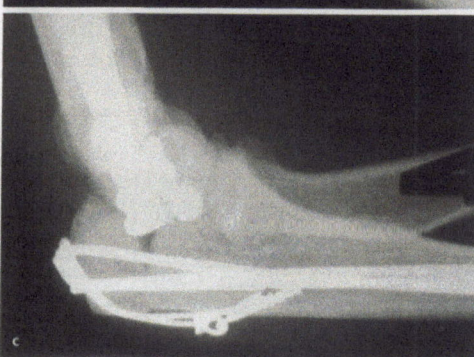

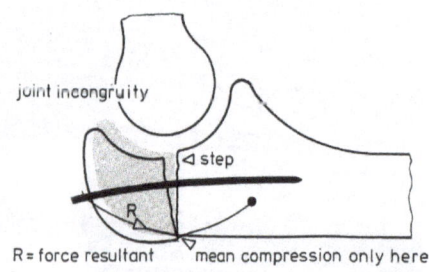

Fig. 82. Biomechanical effects of eccentric tension banding at rest, provided infact that strain is exerted over the cerclage wire: gap, step, joint incongruity and possible complete distraction

4.6.3
Bilateral Cable Tension Band for Olecranon and Proximal Ulna Fractures

Bilateral cable tension banding is a static procedure that was conceived in 1974 [197]. It applies undiluted technical principles from construction engineering to bone healing. This is achieved through the directed introduction of forces into the fracture using bilateral pre-tensioning. The tension forces to be expected from moving muscle force become overstressed and thus ineffective. In 1977, Schmelzeisen

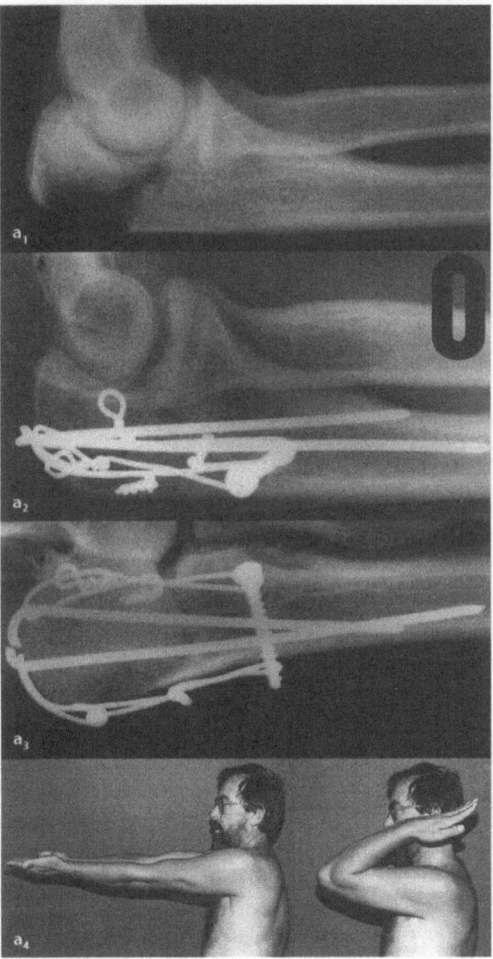

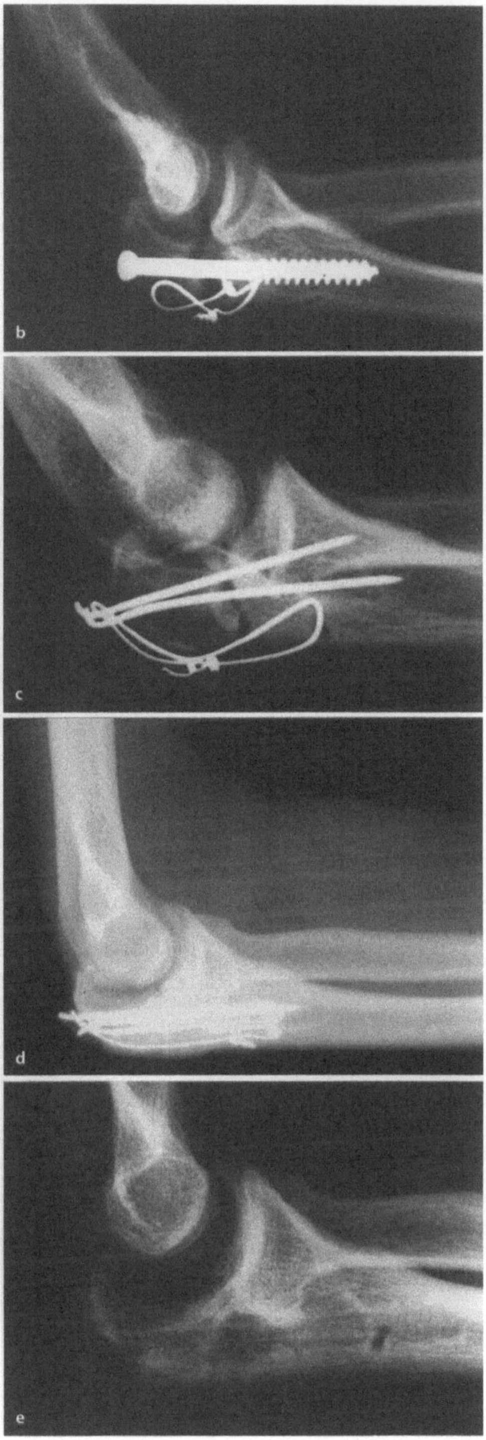

Fig. 83. Wire forerunner of bilateral cable tension banding (1976). **a** Fresh fracture. **b–e** Non-union after two conventional wire tension bendings, healing with the new technique without any problems

[343] recognized that "its principle, seen statically in accordance with interfragmentary compression, is plausible." Rüter and Burri [330] and Burri et al. [40] on the other hand unanimously asserted: "The double-sided technique proposed by Labitzke does not fulfill the principle of tension banding. It admittedly produces a more solid fixation but true advantages compared with the traditional technique are not verifiable in practice." This assertion is both biomechanically and clinically incorrect: 31 olecranon fractures, amongst which were 4 non-unions and 3 secondarily dislocated osteotomies following conventional tension banding (23%), healed without a problem using bilateral wire tension banding [205]. As an example, a professor in mechanical engineering had by chance read about this procedure in a popular scientific newspaper and naturally understood it straight away. When he himself sustained an olecranon fracture he remembered it and traveled to our clinic for the operation. Here is the series of his X-rays as well as a clear example of the healing of a twice operated non-union (Fig. 83).

Principle of Operation

Two lateral cable tension bands are stretched between the two intra-medullary Kirschner wires laid parallel in the center of the ulna and a foundation screw passing transversely through the ulna shaft. They produce high static compression over the entire fracture area. Limited by the anatomy they lie more often than not somewhat to the extensor side, which is still perfectly acceptable as regards absorbing forces. Traction forces of the triceps and the flexors (which strain fracture types C and D) are neutralized; harmful shearing and bending forces or turning moments do not arise (Fig. 84). Therefore reconstructed joint anatomy is protected from secondary shifting. Additional screws may be helpful for oblique fractures.

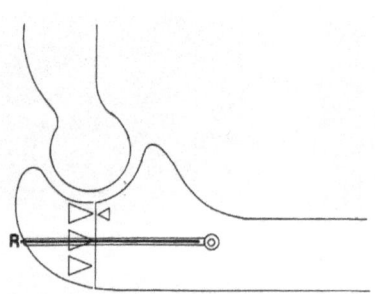

a   R = force resultant

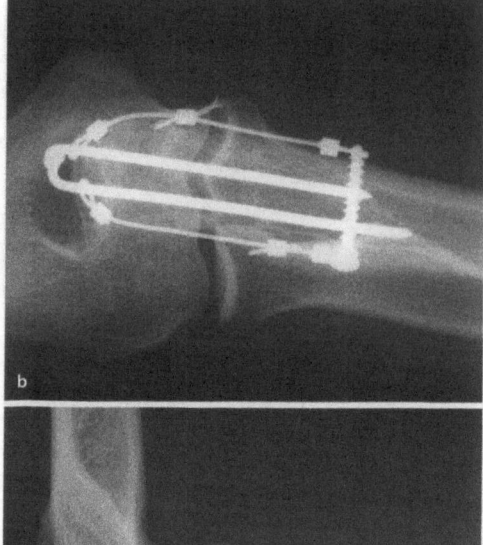

Fig. 84. Principle of operation

Advantages and Disadvantages

+ Immediately and permanently effective cable tensioning needs no additional introduction of "dynamic" forces in order to compress the fracture.

+ Exercise can usually be taken immediately without the risk of dislocation.

+ In case one of the cables should loosen there is still the other to provide enough stability for undisturbed healing.

+ The degree of difficulty of the operation is not increased by the additional insertion of a foundation screw and the double tension banding; the incision is not extended.

+ Metal removal is no more involved than in Weber's tension banding. Provided that one does not wish to re-open the whole scar, it can be performed via three small incisions: the cable is cut next to the head and thread passage of the foundation screw so that both distal loops and the screw can be removed effortlessly. The Kirschner wires with the rest of the cables are accessible over the tip of the olecranon. Withdrawing the cable together with the crimp is not traumatic.

− Disadvantages were not observed

Indications and Contraindications

• Olecranon fractures in accordance with the anatomical-biomechanical definition – cf. Fig. 84.

• Oblique fractures, distal pseudo-olecranon fractures of types C and D, i.e., intra- and extra-articular proximal fractures of the ulna shaft, occurring in isolation or together with Monteggia's injury. They can be well combined with Kirschner wires, screws, or a short neutralization plate.

+ Re-interventions in delayed healing and pseudarthroses after previous operation.

• Olecranon osteotomy in ventral position in order to improve insight into distal intraarticular humerus fractures (Fig 85, 86).

− Minimally dislocated tip fragments and intra-periostal stable fractures with preserved extensor function.

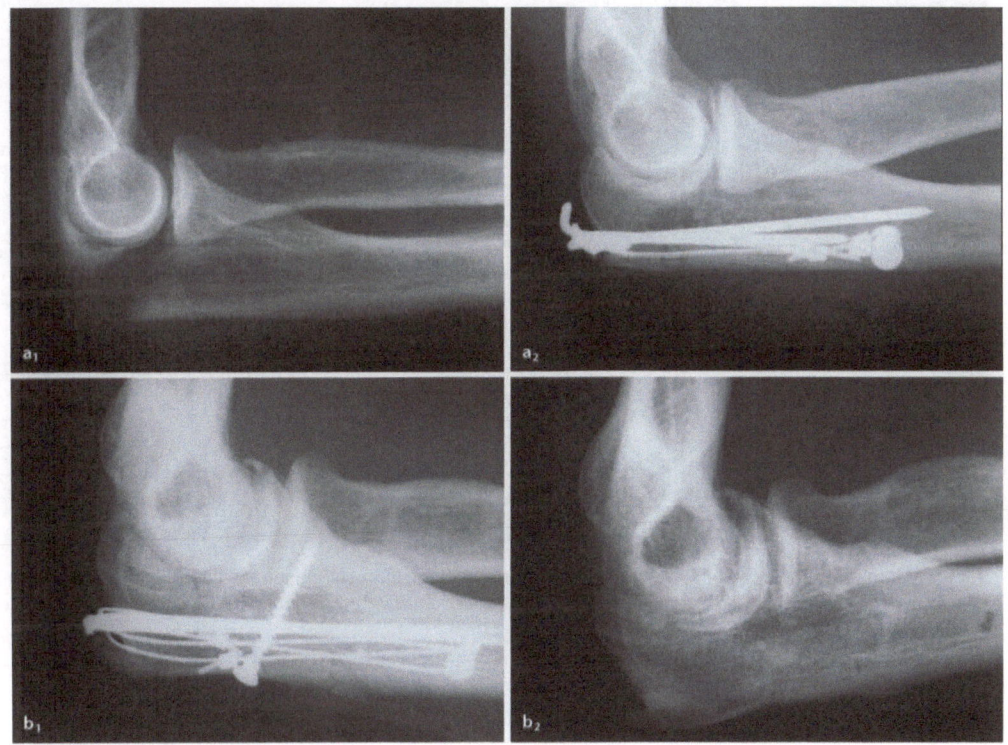

Fig. 85a – c. Indications: **a** simple transverse fracture extending into the distal half of the joint; **b,c** combined transverse, oblique and comminuted fractures extending into the proximal region of the shaft (proximal ulna fracture)

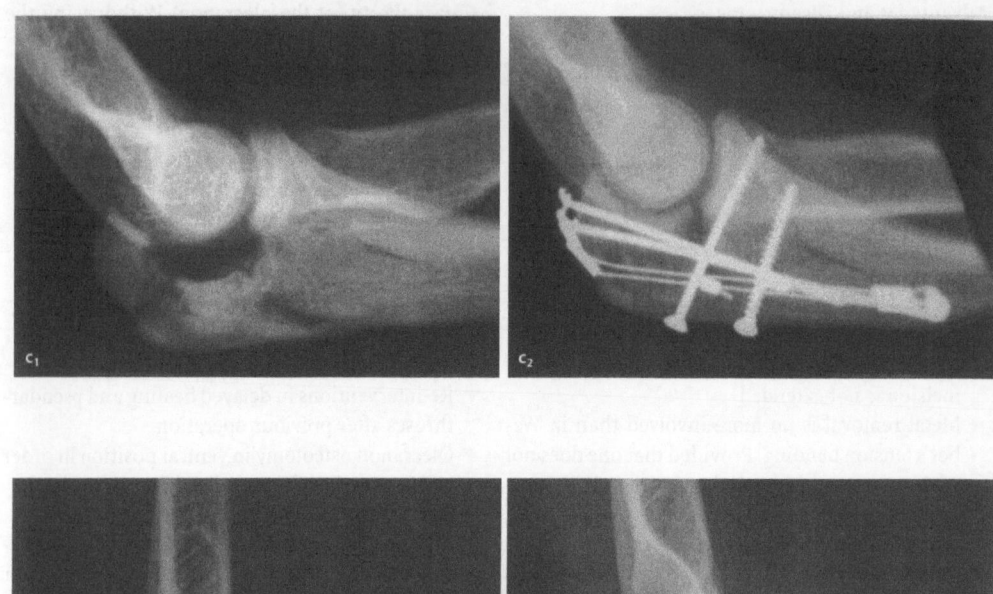

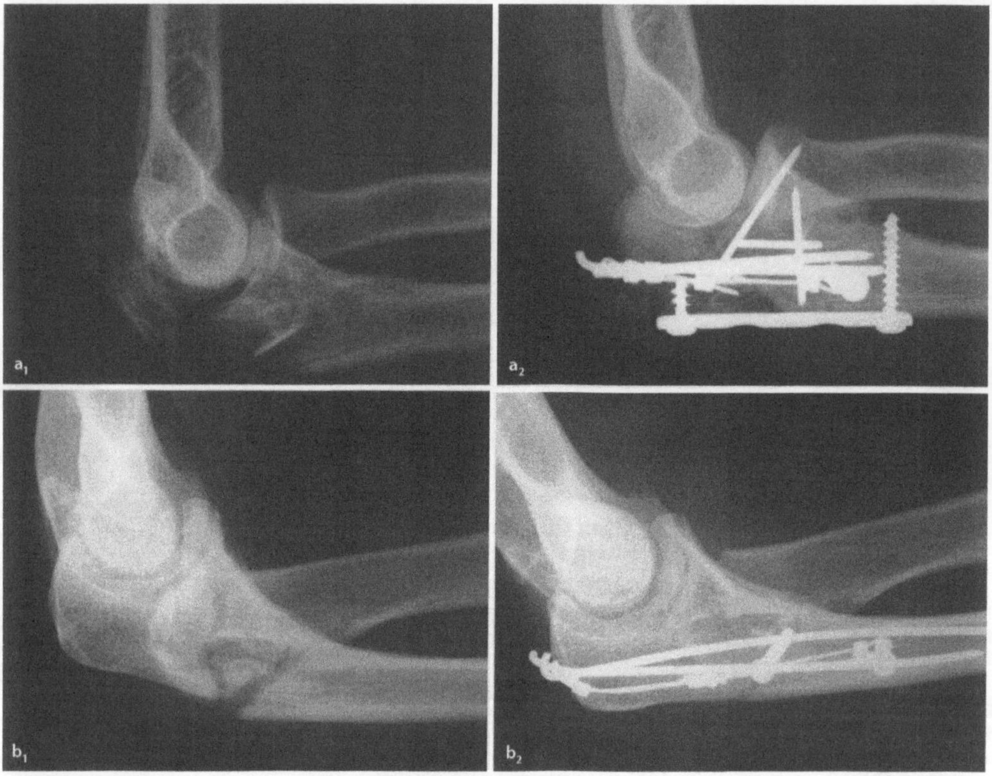

Fig. 86. Indications: **a** combined intra- extra-articular comminuted fracture of olecranon and ulna. Bilateral tension banding, K-wires and neutralisation plate; **b** proximal extra-articular ulna fracture, comminuted fracture of the head of the radius (Monteggia's injury)

Positioning
- Supine
- Surgeon and first assistant stand homolaterally, the second assistant holding the wrapped arm across the thorax stands on the opposite side

Instruments
- In addition to the special cable instruments on the table there should be an electric drill, drill sleeves, Kirschner wires (2.0-mm), cable scissors, curved pins, pointed and flat pliers or curved Zimmer forceps, small Hohmann retractors, two small pointed repositioning forceps, raspatories, and small fragment instruments.

Operation Technique
- Generous transverse incision above the fracture or dorso-radial access according to Boyd. It begins 2–3 fingerbreadths above the joint, goes around it radially, and ends a few centimeters further on distally directly next to the edge of the ulna. After separation of the skin and blood-rich subcutaneous tissue there is generally a clear view into the internal joint because the olecranon, attached to the triceps, is pulled upwards.
- The joint becomes even more visible with incision of the radial joint capsule directly next to the triceps tendon. The trochlea of the humerus lies free; the joint can be lavaged and cleaned of splinters. The olecranon is repositioned in the extension position and held with one or two pointed repositioning forceps. Visual control of the joint surface from the radial side (Fig. 87).

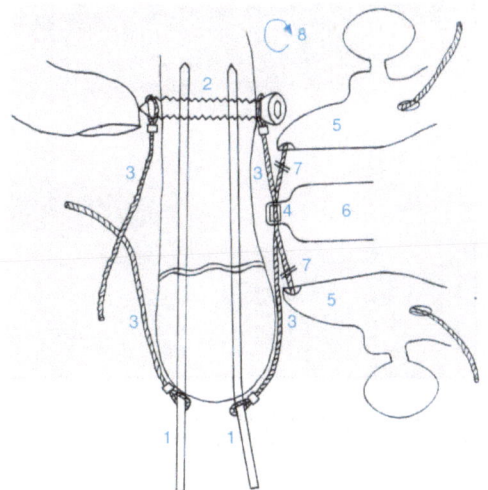

Fig. 87. Operation technique

- The triceps reflector is incised with a pointed scalpel directly at the olecranon, two 2 mm Kirschner wires (1) are guided through it and drilled in as parallel as possible through the fracture into the ulna shaft. The wires should touch the center of the ulna or lie very slightly on the extensor side.
- With the straight awl each of the cables (3) hooked respectively over a Kirschner wire, is guided laterally beneath the triceps and, without interposing soft tissue, directly along the lateral bony surfaces of the ulna. If the awl does not go through the tendon tissue easily it can be held on the compact shaft with flat pliers.
- Now the muscles are pushed away from the posterior edge of the ulna towards each side as far as the middle of the bone. A small cortical screw (2) is inserted through the loop of a ready-made cable (3) and then 3 cm distally to the fracture transversely through the ulna. It has to be 1–2 thread twists longer than the measured width of the ulna so that it can grasp the cable on the opposite side.
- With the index finger the loop of another cable (3) is now held above the screw just perforating the opposite cortical layer so that its threads can be directly screwed into the loop. This technique is simpler than manipulating the loop from behind over the protruding thread.
- Both cable ends, running in opposite directions, are now placed through a crimp (4) and fixed in the cable tensioner (5). The apparatus is drawn far enough away from the upper surface of the bone so that the crimp pliers (6) can grasp the crimp effortlessly and correctly in its jaws. On the ulna side of the joint the ulna is usually concave so that the crimp can be squeezed in the free space.
- Both pairs of cables are tightened one after the other until each Kirschner wire is bent over by approximately 10 °.
- Now the crimp pliers are quickly and firmly pressed together for 1–2 s until there is contact between the force limiting knobs, so that the crimp can shape itself.
- Finally the cable tensioner is loosened. The excess wire cable (7) is cut off, the Kirschner wires are shortened, bent inwards, and finished off. By tightening the foundation screw (8) additional tension is achieved on the side of the head – cf. Fig. 35.
- Closure of the muscle fascia, strain free atraumatic, cutaneous and subcutaneous suturing, neutralizing clip plaster or Medi-Zip wound closure.

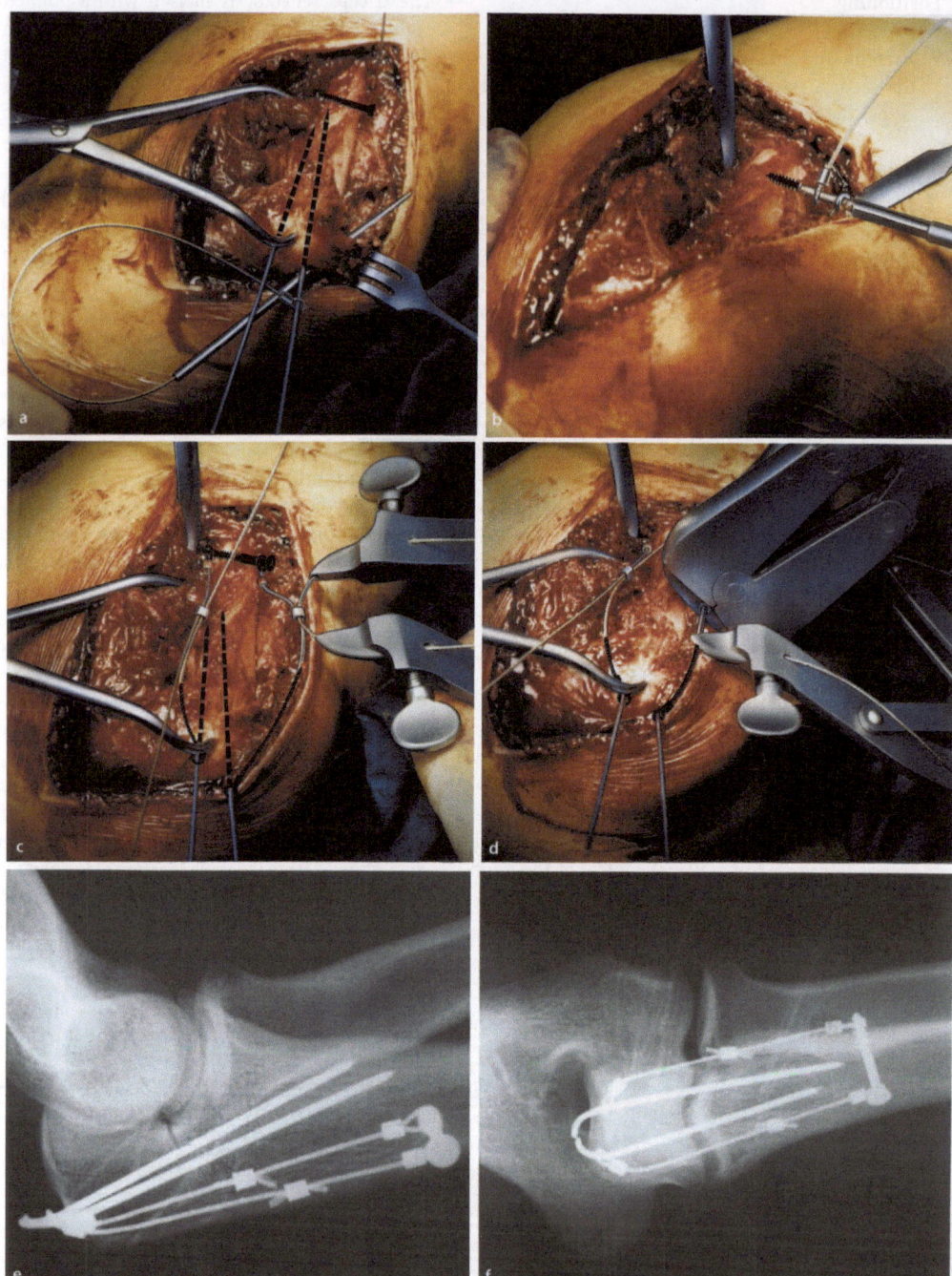

Fig. 88. Course of the operation and X-ray results. Kirschner wires and cables were introduced divergently intentionally for this series in order to avoid disruptive overlapping. (The operation photographs have been taken provided by Mr. Leibinger, by kind permission of Aesculap AG Tuttlingen.)

Steel wool compression bandaging. For comminuted fractures with severe soft tissue damage, temporary dorsal synthetic splints (Fig. 88).

Operative Peculiarities and Variations

- In order to obtain a good overall view of the olecranon joint surfaces and to be able to control repositioning visually and palpably, the radial capsule incision is recommended.
- As in the patella, a cable positioned slightly on the extensor side which just reaches the central cross-sectional area is biomechanically sound. This is almost always achieved because of the triangular form of the ulna – cf. Fig. 84.
- Before an olecranon osteotomy, the Kirschner wires are pre-drilled. That makes refixation without a step easier at the end.

Complications, Mistakes, and Dangers

- It is biologically and mechanically wrong to stretch cables hooked on the Kirschner wires *over* the triceps tendon. That would not be a strong foundation and would cause disturbance to blood flow and loss of tension.
- Squeezing the crimp should always take place in the free space above a bony concavity so that high compression develops – cf. Fig. 32.
- On no account is a cable drawn through a bore canal, as practiced following the old method; it would cut in immediately and tension would be lost. The foundation screw is essential!
- The Kirschner wires should be 2 mm thick; thinner ones are too weak for cable tensioning and for the absorbing transverse forces. – cf. Fig. 81 b.
- Parallel Kirschner wires, placed widely apart, allow the olecranon to slide as if on a runner and are stable to rotation; crossed Kirschner wires block and wrench the fragments.
- Tight bandages lead to constriction and pain, forced passive movements provoke swelling, compartment syndrome, dislocation and peri-articular ossification.

Post-operative Treatment

- Almost always free of plaster; arm sling, swelling reduction measures.
- From day two, independently organized movement exercises along physiotherapy guidelines for the elbow and shoulder joint. If available, electric movement splint.
- In cases of dubious stability, open upper arm plaster, the arm to be exercised out of it.

Results

Up to the end of 1995, 81 olecranon fractures were treated with lateral cable tension banding. In 18 cases a temporary plaster was applied for 2–4 weeks. The average age was 52 (16–88 years of age), with a slight predominance of women; 73 fractures were closed, 8 open of which three were second and third grade. There were 33 transverse and oblique fractures (including 3 cases of polytrauma), 48 multifragment and comminuted fractures. In nine cases the situation was complicated due to concomitant fractures near the elbow: three cases involved the distal humerus, five the proximal radius, one was a war injury with shot wound and stiffening. Apart from that, three Monteggia injuries were treated. These 12 and a further 7 cases, about which no adequate information could be gathered, are not considered.

The X-ray series and completed outpatient notes of 62 cases were evaluated. The end result and function were noted. A very few incomplete case notes were completed after further follow-up investigations. All 62 fractures had complete osseous reconstruction, and no non-union developed. Three cases of a cable loosening on one side healed without further ado, the tension of the opposite side stabilizing the fracture adequately enough. The comminuted fracture of a 56-year-old woman had to be re-operated on due to complete distraction. One deep and four superficial secondary healings were noted; fully healed (Fig. 89).

> ▶ Of the 62 cases, 54 (87%) were rated as very good (free function, unremarkable X-rays, no pain) and good (final degree of movement limitation up to ≦10 ° and/or minimal deviation on X-ray, hardly any complaints), 8 (13%) as satisfactory (extension and/or flexion deficits ≧10–20 ° and/or slight arthrotic signs on X-ray with complaints). There were no poor results with greater deficits and/or more advanced arthroses.

A comparison with the final results of conventional tension banding turned out to be just as unambiguous for the olecranon as for the patella. However 97% excellent results [429] are not attainable; the good results – although often not quite comprehensible – ranging between 55% and 80%, were surpassed. Loosening of the osteosynthesis with displacement and loss of joint alignment [271], joint steps, non-unions, high and often painful movement deficits are largely avoided with stable cable tension banding.

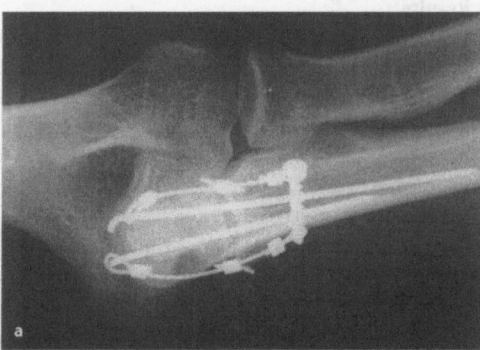

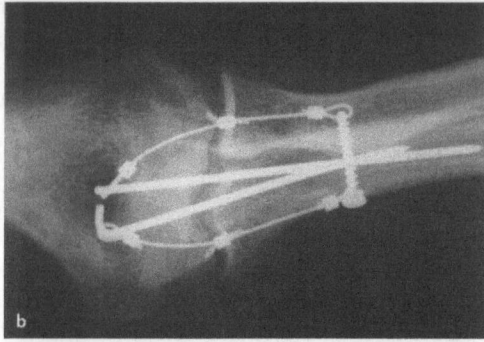

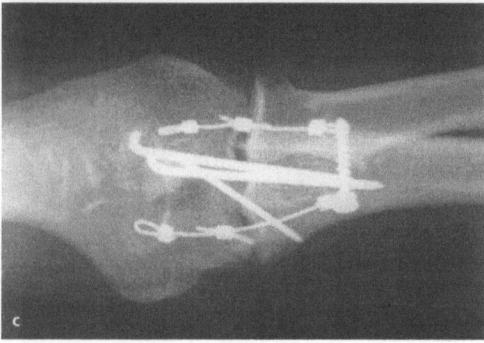

Fig. 89. Cable loosening in three cases

Contemporary Alternatives and Conclusions

Although its biomechanical weaknesses are repeatedly discussed [86, 127, 196, 270, 322, 327], AO tension banding is also the most frequently used method of operation for olecranon fractures. Indeed, how to do it is still discussed 35 years after its inauguration – only passing through tendon insertions, combined with Kirschner wires, screws or Rush pins, figure-of-eight or O-shaped cerclage, stiff, thick or thin more flexible Kirschner wires, one or two twists [138, 153, 270, 284, 327, 330, 339, 429] etc. etc. – but predominantly good results are described.

Frequently the problems of olecranon fractures are underestimated: that can be deduced from the undifferentiating recommendation of completely different treatment techniques.

"Open reduction and internal fixation with tension band, screws, plate and screws, or band and plate can be relied upon for satisfactory end results", so Horne 1981 [136].

"The AO cancellous screw alone and, in severely comminuted cases, in combination with tension band wiring were found to be an excellent fixation device for olecranon fractures" stated Johnson 1986 [155].

"The standardized wire tension band osteosynthesis is easy to learn and permits very early functional post-operative treatment, which is why the indications for dislocated olecranon fractures according to AO classification of types B1, B3 and C1-C3 can be extended" says Jockheck in 1995 [153].

In 1990 Parker et al. [291] thought that the conventionally achieved results with early function "compare favorably with cases treated by operation" – not a particularly good evaluation of surgical methods!

The disadvantages of wire tension banding are not only seen on genuine olecranon fractures but also and particularly on proximal intra- and extra-articular ulna shaft fractures which belong to the olecranon. Here tension banding on the extensor side is *contraindicated* because it intensifies the traction strains of the flexors arising ventrally – cf. Fig. 80. In these cases plates are recommended [86, 184, 242, 306], which are to be used with care because of the sparse and often contusioned soft tissue, and are best indicated in extended proximal ulna fractures.

In 1992 Rowland and Burkhart [327] reconsidered the stability of the traditional tension band in question and published an alternative solution. They tried to improve it using wire cerclage which is placed through the distal ulna shaft, *ventrally* to a Rush pin (which is inserted instead of Kirschner wires). This method was to reduce gaping. The non-biological method of driving a thick pin through the olecranon and medullary cavity (which is technically difficult where there are smaller fragments) can hardly have found supporters. It is rejected by engineers on account of mechanical considerations: "The technique should not be used" Roe [322] claimed in a reply.

Helm et al. [127] summarized their experiences with conventional wire tension banding in a statement which is irrefutable: "The technical quality of the fixation was open to criticism in half the cases."

Medullary cavity screws, thread pins, and Rush pins are probably only used in exceptions. They loosen with plaster-free post-operative treatment.

The plate can be indicated simply in intra-extra-articular fracture combinations. For us it is the only conceivable alternative (or a rare additional measure) to the bilateral cable tension banding for extended comminuted fractures.

▶ It may be concluded that for olecranon and proximal ulna fractures near the joint, on bio-mechanical grounds there are (almost) no alternatives to bilateral cable tension banding. It produces – even in proximal shaft fractures! – elastic interfragmentary compression according to construction engineering rules over the whole region and does not disturb blood flow. Low risk post-operative treatment with free joint mobility is the rule.

4.7
Ankle Joint and Pilon Fractures

"The orthopedic specialist is confronted almost daily with poor results from conventionally or surgically treated malleolar fractures. He becomes aware of how meticulously exact treatment of these injuries must be, so that later on they do not develop into a painful post-traumatic arthrosis deformans" wrote M. E. Müller in 1966 in his foreword to Weber's monograph [409].

At the time of L. Böhler [20] most fractured ankles were still conventionally treated: "With common ankle fractures there is almost always success when setting them under good anesthesia followed by holding the fractured pieces in the right position with an unpadded plaster cast. Surgical re-alignment and fixation of the re-set bone with screws or wires is superfluous."

Jahna et al. [147] also reported good results, though Nonnemann and Plösch [280] had previously listed 8% non-unions as well as many anatomical defects. The transition from non-surgical retention in plaster to surgical intervention was introduced with the wire extension method which is associated with the names Kirschner and Klapp [166, 170]. In 1875, v. Volkmann refixed a ventral heel fragment by suturing; systematic surgical intervention began with Lane and Lambotte. In 1948 Danis was the first to operate on fibular as well as tibial lesion (quoted from [409]). With the AO Group came the navicular screw for the medial malleolus; Weber introduced tension banding. It was performed with a cerclage wire that was threaded between Kirschner wires and a sagitally drilled canal through the tibia. Later instead of the bore canal Brunner and Weber [33] indicated anchorage with screws, which is essential for effective wire tension.

In our own trauma surgery unit ankle fractures are amongst the "most frequent types of bone fractures" [249]. They are present in all degrees of severity from a simple avulsion of the lateral malleolus, Weber type A, to tri-malleolar dislocation fractures extending into a tibial pilon fracture. With few exceptions they are operated on because, for pain free function, the anatomically correct realignment of the weight-bearing column of the shinbone and the mortise recess of the ankle joint is of vital importance. For biological osteosynthesis of this muscle-free, easily infected region, sound minimal intervention by means of cable tension banding is more physiological than screws or plates [9, 274, 355], which for years we have only used on the tibia in exceptional circumstances.

In the region of the ankle, the medial malleolus is the obvious site for tension banding. For this reason fractures in this area shall serve as an example of how to carry out tension banding. But even extreme distal tibial breaks, with spurs into the joint for which interlocking nails are only partially suitable, and large pilon fragments can be positioned correctly, and cable tension can be applied. Lateral malleolar fractures are, on the other hand, regularly plated or screwed; tension banding is suitable for Weber type A avulsion fractures or for special cases. The posterior Volkmann triangle is usually screwed from the front. Here tension banding does not achieve its goal.

4.7.1

Cable Tension Banding on the Medial Malleolus

The medial malleolus is only occasionally involved in fractures of the ankle joint because it is predominantly the supination trauma in which the lateral malleolus and syndesmosis are the main victims. Isolated medial malleolus fractures are seen as the result of an eversion-pronation impulse; frequently in the presence of bi- or tri-malleolar (dislocation) fractures it fractures as well. In our clinic it is always treated using cable tension banding. It is effective and compact.

Principle of Operation

> Osteosynthesis is achieved with a tension cable running between two Kirschner wires screwed through the break surface and a proximally placed foundation screw (Fig. 90).

Note the exact course of the wire, the crimp placed in the concave area, and the bowing of the Kirschner wires and the foundation screws as indicators of high interfragmentary compression. A slightly upward sloping foundation screw is best because it raises interfragmentary compression on tightening. The attendant tibial fracture is stabilized biologically with an EndoHelix [218].

Advantages and Disadvantages

✚ A small skin incision is enough; little extraneous material is required.

✚ Very sound osteosynthesis which counters the pull of the deltoid ligament with a highly compensating flexible device. Using this method, treatment is without plaster and allows early partial weight bearing.

✚ The risks of cerclage wire and screw osteosynthesis, such as loosening, shifting of fragments, and calcification are largely avoided.

━ No disadvantages observed

Indications and Contraindications

✚ Dislocated medial malleolus fractures, isolated and combined with injury of the ankle joint. Small fragments – even the Tubercle de Chaput – are better held with tension banding than with a screw. An additional chisel component is screwed transversely [22].
Medial malleolus osteotomy to expose the talus.

✚ Medial malleolus non-union

✚ On the lateral malleolus: bony ligament tears and Weber type A avulsion fractures. Wire cerclages [249] are obsolete (Fig. 91).

✚ Corrective osteotomy after wrong positioning.

━ Isolated chisel fractures with vertical fracture faces.

━ Non-displaced isolated fractures especially in children and the elderly.

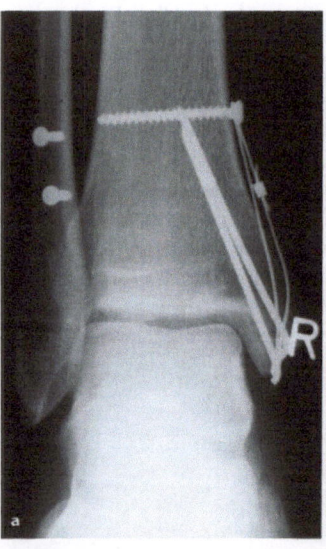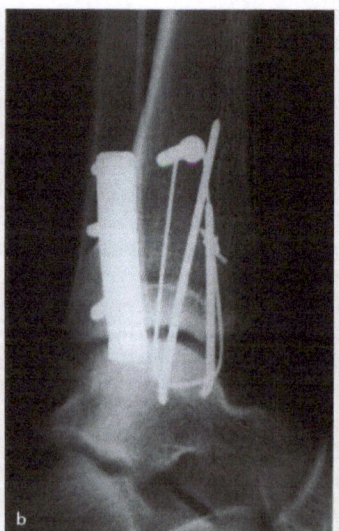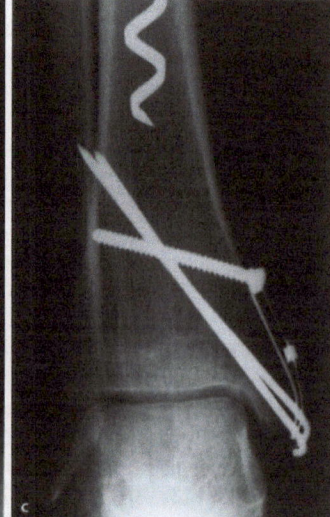

Fig. 90. Principle of operation. Compared with **a, c** shows the more favourable position of the foundation screw – cf. Fig. 38

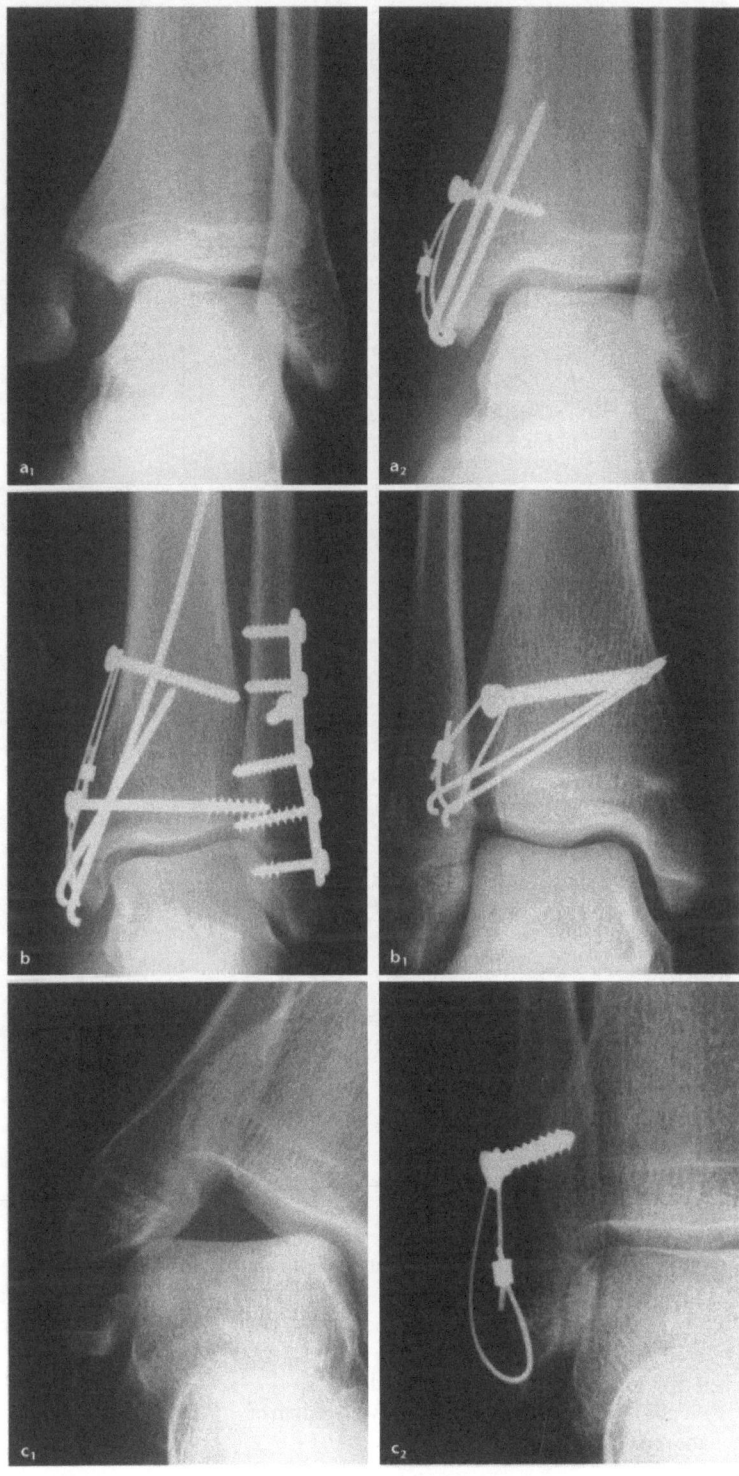

Fig. 91a–e. Indications **a** Isolated inner ankle fracture. **b** The vertical component of the inner ankle fracture is stabilized with an additional horizontal screw. b_1 Bony avulsion of syndesmosis. **c** Bony external ligament ruptur

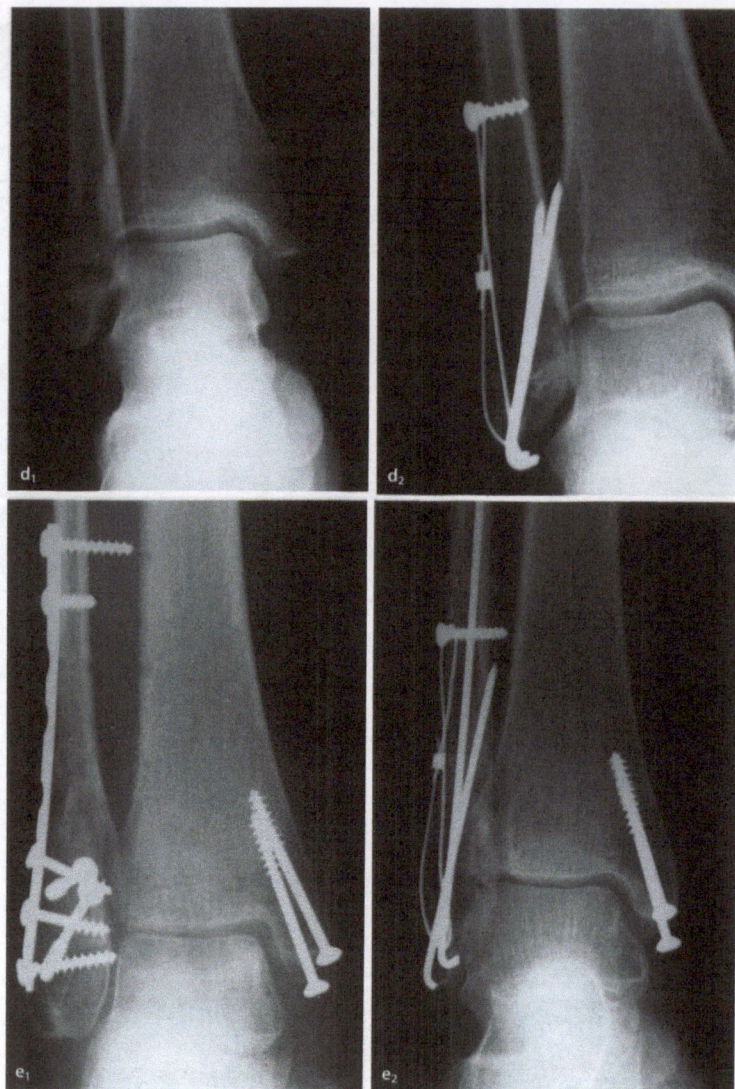

Fig. 91.d Weber A fracture.
e Corrective osteotomy of a non-union in rotational malposition after Weber A fracture

Positioning

- Thermal mat, supine position, right and left side supports.
- Cover to beneath the knee. The forefoot is covered with a rubber glove fixed with a tape.
- Foam rolls under the knee and ankle.
- Gentle lowering of the other leg allows freedom of movement for the surgeon.

Instruments

- In addition to the special cable instruments there should be on the table an electric drill, drill sleeves, 2.0 mm Kirschner wires, side cutters, curved pins, curved Zimmer forceps or pointed and flat forceps, and two small pairs of pointed repositioning forceps.

Operation Technique

- In bi- and tri-malleolar fractures first deal with the lateral malleolus and the syndesmosis by means of longitudinal incision running diagonally. Anatomical position is maintained using a small plate or tension screws, exceptionally also using cable tension banding. Access to the inner side of the joint varies with each injury. A clean break of the medial malleolus is exposed using a short oblique longitudinal incision which runs from above the fracture to the level of the deltoid ligament. If, in addition, a posterior Volkmann triangle requiring treatment is present, the incision is extended upwards to the posterior edge of the tibia in order to give a better overall view and make repositioning easier. In pilon fractures it may be necessary to make a more anterior incision. Hockey-stick shaped curved incisions are unsuitable as they do not always allow the resulting flaps to heal undisturbed (Fig. 92).

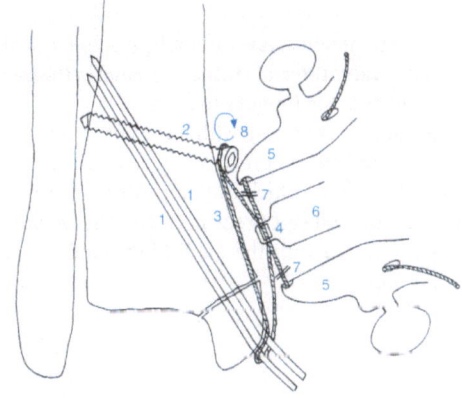

Fig. 92. Operation technique

- Presentation and lavage of the fracture. The inwrapped periosteum is removed and the fracture cleaned.
- Two Kirschner wires (1) running as parallel as possible are positioned and drilled through the malleolus, held in place using one or two pairs of pointed repositioning forceps, so that they are driven through the fracture area transversely and just through the opposite cortical layer of the tibia. In this way they have a better hold.
- At a position 2–3 cm above the fracture a small cortical screw (2) is screwed through the tibia

crosswise or sloping slightly upwards, as a proximal stopper for the cable, until its head just reaches the cortical bone.

- Using the straight or curved awl, a cable approximately 20 cm in length is cut from the roll (3) and threaded through directly between the two Kirschner wires and the head of the medial malleolus *under* the deltoid ligament and positioned in an O-shape around the foundation screw.
- Both cable ends are now put through the crimp in opposite directions and fixed in the tensioner (5).
- The still slack cable is drawn away from the bone under gentle tension, the crimp in the region of the concave tibial mortise recess is grasped with crimp pliers (6) and handed to the assistant. The construction is then tightened by turning the handle of the cable tensioner until the Kirschner wires have been drawn through a good 10 °. That is the visual indication of sufficiently high pretension.
- Now the assistant squeezes together the crimp pliers until contact is made with the force-limiting notches for just 2 s, so that the crimp has time to become distorted.
- The rest is routine. The excess cable is cut off (7) the shortened Kirschner wires are bent inwards so that the cable does not slip.
- The foundation screw (8) is tightened as far as possible so that additional tension is gained.

Operative Peculiarities and Variations

- The foundation screw need not necessarily perforate the cortical bone on the opposite side, a short screw provides sufficient hold for small fragments.
- In multi-fragment fractures with a chisel component the vertical fracture plane is fixed with 1–2 transverse screws.
- Foundation screws screwed slightly upwards provide a double gain in tension which stems from the lengthening and sliding of the cable onto the semi-spherical head of the screw. The slant however holds the danger of the cable slipping if it is turned too steeply upwards. Washers are not needed; they may damage the cable with their sharp edges.
- The Kirschner wires should meet in the middle of the fracture surfaces, lying as parallel as possible and, in order to anchor them particularly firmly, should perforate the opposite cortical layer of the tibia. However this is not essential.

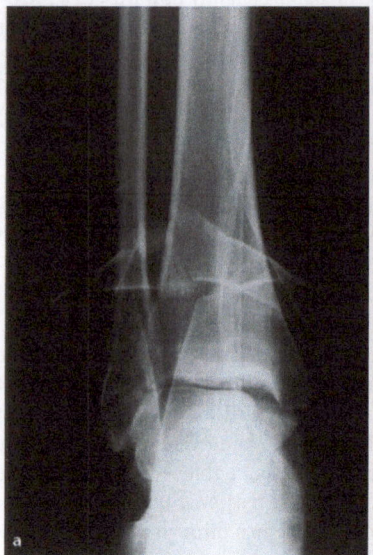
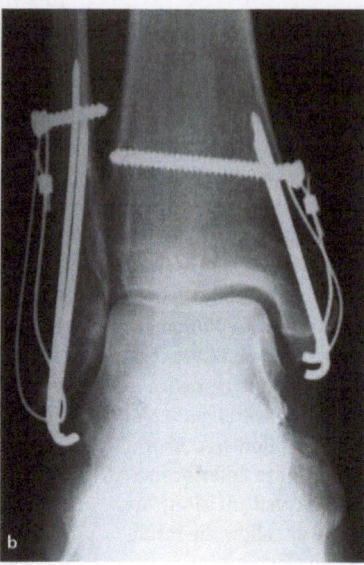

Fig. 93. Atraumatic biological osteosynthesis in a 2nd degree open luxation fracture. Free function, no pain

In this (dislocated) eversion-pronation trauma with syndesmosis rupture and severe soft tissue damage double cable tension banding is used for biological osteosynthesis. No plaster. Mobility without support from the seventh week (Fig. 93).

Complications, Mistakes and Dangers
- The O-formed tension band is best; crossed wires absorb rotation forces poorly.
- In order to maintain high tension, pressure to the crimp is not exerted directly onto the bone, but over its concave upper surface in the free space.

- The foundation screw cannot be dispensed with, since a cable threaded through a canal in the bone would bite into it under tension.
- Atraumatic operating with loose cutaneous-subcutaneous sutures prevents circulatory disorders and infections, which can quickly occur through skin-edge and soft tissue necrosis. The wound is gently closed with the Medi-Zip wound closure (Fig. 94).

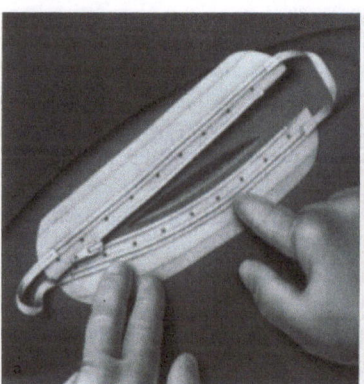
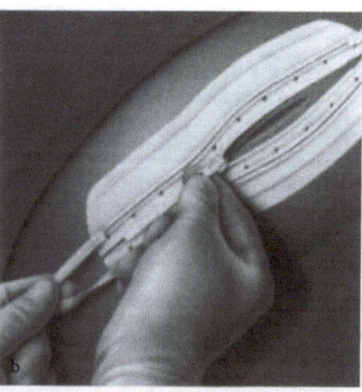

Fig. 94. Atraumatic wound closure with Medi-Zip

Post-Operative Treatment

- Raised position for a few days, immediate electric movement splints, bed exercise-cycle or pedal-roller, compression stockings, no plaster.
- Early partial weight bearing is possible for clean breaks. In compound injuries including the tibial pilon six weeks non-weight-bearing in a support dressing or brace is required for cartilage regeneration.
- Even partial weight-bearing walking benefits circulation, sitting and standing result in swelling due to elevated hydrostatic lymph pressure.

Results

Up to the end of 1995, 294 ankle fractures were treated with cable tension banding. As has been demonstrated on the medial malleolus, its efficiency is to be confirmed by its results.

X-ray series and outpatient clinic notes covering 1992–1994 were evaluated for 50 successively operated isolated medial malleolus and bi-malleolar fractures (in which the lateral malleolus was screwed or plated). Complex injuries treated during that period were not included.

> ▶ All 50 medial malleolar fractures rebuilt strong bones in anatomical positions within a few weeks. Functional losses which result in disability are not noted.

Although in one case a cable loosened, in one tension was no longer distinguishable radiologically, and a third was torn away from the Kirschner wire for unknown reasons, no dislocation, delayed healing, or non-union occurred (Fig. 95). A plaster was only considered necessary in three cases.

After checking the X-rays and outpatient clinic notes of almost all ankle fractures it can be said that the more closely the carefully attained reconstruction is followed up, the more robust the osteosynthesis achieved, with the least material possible, and the earlier post-operative treatment with complete joint flexion is possible, the better the cartilage regenerates ad integrum. Particular stress is to be laid on the exact reconstruction of the syndesmosis, which ensures a correct and stable mortise recess, and thus counteracts subsequent naturally occurring arthrosis [51]. In pilon, bi-, and tri-malleolar dislocation fractures cartilage trauma must not be underestimated. Unfortunately arthroses can also appear here, which however were not necessarily to be expected following the first post-operative X-rays. Two arthrodeses were the result of these complex injuries and are dealt with in Chap. 4.10.1.

Contemporary Alternatives and Conclusions

The most frequently practised osteosyntheses on the medial malleolus are screwing, by means of a navicular or cortical screw and wire tension banding. Both have, as eight different examples demonstrate, mechanical and operative disadvantages (Fig. 96).

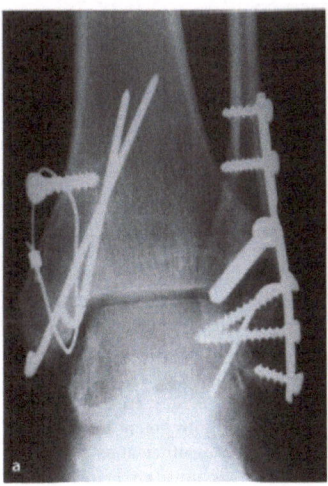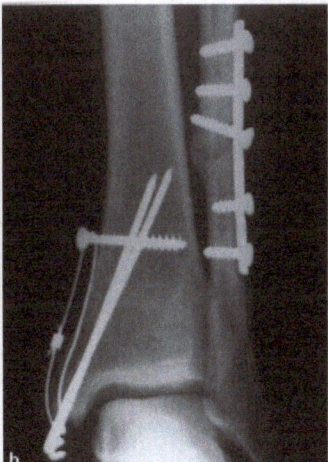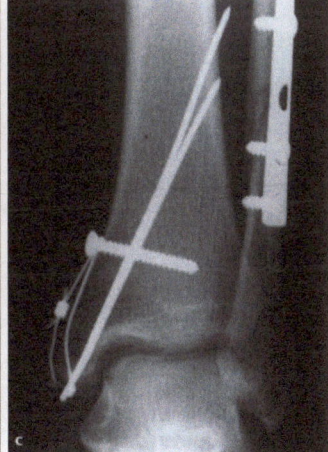

Fig. 95. Healing despite cable loosening, three cases

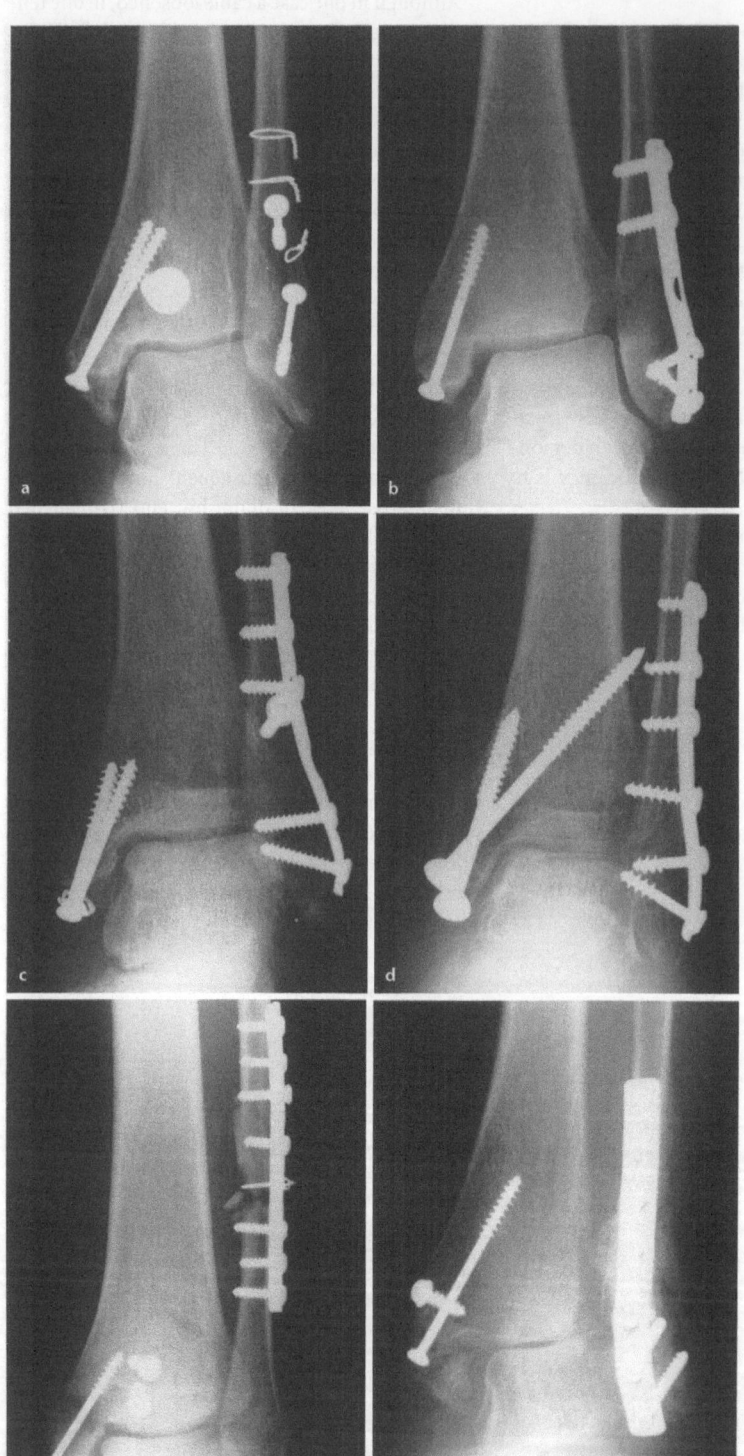

Fig. 96a–h. Disadvantages of screw osteosyntheses. **a, c** Calcification of the inner ankle tip. **b, c** tilting of the inner ankle due to dividing of the screw force into a compression and shearing component. **d** demineralization following the rigidity of two malleolar screws. **e** insufficient minifragment screw. **f** totally insufficient osteosynthesis, inner ankle fragment not fully grasped

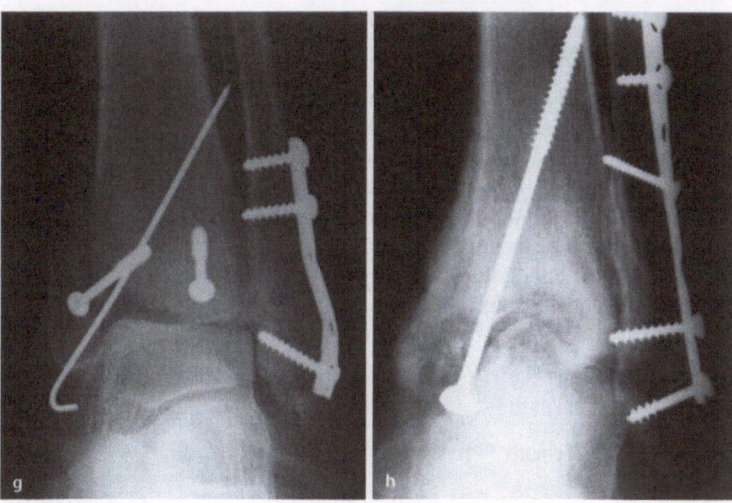

Fig. 96. g, h. Osteosynthesis efforts, two contemporary cases leading to arthrodesis

Cerclage wires, possibly even pulled through a bone canal and not fixed to a screw, permit no tension banding per se in the technical sense. Rush rods, navicular, and other screws [307, 313] are not to be trusted. They are not stable enough for flexion, slipping of fragments, and calcifications occur; for small fragments they are too large-scale. In some cases loosening, dislocation, delayed healing, and non-unions are observed [280]. The stress protection which arises results in demineralization. Introducing screws via point incisions in open fractures [128] is also not advantageous: repositioning cannot be accurately judged. The wound can almost always be included in the modified incision without additional damage.

Frequently osteosyntheses of the upper ankle joint are not correctly performed and the results that arise are not always acceptable to the patients. As an official assessor, the author was confronted with osteosyntheses which showed complete lack of understanding of the biomechanics of the ankle and

a lack of manual skill. Many poor results put down to post-operative trauma are in reality the consequences of unprofessional osteosyntheses. Better results can only be expected if this fact is acknowledged.

▶ Yet in 1999 Schmitz et al. [345] recorded: "Radiological signs of arthrosis of the ankle joint and significant load differences" were discovered from gait analyses in *half of the cases* three years post-operative.

▶ It may be concluded that cable tension banding with Kirschner wires and foundation screws is a very stable method of osteosynthesis for the upper ankle joint, in particular for the medial malleolus. It allows early functional post-operative treatment and leads to very good results. Complications, which are common in conventional procedures occur to a much lesser degree. Biomechanically it is also the method of choice for this region.

4.8
Osseous Prominences

Trochanter major femoris, tuberculum majus, the (epi-) condyli humeri and the base of the fifth metatarsal form extended levers as bony projections for the muscles inserted. As a rule damage to them will result in dislocation. Accordingly, correct anatomical restoration is of functional significance, a fact that is not to be underestimated. Surgery is therefore indicated in most cases.

4.8.1
Trochanter Major Femoris

Significant avulsion to the trochanter has been witnessed since the introduction of hip endoprostheses. Böhler [20] does not mention it, but it is not rare [123, 318] and also not easy to treat. As can be deduced from analyzing various procedures, its osteosynthesis is problematic [6, 49, 259, 335, 350].

Exact anatomical refixing of the trochanter major is demanded because it forms a spatially three-directional lever system for the hip muscles with which to balance the upper torso on the respective leg whilst standing. This is the most complex of its various tasks. The (maximum?) traction of the abductors should be approximately "2200 N in a person of normal weight" [135]. Their force can develop fully using long levers, because muscles work efficiently [366]. The static and dynamic strain on the hip joint which arises from different rotating moments of the body weight and the opposite rotating moments of the equilibrating muscles is minimized through them just as much as the consumption of muscular energy.

The *frontal* distance of trochanter major – the distance from its tip to the middle point of the head of the femur – amounts to approximately 6 cm in a person of 1.80 m in height. Thus a virtual lever of 4–4.5 cm results for the abductors. In 1933, Storck [367] indicated it at 3.5 cm for a person of 1.70 m in height. Using it the abductors, which are almost exclusively active during the standing phase, stabilize the pelvis together with the upper torso on the supporting leg against the rotating moment of the body weight. The center of gravity of this partial body weight is named by Pauwels [293, 296] as S5 and correctly pinpointed. It was calculated under resting

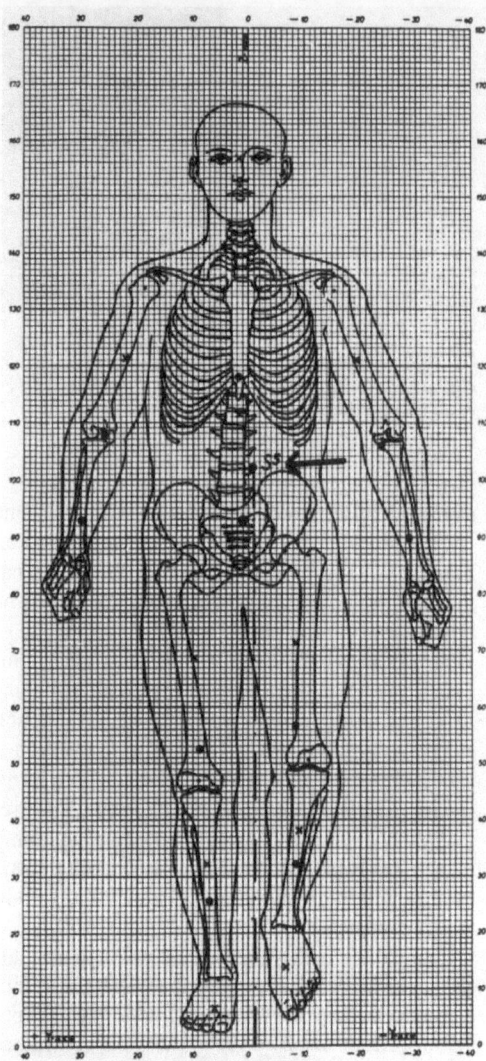

Fig. 97. Pauwels' construction of the partial centre of gravity S5. It forms the basis of his model of hip loading (from [296])

conditions and is only valid for a suspended partial body from which a leg has been removed. It has therefore shifted slightly from the center of the body to the side of the remaining leg, in Pauwels' diagram, therefore, towards the free leg; indeed the supporting leg is ineffective as a partial weight influencing the center of gravity. In his consideration of load on the hip during walking he admittedly left the position of S5 unchanged on the side of the leg in play. That would increase body rotating moments on the supporting hip and thus result in a pointless increase in the work of the abductors. According to Pauwels an "extraordinarily high pressure load" on the hip would arise, comparable with a "hammering" which he by far overestimated at 4.5 times the body weight. Storck, however, calculated the hip load as only twice the body weight which was far more realistic [204]. Nature does not work uneconomically. In addition Pauwels' weighed person, without the support of the balancing leg, would of course immediately tip over to the side. In order to counter this, the partial center of gravity S5 has to be positioned by *lateral movement* of the upper body, naturally to the side of the respective *supporting leg*. The distance of movement is different, depending on whether one is standing or walking. The quicker the successive steps, the closer the center of gravity of the upper body remains to the mid-line, since it has always to be positioned over the corresponding foot, on changing the supporting leg. That is why the projections of the body are different when standing and walking (Fig. 97).

A further error of Pauwels is derived from the first, namely his curve for the position of the center of gravity on walking which had much too wide a distance during a half step (a change of supporting leg) and shows a "jerkiness" which, were it to be correct, would make the human gait resemble that of a wooden puppet. The acceptance of this thesis in secondary literature as acknowledged fact [265] is astounding (Fig. 98).

In order to keep the shift in the center of gravity to the respective supporting leg when walking as low as possible, human femurs (and similarly those of most animal species) show adduction of around 9°, which corresponds in the frontal plane to their "neutral position" [204]. Despite this anatomical adaptation of our skeleton to forces that have to be dealt with, a lot of support work is still necessary which is made easier for the abductors particularly by means of the long frontal trochanter lever.

By means of a *sagittal* lever of approximately 3 cm in length, orientated from the head of the femur dorsally, which arises from the posterior position of the trochanter towards the neck of the femur of 25° and from the ante-torsion of the hip of 12°, the pelvis is stabilized sagittally, especially against dynamic influences in walking and running, whilst the moment

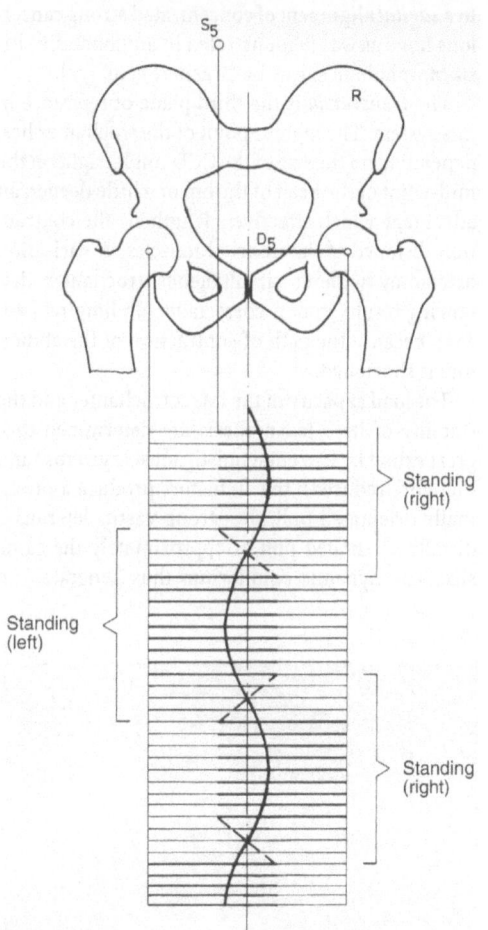

Fig. 98. Pauwels' representation of the shift in the center of gravity during walking (from [296]). The center of gravity always lies, according to him, on the side of the *moving leg* – the person would fall over. The short diagonal connections drawn in show the jerky change of center of gravity in such a system; the wavy line also added describes the actual course of the center of gravity (from [204]).

of tilt, orientated towards the front, which, by inertia, develops through the forward motion of the upper body at the beginning of the standing phase at the moment when the heel starts to touch the floor, is curbed by the abductors. At the end of the standing phase they also support the leverage capacity of the extensors by the same means.

The forces to be absorbed during walking by the center of rotation in the head of the femur have led to a *sagital* alignment of concentrated strong cancellous bone as was demonstrated in an impressive histomorphological way by Draenert et al. [78].

The *transversal* is the third plane of reference in this system. The highest point of the trochanter lies, depending on the size of the CCD-angle, right on the mid-point of the head of the hip or a little deeper, an advantage which effectively lengthens the contraction distance of the inserted muscles. A variasation osteotomy without simultaneous trochanter distancing results in non-correctable hip limping [101, 265], because the path of contraction of the abductors is shortened.

The load capacity of the intact trochanter and the stability of its osteosnythesis are determined to a great extent by two antagonistic muscle groups (and therefore reduced): the abductors produce a proximally orientated pull, the strong vastus lateralis a distally orientated pull of approximately the same size. The dynamic equilibrium thus generated on the trochanter is disturbed by surgical detachment of the vastus as well as by a trochanter fracture. Because of this special emphasis must be laid on secure reparation of both [318, 349].

In all planes the trochanter forms levers in relation to the mid-point of the hip-head which increase the efficiency of the hip abductors in three dimensions. Its exact refixing and transposition in the case of dysplasia is not only necessary, but also an imperative pathophysiological requirement. Slipshod anatomical handling negates the effect of the abductors, the most important hip stabilizers, and provokes severe pain which is very difficult to get under control. A safe fixation of them is therefore necessary [101].

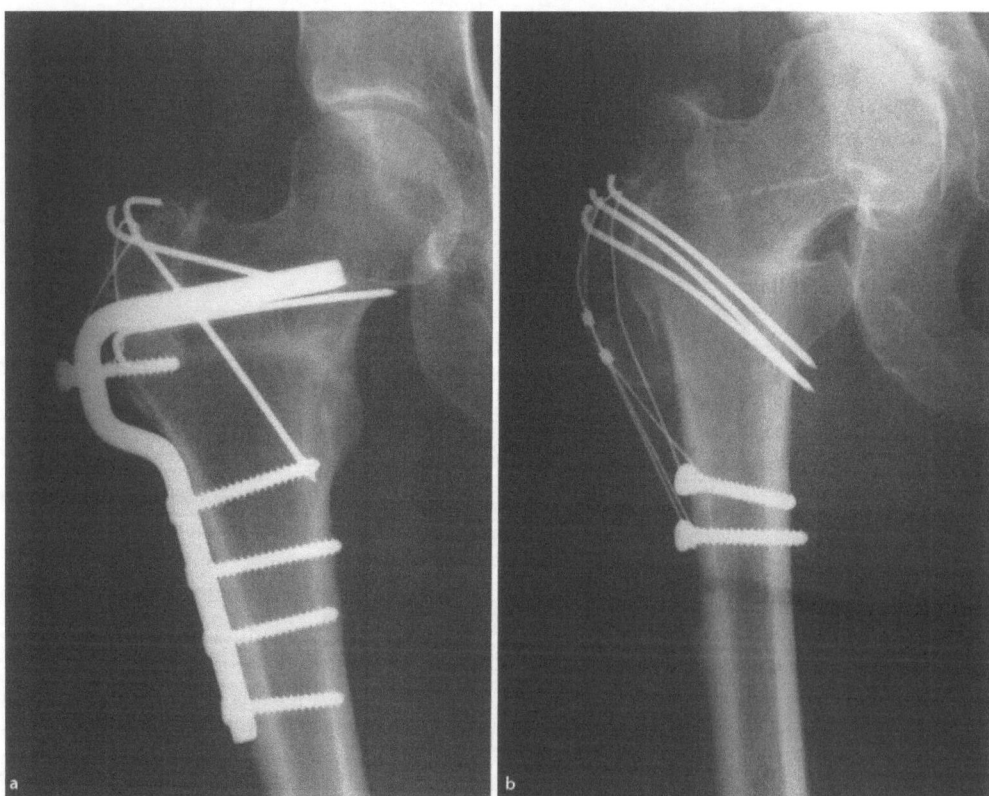

Fig. 99. Principle of the operation. Primary (**a**) and secondary (**b**) trochanter distalization, the latter because of painful hip limping after mere variasation osteotomy. Note the cable tension indicators

4.8.1.1
Trochanter Cable Tension Banding

Principle of Operation
Interfragmentary compression and securing against distraction by the abductors of the exactly repositioned trochanter is achieved by a wire tensioning between two or more 2.0-mm Kirschner wires inserted obliquely downwards, and a foundation screw pointing slightly downwards. Both Kirschner wires and screw have to be anchored in the opposite cortical layer so that they can withstand the high muscle tension (Fig. 99).

Advantages and Disadvantages
+ The stability of the construction surpasses the conventional wire procedure because the tension band cable can take a great strain and be anchored perfectly.
+ Safe osteosynthesis and, as regards volume of material and price, an economically viable method.
+ Metal removal optional.
– In comminuted fractures the cable can loosen if the patient is put under full strain before six weeks have elapsed.

– Independent of the type of osteosynthesis chosen, torn muscle parts near the joint have a tendency towards calcification, myositis ossificans.

Indications and Contraindications
• Trochanter avulsion fracture on changing prosthesis.
• Re-dislocation after wire fixation.
• Trochanter distancing in the context of varisation adjustment osteotomy or hip re-mobilisation by TEP after arthrodesis.
• Trochanter projection in hip dysplasia with painful limping.
– There are no contra-indications. Refixation is necessary in all cases (Fig. 100).

Positioning
• Thermal mat, supine position, right and left side supports.
• Wash from umbilicus to below the knee. A narrow wedge under the pelvis facilitates access to the trochanter, which lies dorsally.
• Wrap the leg to above the knee, cover with an U-drape leaving the hip exposed.

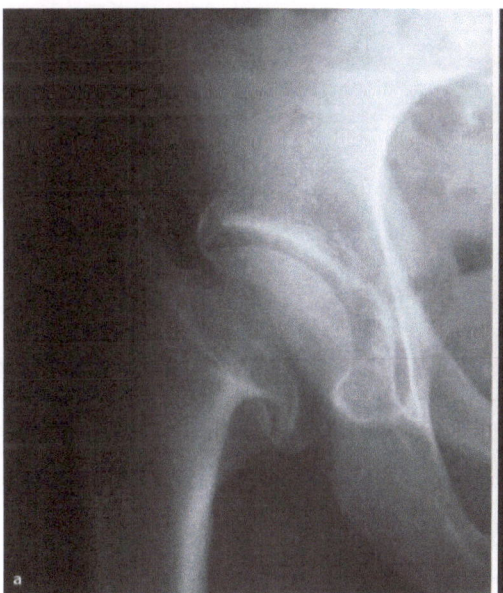 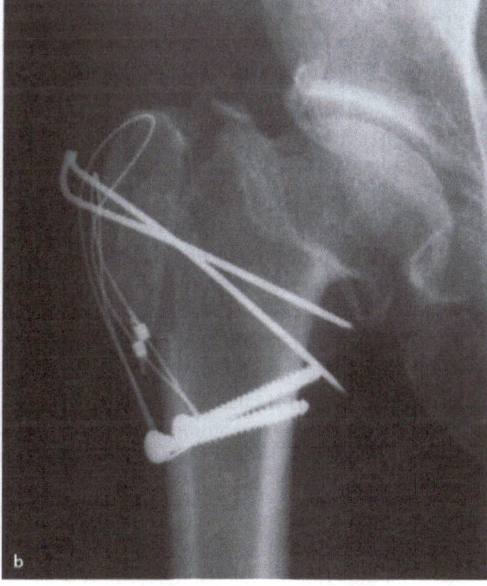

Fig. 100a – d. Indications. Hip dysplasia after childhood epiphyseolysis. Removal of the painful limp by trochanter distalization and lateralization (case one)

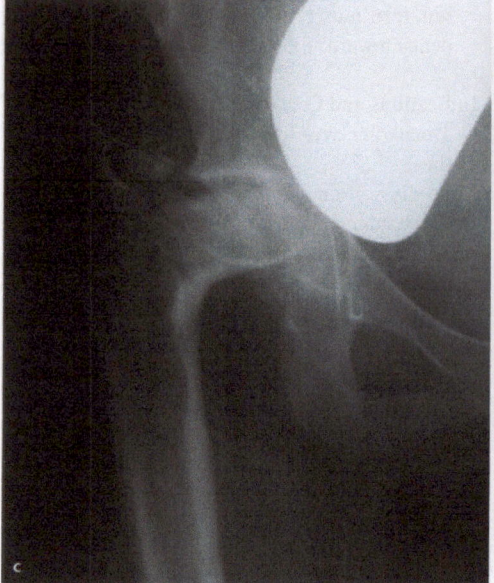
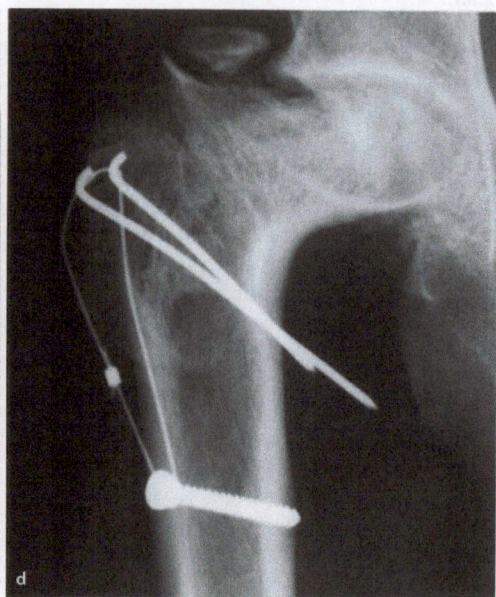

Fig. 100c, d. Case two

Instruments

- In addition to the special cable instruments there should be on the table an electric drill, drill sleeves, 2.0-mm Kirschner wires, side cutters, curved pins, pointed and flat pliers or curved Zimmer forceps, large pointed repositioning forceps as well as blunt and pointed Hohmann retractors.

Operation Technique

- Longitudinal incision in height of the proximal femur, extending 5 cm upwards above the trochanter; otherwise access is determined by the prosthesis technique. The subcutaneous tissue is separated using an electric knife, the fascia lata between tensor and gluteus maximus is slit longitudinally (Fig. 101).
- The vastus lateralis is pushed away with a large raspatory so that the osteotomized or fractured trochanter can be gripped with suitable repositioning forceps.
- It is exactly repositioned and fixed with at least two Kirschner wires (1) which are twisted from posterior superior lateral to anterior inferior medial until in the opposite cortical layer.

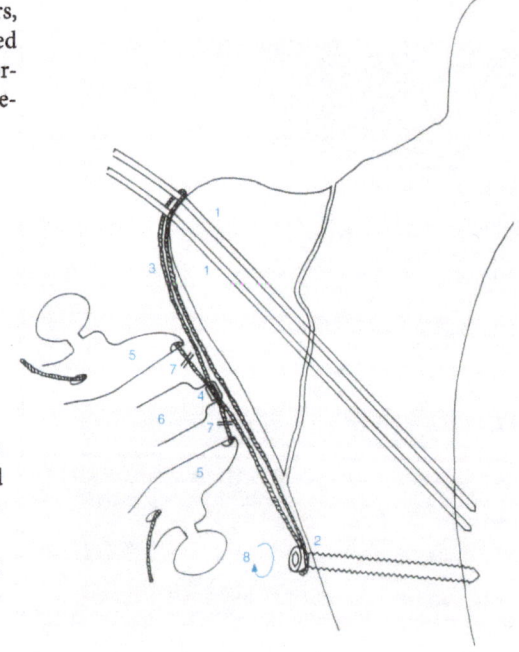

Fig. 101. Operation technique

- A large cortical screw (2) is inserted beneath the fracture slightly diagonally downwards or cross-wise through the shaft of the femur and the opposite cortical layer. Its head should just touch the upper surface of the bone. It forms the distal stopper for the cable.
- Using the awl, the cable (3) is passed *under* the abductor tendons without any soft tissue being interposed, directly onto the bone, and around the Kirschner wires, so that it is securely anchored.
- The cable coming from behind is passed around the foundation screw from behind, both cable ends running in opposite directions are passed through the crimp (4) and fixed in the cable tensioner (5). The assistant grasps the crimp with the crimp pliers (6), the surgeon tightens it until the Kirschner wires have been drawn through a good 10°.
- Pressure is applied in the free space within the concave section of the bone so that on removal of the pliers there is no loss of tension.
- After the tensioner has been slackened, the excess cable is cut off with cable scissors (7) immediately next to the crimp, the Kirschner wires are bent upwards away from the cable and finished off. To conclude, the foundation screw (8) is tightened in order to gain additional tension.

Operative Peculiarities and Variations

- In comminuted fractures individual fragments are dealt with using further Kirschner wires. In this case an additional cable cerclage around the fragments or a second tension band placed somewhat deeper or in a figure of eight, can be useful.
- Before a trochanter osteotomy a long notch is chiseled out to start with to mark the positioning for correct rotation.
- In dysplastic trochanter projection the anatomically normalized position improves the levers for the abductors. Its position is optimized, by moving it far enough distally, dorsally and laterally by padding with a corticospongeous wedge – cf. Fig. 100.

Complications, Mistakes, and Dangers

- Osteosynthesis has to be performed carefully encompassing all fragments so that it stands up to strong abductor tension.
- Tension banding must never simply be placed alone around the tendon insertions without the Kirschner wires, and soft tissue must not be interposed between a Kirschner wire and the cable.

Only in this way can blood flow and tension be maintained post-operatively.

- The Kirschner wires must perforate the opposite cortical layer and be bent upwards so that the wire does not slip.
- A foundation screw, which only involves one cortical layer, yields to wire tension. Using screws drilled in upwardly results in loss on tightening.

Post-operative treatment

- Electrical movement splints until bony reconstruction is complete.
- In stable conditions movement on level stretches with weight relief for the leg using crutches for three weeks, after which weight bearing is increased.

Results

Up to the end of 1995, 48 trochanters were repaired with cable tension banding. 30 cases concerned a change of prosthesis, 9 cases an adjustment of the coxa valga with distalization of the trochanter, when it had been split by means of the condylar plate or when the fixation did not appear secure enough. In another 9 cases an isolated trochanter projection, which was responsible for painful hip limping, was operated on in order to normalize abductor action.

With the exception of planned distalization in the case of isolated projection, trochanter tension banding is becoming a necessary intra-operative additional measure. On account of this only the results concerning bony reconstruction can be considered; the subjective picture of pain arises to a large degree from the underlying hip complaint and the main operation.

> Of the 48 osteosyntheses, 43 (90%) resulted in bony reconstruction. In endoprostheses 4 secondary dislocations were observed which made a walking stick necessary. The patients were nevertheless satisfied as they had been freed of their coxarthrosis pain by having a total hip replacement. Eight patients were free of pain after varization, in one 48-year-old woman the tension banding was removed alio loco after three months; the further course of events is unknown.
>
> Trochanter distalization resulted in patients being free of pain. The nine still young patients are again working and very satisfied with a hardly perceptible or even complete loss of limp.

Contemporary Alternatives and Conclusions

There are several competing osteosynthesis procedures as experience shows. Bernard and Brooks [15] expressed it thus: "Problems with the reattachment of the trochanter are well recognised." Savvidis [335] stated: "Osteosyntheses of the trochanter major suffer a high failure rate due to breakage of the osteosynthesis materials – (between 17% and 32% [52]) – as well as through the formation of non-unions. Clear relative movements in the fracture, or rather the osteotomy gap during even relatively light loading of the trochanter major are responsible for this. Therefore different osteosynthesis techniques are proposed: simple wire cerclage, figure-of-eight wire cerclage, osteosyntheses using tension screws, hook plate osteosyntheses."

Unfortunately these lack the necessary stability [58, 336]. As early as 1985 Hopf and Brill [135] ascertained: "By combining threaded wire osteosynthesis with a tension band cerclage with twisted fixation only a small interfragmentary compression force exists in principle, which leads even with relatively slight strain between the osteotomy surfaces to a lack of complete contact."

Tension screws, too, are subject to biomechanical objections. Because their position is always at a precise acute angle to the direction of action of the abductors, they are also always required for flexion, which they can often not withstand; they loosen or break as comparable examples show (Fig. 102). Savvidis et al. [336] compared the smallest resistance on the trochanter in the destruction of eight different types of osteosynthesis for cortical double screws.

The tension band plate for the neck of the femur [121] was developed for unstable per- and subtrochanteric fractures. It is not suitable for endoprostheses.

The cable-grip system for the reattachment of the greater trochanter by Dall and Miles [58], used since 1983, and meanwhile for cerclages improved, was the first example of application of a cable technique following the publications of the author. Results were superior to those of the commonly used cerclage wires. The almost predestined wire breakages were reduced to 3.1% in 321 cases by means of the 1.6 mm or 2 mm wire(for heavy patients) running through a metal bridge.

> ▶ It may be concluded that trochanter cable tension banding with Kirschner wires and foundation screw is a flexible, firmly anchored osteosynthesis which neutralizes abductor rotating moments by means of a high degree of tightening. It effectively prevents loosening and distraction without the danger of metal breakage which characterizes the cerclage wire technique. Biomechanically it is also the osteosynthesis of choice for the trochanter.

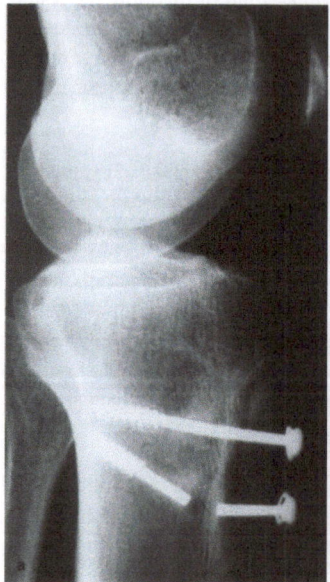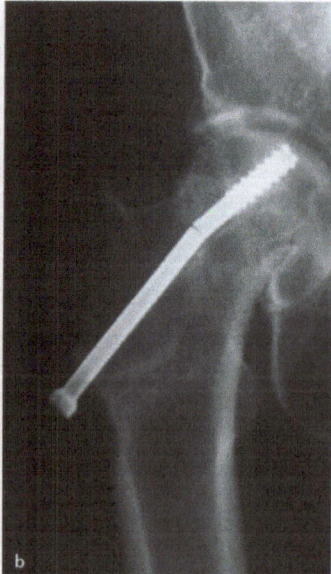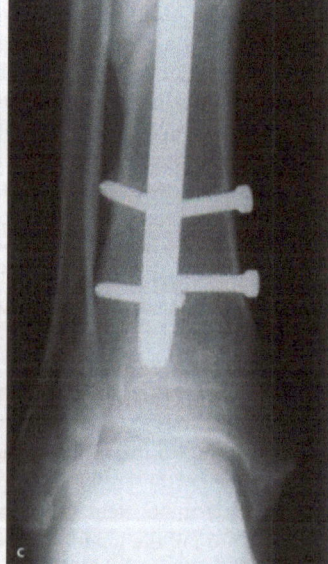

Fig. 102. Screws under flexion strain

4.8.2
Proximal Humerus and Tuberculum Majus

For decades, fractures in this region have been treated conventionally with dressings, splints, and using traction [20, 90, 116, 126, 129, 232, 298]. From the 1920s onwards, bone sutures became popular for dislocation fractures – a technique used to the present day [57, 64, 221]. The AO published guidelines concerning the indications and surgical procedures with plates, screws, Kirschner wires, and wire tension banding [266]. Nevertheless, because of the diversity of fracture types one has always to proceed on an individual basis in order to meet the challenge of fitting together like the pieces of a puzzle the shattered head of a humerus. The difficulties are reflected in post-operative X-rays, which in most cases only show an approximation of what one actually wanted to achieve. Recommending endoprosthesis in the case of comminuted fractures [255, 390] therefore seems to be an expression of resignation; its functional results are often only moderate [362].

In the classification of fractures the divisions A–C of the AO and 1–6 according to Neer have become generally accepted [72, 276].

The therapeutic problems of subcapital fractures of the humerus can even be expressed statistically: at present 80%, including comminuted fractures, are treated conventionally [255, 384]. For the latter, however, minimal osteosynthesis is also recommended [61, 161, 190, 221]. The particular worry here is the preservation or restoration of the blood supply to the head to avoid necrosis [362]. An adequately stable osteosynthesis with little metal causing no additional devascularization supports the favorable healing tendency of this cancellous region. Therefore initial stability [54] has to be attained in every case. Here screws and plates are also justified [59, 161, 255, 370] along with the classical minimal implants of Kirschner and cerclage wires. We are currently compiling data from trials using the combination of a longitudinal stabilising EndoHelix [216, 218] and cable tension banding – cf. Fig. 106.

Isolated tuberculum fractures are relatively rare. They dislocate easily. The external rotators of which the supraspinatus muscle produces more than half the total force, are attached to the large tubercle of the humerus. Impulse-like forces, such as those arising in dislocation or jerky internal rotation and through direct trauma with subcapital fracture, cause it to tear away in isolation or additionally break off. The tuberculum can be proximally distorted by muscle tension, so that on elevation of the upper arm it is positioned like a wedge between the head of the humerus and roof of the shoulder and causes impingement syndrome with pain and limitation of movement.

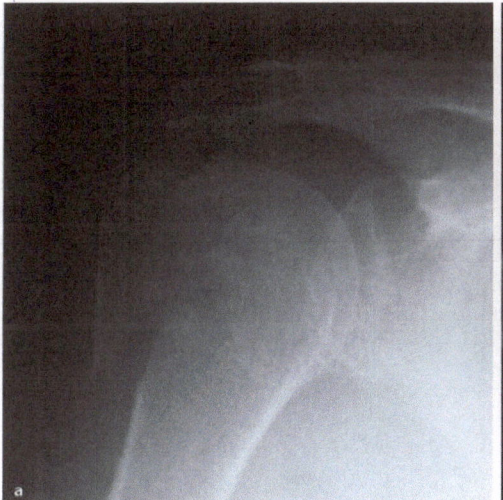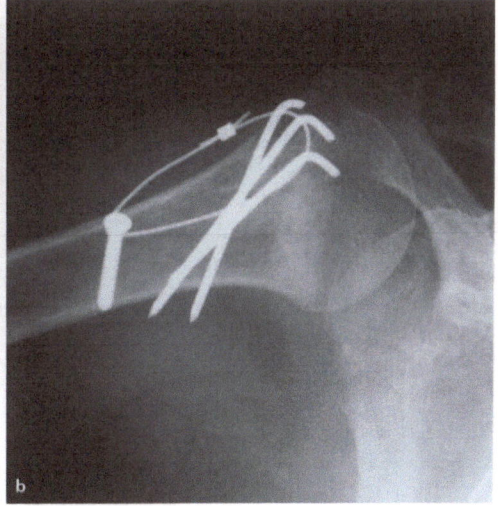

Fig. 103. Principle of operation

4.8.2.1
Cable Tension Banding on the Head of the Humerus and Tuberculum

There is not much room for osteosynthesis material. Repositioning and fixation of the frequently dislocated head or of the whole tuberculum torn off as a block is not always simple. With large fragments the tension banding can be varied by replacing the Kirschner wires with screws. They strengthen interfragmentary compression whilst the cable neutralizes muscle strain. Smaller fragments are pinned with some shortened Kirschner wires or small screws. The encircling tension banding wire helps to hold everything together like a packet.

Principle of Operation
Interfragmentary compression is achieved (as in the trochanter) with cable tension between two or more 2.0-mm Kirschner wires or screws inserted obliquely from the collum anatomicum or from the tuberculum downwards to the opposite cortical layer and a foundation screw angled slightly downwards (Fig. 103).

Advantages and Disadvantages
✚ Stable construction, because the firmly anchored cable absorbs strain well.
✚ Small volume, little iatrogenic trauma.
✚ Optional metal removal.

━ Comminuted fractures can fuse together. This danger is, surprisingly, almost as great in the shoulder as it is in the trochanter major, although the forces are weaker here.
━ Independent of the type of osteosynthesis chosen: torn muscle near the joint is prone to calcification, myositis ossificans.

Indications and Contraindications (Fig. 104)
✚ Isolated tuberculum break with projection which blocks abduction movement and consequently leads to impingement.
✚ Subcapital (dislocation) fractures with or without tuberculum breaks, but without larger comminuted zones. The head fragment has to be securely repositioned on the shaft. The subcapital bore canal (Fig. 104, a_2) shows the transosseus fixation of long biceps tendon [217] which was torn at a sharp fragment.
✚ Complex fractures with tuberculum destruction used in conjunction with a plate if need be.
✚ Subcapital oblique fractures must be fixated with additional interfragmentary tension bolt.
━ Non-dislocated fractures.
━ Comminuted fractures with subcapital instability.

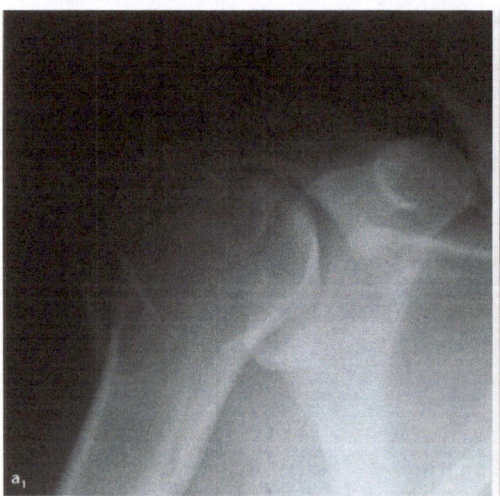
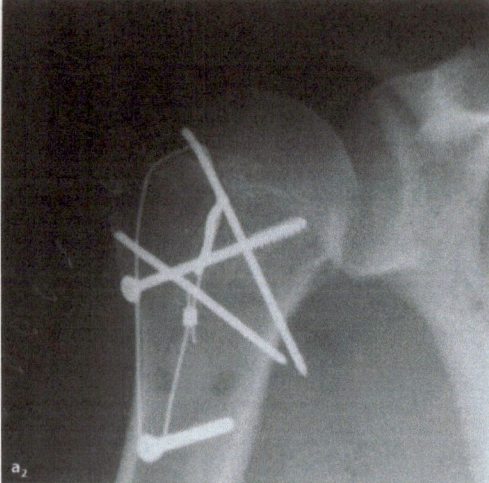

Fig. 104a–d. Indications (see text)

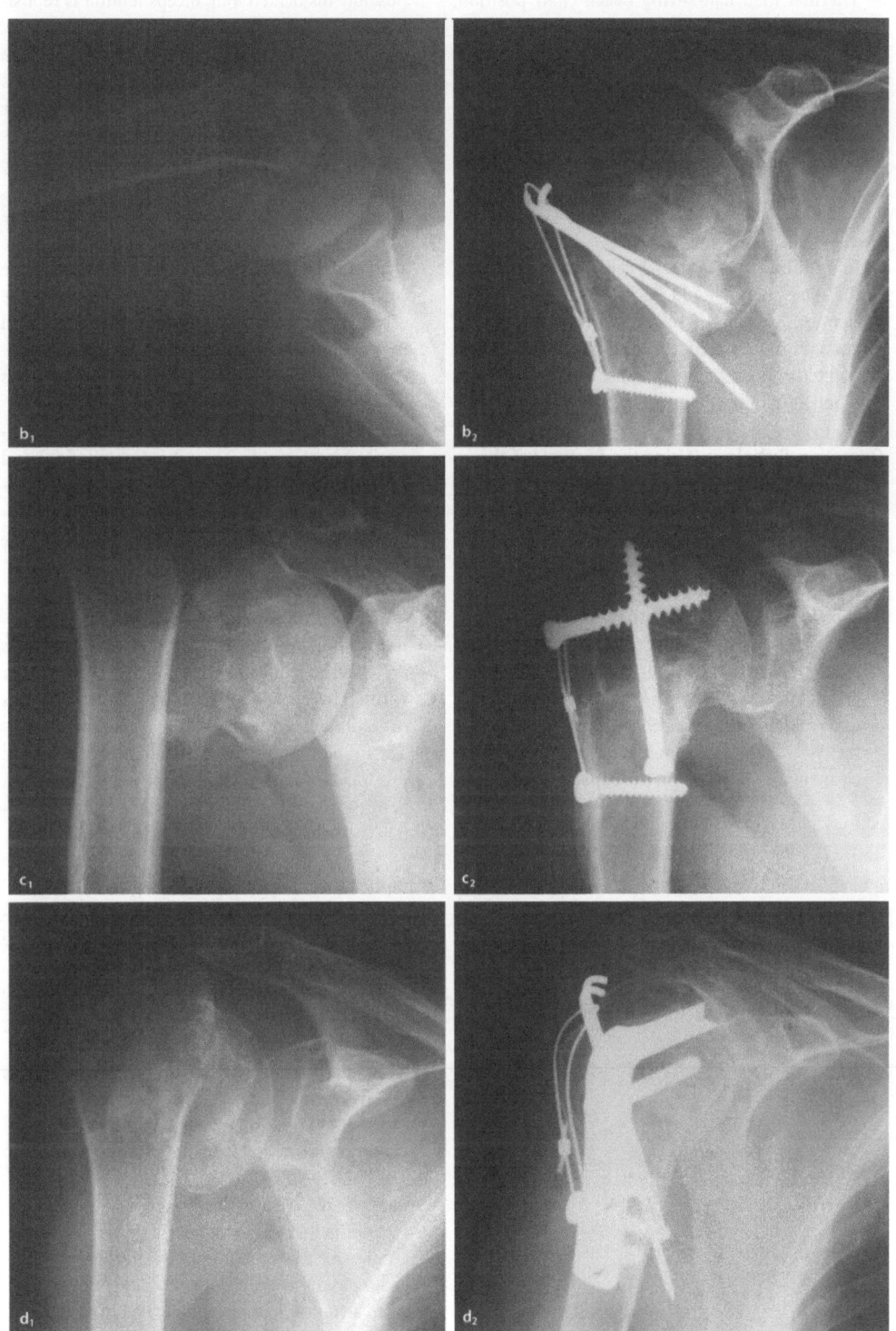

Fig 104. Indications

Positioning

- Thermal mat, half-sitting beach-chair position. The upper arm extends out over the edge of the operating table and is placed in an arm support. Cover with drapes leaving the shoulder and elbow joints free. Lower arm and hand are wrapped. Thus, a good area of movement is obtained for the extremity. Foil covering is not necessary.

Instruments

- In addition to the special cable instruments on the table there should be an electric drill, drill sleeves, 2.0-mm Kirschner wires, side cutters, curved pins, pointed, flat, or curved pliers, small pointed repositioning forceps, and pointed and blunt Hohmann retractors.

Operation Technique (Using the Example of the Tuberculum Majus)

- Straight or slightly S-shaped incision approximately 8 cm long, beginning two fingerbreadths laterally at the level of the coracoid process and going over the deltoid muscle distally to the lateral bicipital groove. After separation of the subcutaneous tissue, incision of the deltoid fascia, after which the deltoid muscle is widely teased apart and held to the sides with long retractors. On medial rotation of the arm the fracture becomes directly visible. The shoulder joint is inspected, cleaned, and lavaged via the capsule over the tu-

berculum which has been torn or incised. The possibly dislocated long biceps tendon is repositioned (Fig. 105).

- The tuberculum majus or the fragments of it are repositioned using pointed repositioning forceps and fixed with at least two Kirschner wires (or one or two screws) (1) which are inserted downwards at an angle, medially until they perforate the opposite cortical layer.
- Then a cortical screw (2) is inserted beneath the fracture slightly diagonally downwards through the shaft of the humerus until its head just touches the cortex of the bone. It forms the distal stopper for the cable. Further action corresponds with "Technical Instructions for Operations" in Chap. 4.2.
- A cable (3) is placed around the Kirschner wires and foundation screw without any soft tissue being interposed and put through a crimp in the opposite direction (4). Then it is tightened (5) and squeezed in the free space within the concave section of the bone (6) so that no loss of tension develops when the crimp pliers are removed. The rest (7, 8) is routine.

Operation Peculiarities and Variations

- In comminuted fractures individual fragments are fixed in addition with shortened Kirschner wires. The cable should as far as possible pass over all the fragments and press on them.
- The foundation screw angled slightly downwards produces a doubled gain in tension on tightening, because the cable slides on its head and the distance is extended.

Complications, Mistakes, and Dangers

- The cable is never only placed around tendon insertions and through a bone canal. This simple tension banding [339] always loosens.
- The Kirschner wires must perforate the opposite cortical layer and be bent upwards so that the cable cannot slip.
- A foundation screw angled upwards leads to loss of tension on tightening.
- A short foundation screw which only encompasses one cortical layer is not stable enough.

Post-operative Treatment

- Pendulum exercises and Specht's after-treatment; an electric movement splint would be advantageous. Excessive physiotherapy encourages capsule atrophy and peri-articular calcification, loosening, and distraction.

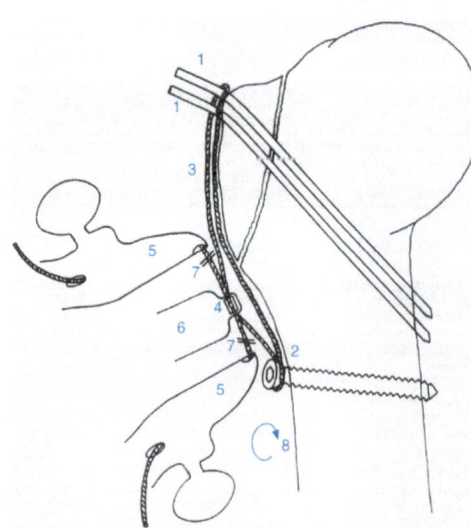

Fig. 105. Operation technique

Results

Up to the end of 1995, 42 per- and subcapital fractures of the humerus were treated surgically: in 7 cases plates were used, screws were used 5 times, 8 times percutaneous Kirschner wires were employed, and in 22 cases cable tension banding was carried out, of which 2 were used in conjunction with plates, 3 with an EndoHelix. The case numbers are too small for statistical analysis.

> ▶ All wire tension bandings showed bony healing except for one case, where a 52-year-old woman had to be operated on twice due to distraction. Necrosis of the head of the humerus was not encountered. Several times loosening of the cables could be assumed radiologically, which is especially problematic in these types of fractures, in particular four fragment fractures [282, 384]. In three cases, owing to this, functionally insignificant dislocation occurred, once with a varus tilt of the head. This was corrected and plated.

Excessive post-operative treatment may have contributed to loss of tension. Since we have become aware of this, we have as a consequence provided for two to three weeks rest in a Gilchrist bandage, with physiotherapy undertaken during its use.

Independent of the surgical procedure frequently an ultimate or severe degree of movement limitation remains which hardly affects the daily life of the mostly elderly people, an experience that is confirmed [59].

Contemporary Alternatives and Conclusions

There is no generally valid osteosynthesis procedure for the proximal humerus. The pattern of injury is too complex. Minimal osteosynthesis is preferred. This is carried out in the form of plain wire cerclage [221], wire tension banding with screws [54, 161], or Kirschner wires [61]. The latter is said to be completely stable during exercise and indicates good dynamic muscular splintage of the shoulder. Apparently, the constant score is surprisingly high: 88 – 90 points [161, 221]. Supposedly, its advantage is the far lower rate of necrosis of the head of the humerus [190]. This however depends not only on the destruction, but also increases with the rate of secondary dislocation. Ochsner and Ilchmann [282] experienced 50% necrosis of the head after using wire cerclage alone and PDS-cords, which without exception followed a secondary dislocation, the cord being "easier to handle and clinging better than cerclage wire to the bone." Therefore, despite its lack of rigid fixation, osteosynthesis which is stable under movement is deemed possible with it [362]. Schweiberer et al. [390] saw no connection between dislocation and rate of necrosis, this being related rather to the number of fragments and (because the blood vessel of the head of the femur may be involved here) the distance of the fracture from the collum anatomicum. The results with 3- and 4-fragment fractures reach scores of 68 and 57 points respectively – a clinically realistic statement.

Even plate osteosynthesis has its place, in particular for metaphyseal comminuted zones and in elderly patients. After early metal removal which, according to Neer, is combined with a division of the coraco-acromial ligament or acromioplasty, "82.6% very good to satisfactory long-term results were achieved" (in our opinion an impermissible summary of different results), 17.4% were poor [59]; 52% good results came from Szyszkowitz et al. [370] with different plates used in 70% of cases; with Schweiberer they remain exceptions.

> We do not use shoulder prostheses and agree with Tscherne et al. [161]: "The very satisfactory results of minimal osteosynthesis show that the anatomical reconstruction of the head of the humerus is preferable to primary implantation" – at 68 points its score is clearly not as good [255].

Among our patients there are two identical cases: dislocation fractures C3/Neer 4 in 72- and 78-year-old women. In the first case, after repositioning of the head of the humerus, an EndoHelix [218], which could still reach the collum anatomicum, was screwed in and the tuberculum majus was secured with cable tension banding. The metal was left in. After more than five years there was no necrosis of the head and a very good functioning.

The 78-year-old patient had been fitted with a total shoulder replacement which ,gives', causing pain in the dislocation position (Fig. 106).

> ▶ It may be concluded that, for tuberculum majus and multiple fragment fractures in the subcapital region of the humerus, which are stably repositioned, minimal osteosynthesis in the form of cable tension banding with Kirschner wires and foundation screws is a good alternative to plates, wires and screws.

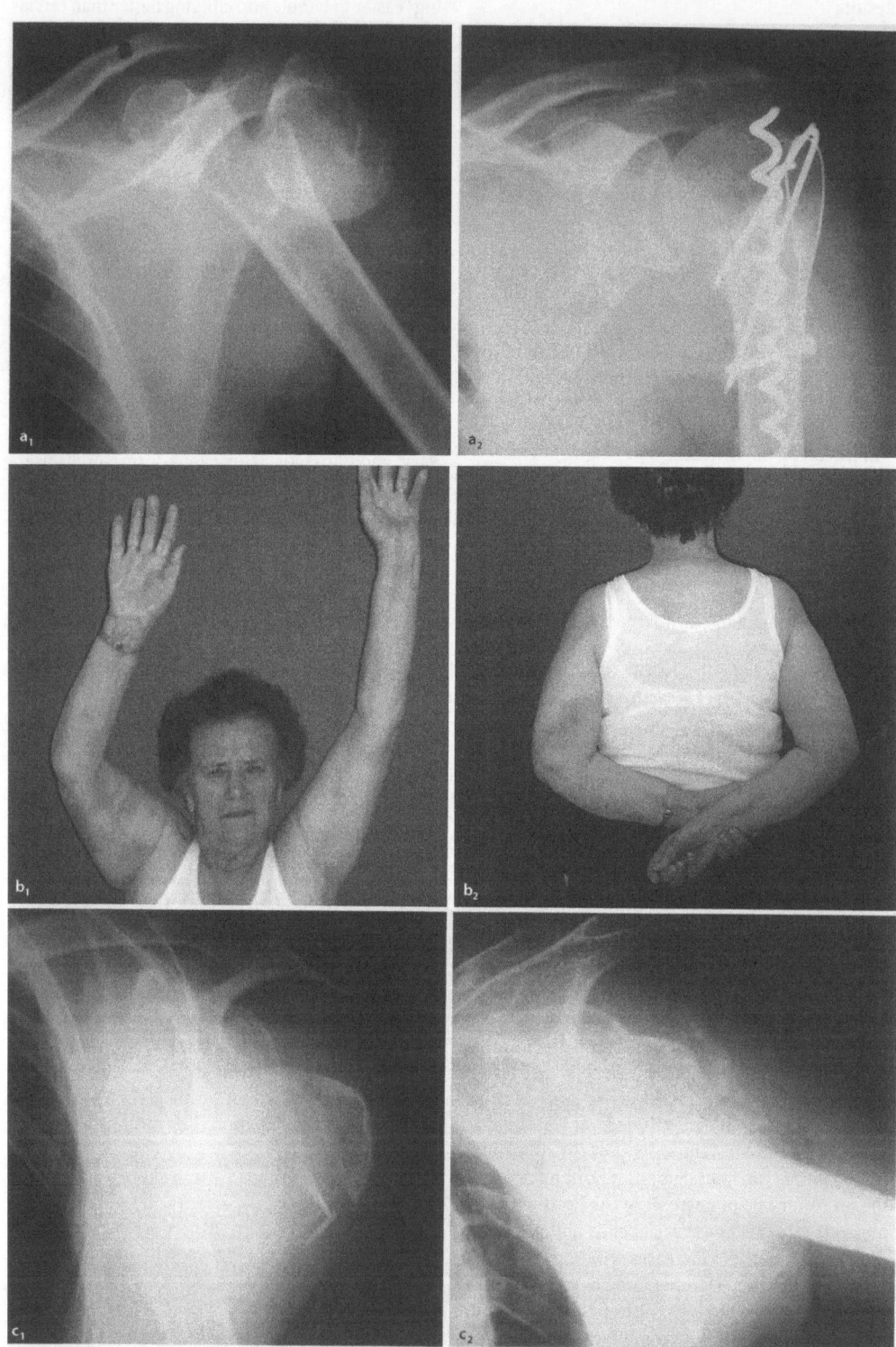

4.8.3
Distal Humerus Fractures

Humerus fractures close to the elbow cover a range which extends from simple extra-articular avulsion of an epicondyle type A1 to complex comminuted fractures type C3 of the AO classification [72]. Apart from epicondyle and supra-condylar fractures, the joint is always involved. Anatomically correct re-alignment is essential. With Böhler [20] almost all fractures were still repositioned and plastered. Only if a fragment "cannot be removed from the joint during the setting procedure one does extract it and place it on the humerus. Put in plaster for three weeks." The small size of the joint anatomy prohibits voluminous implants. On the other hand because of the high strain on the elbow which is initiated over the upper and lower arm, stable osteosynthesis is necessary. This dilemma often makes it difficult to decide as to which form of treatment is the best.

4.8.3.1
Cable Tension Banding Shown on Epicondylus Ulnaris Avulsion

Because of the traction forces during a fall and in dislocation of the elbow the avulsed (epi-) condyle is frequently tilted and twisted and cannot be conventionally repositioned and maintained in place. Therefore, operations are carried out – on both children and adults.

Interfragmentary compression is achieved by using a cable that (as in the medial malleolus) is stretched between two Kirschner wires (1.6–2.0-mm), placed crosswise through the fracture plane, and a small proximal foundation screw.

Muscle tension is neutralized, iatrogenic trauma is slight and does not alter circulation. There are no disadvantages (Fig. 107).

Operation Technique
- The operation is performed in the supine position with the upper arm in a blood-reducing cuff on a hand table. The arm, washed as far as the shoulder, has only the elbow exposed.
- In addition to the cable instruments we use small Hohmann retractors and two small pointed repositioning forceps.
- The slightly curved incision begins three finger-breadths above the epicondylus ulnaris and extends to the level of the joint gap. Directly on the lateral side of the bone the fascia is separated and the fracture exposed. In extra-articular avulsions the joint remains closed, in intra-articular fractures it is opened, lavaged, aspirated, and inspected (Fig. 108).
- The joint surfaces of the humerus are repositioned under visual and palpatory control, the condylus is fixed with small repositioning forceps, and two 1.6–2.0-mm Kirschner wires (1) are inserted parallel through the epicondyle and the fracture plane as far as the opposite cortical layer.

◁

Fig. 106. Superiority of a biological osteosynthesis (**a, b**)

Fig. 107. Indications (**a, b, c**) and contraindications (**d**). Cable tension banding is *indicated* in isolated dislocated epicondylar avulsions A1 and transcondylar fractures B1 and B2, more rarely in C fractures; in re-dislocation delayed healing and non-union. It is *not suitable* for vertical fractures

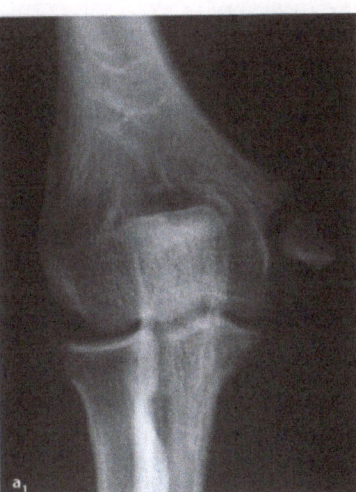
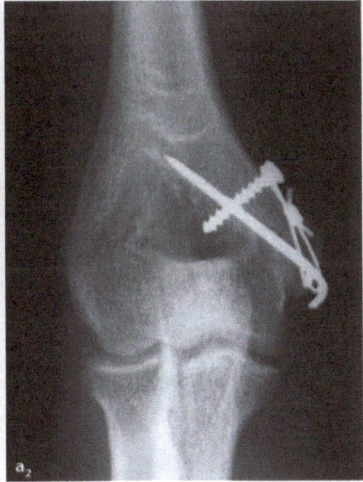

a₁ a₂

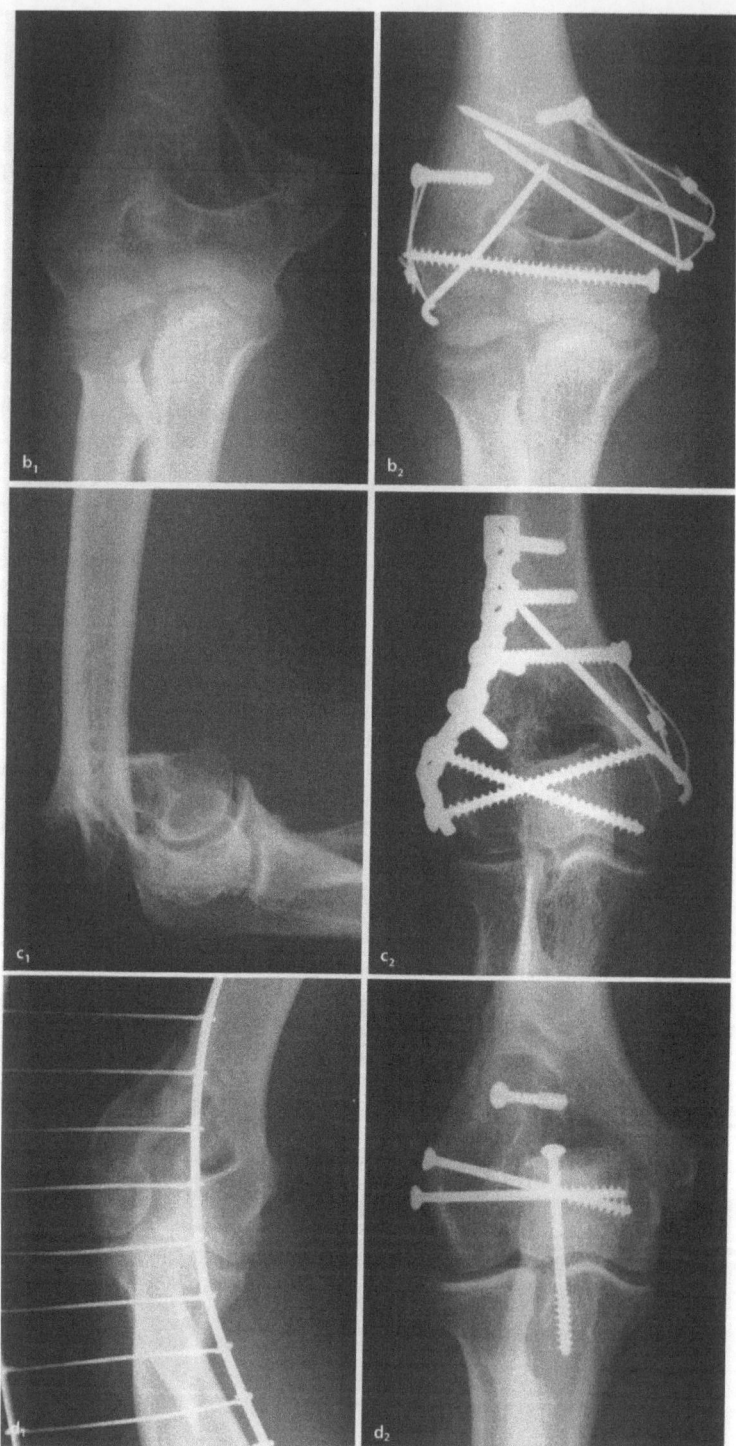

Fig. 107

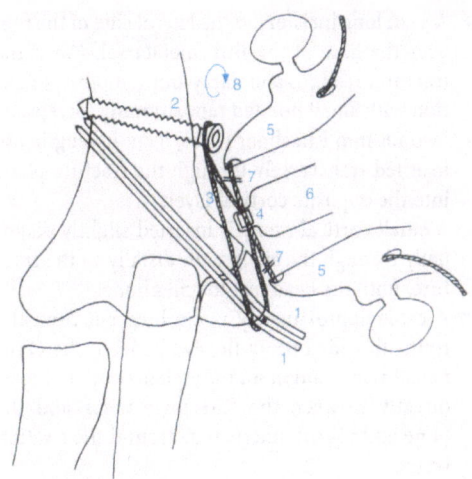

Fig. 108. Operation technique

- In a position 2–3 cm above the fracture a small cortical screw (2), sloping slightly upwards, is inserted and in adults screwed as far as the opposite cortical layer. The cable (3) cut from the roll and of a suitable length is threaded using an awl directly on to the bone-Kirschner wires contact position and from there on around the foundation screw. Soft tissue must not be interposed, in order that good anchorage develops.
- Then a crimp (4) is slipped on, tightened (5), squeezed (6), and the excess cable is cut off (7). After the Kirschner wires have been bent around and finished off, the foundation screw (8) is tightened to increase the cable tension still further.

Post-operative isotonic movement exercises. Sensitive physiotherapy to avoid peri-articular calcification.

Results
Up to the end of 1995, 32 distal humeral fractures had been stabilized with cables (some combined with a contra-lateral plate or an external fixator). Of 17 epicondylar avulsions 85% concerned the ulna. In five young people and eight adults cable tension banding was used, in four small children only Kirschner wires.

▶ Of the 32 cable tension bandings, 31 (97%) healed primarily in anatomical positions, those concerning epicondylar fractures without reduction in movement. In a 29-year-old man, in whom non-union had developed after plaster treatment as a youth, the tension banding loosened over the spongiosa concerned. Re-operating with a block of cortico-cancellous bone resulted in healing with free function.

Contemporary Alternatives and Conclusions
Distal humeral fractures are difficult to stabilize. Minimal osteotomy is biologically sound but often not sufficiently strong. Nevertheless it may be indicated in comminuted fractures, but must then always be protected with plaster or an external fixator spanning the joint.

For epicondylar avulsion wire tension banding or screws are recommended [39, 138]. We reject screws on grounds which have already been discussed in trochanter and medial malleolus fractures; often the fragments are also too small for them. Cerclage wire does not compress and plates are unsuitable for these special types of fractures.

The plate has found its place for complex injuries of the joint-bearing part of the distal humerus. The long levers of the upper and lower arm require at least one firm pillar. On the opposite side it can well be used in conjunction with cable tension banding. Double-sided tension banding, described as stable, [139] should remain reserved for exceptions.

▶ It may be concluded that cable tension banding is an optimal procedure for (epi-)condylar avulsions in adults and children and for simple distal humeral fractures. A high degree of interfragmentary compression, neutralizing muscle tension, is achieved using very little metal. It has also been proved to be beneficial when used in conjunction with a plate or fixator in compound fractures.

4.8.4
Avulsion Fracture at the Base of the Fifth Metatarsal

The base of the fifth metatarsal forms a projection on which are inserted the peroneus brevis tendon and the lateral part of the plantar aponeurosis. Rare fractures develop due to avulsion during an impulse-like inversion and plantar flexion [316]. For Rabl [308] it was always "pointless operating on it." He treated it with restraining plasters, whereas Böhler [20] always indicated an unpadded walking plaster cast for three weeks. Even today, conventional treatment is almost always sufficient.

Re-fixation is indicated – though this is rare – in coarse dislocations, particularly where there is wrenching of the avulsed fragments and only where there is a step in the joint of more than a few millimeters [35, 227, 250]. Since the tension, which is proportional to the load and introduced on walking, above all through the plantar aponeurosis, is to be neutralized, tension banding is a favored procedure, which we prefer to screw osteosynthesis. In 16 tension bandings Bauer et al. [10] found – on average 4.5 years after operation – only moderate interference with walking.

> Interfragmentary compression is achieved using a cable stretched between two 1.6-mm Kirschner wires and a small cortical screw (Fig. 109).

Operation Technique

- Supine position without blood-flow restriction. In addition to the cable instruments there should be two Hohmann toe retractors to keep it open. Re-alignment is maintained with small pointed repositioning forceps.

- A 5 cm long incision on the lateral side of the foot over the base of the fifth metatarsal. Clean the fracture, realign, and carry out temporary fixation with small pointed repositioning forceps.
- Two 1.6-mm Kirschner wires, 8 cm in length, are inserted transversely through the fracture plane into the opposite cortical layer.
- A small cortical screw is inserted slightly diagonally through the shaft 2 cm distally to the fracture, until the head just touches bone.
- A cable approximately 15 cm long cut from the roll is threaded using the awl beneath the peroneus brevis tendon and the plantar aponeurosis directly between the Kirschner wires and the bone and placed, uncrossed, around the fixation screw.
- The crimp is then slipped on, tightened, squeezed, and the excess cable cut off. After the Kirschner wires have been bent around and finished off, the foundation screw is completely tightened up to increase cable tension still more. Post-operative increase in load is soon allowed because the tension banding is adequately stable.

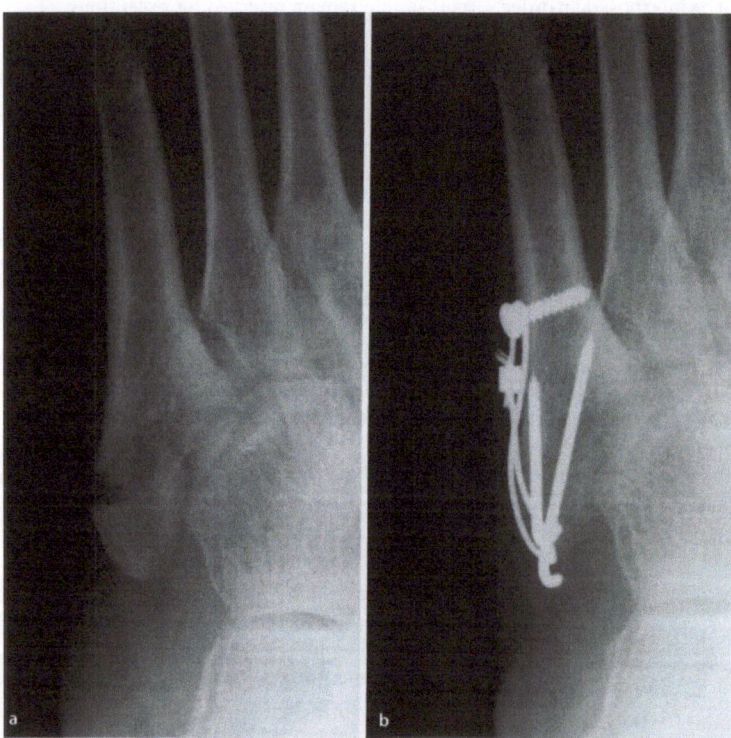

Fig. 109. Principle of operation

▶ Results
We have operated on 12 fractures of the base of the fifth metatarsal with cable tension banding, the last in 1992. All show complete bony reconstruction; nothing is noted about complaints.

▶ Conclusion: In dislocated avulsion fractures at the base of the fifth metatarsal the cable tensionbanding is the method of choice.

4.9
Compression Cable Osteosynthesis

This concept encompasses osteosyntheses which bring about pressure-resistant connection of bone surfaces using cable tension forces. The muscle tension which puts a strain on bony projections such as the trochanter or olecranon is absent here. Flexion forces, which develop due to body weight, acceleration, and deceleration during impulse-like movements are at work distractingly. They have to be neutralized by cable tension in the same way as muscle effort in other situations.

Two indications have become clear:

1. Breaking off of the rim of the acetabulum and column fractures through the hip joint.
2. Tibial head osteotomy to correct the axis of the leg.

4.9.1
Acetabulum Fractures and Dorsal Socket Avulsion Fracture

There is agreement that after an acetabulum fracture the prognosis is dependent on the primary damage caused by the accident on the one hand, and on the other hand to a great extent on the precision of the reconstruction, and that the best possible results can only be achieved in trauma centers with appropriate experience.

In this respect, we are only able to contribute a few cases, which show, however, that here too the use of cables is advantageous. Since 1975, Jungbluth [156] has been using cerclage wires on the acetabulum fixed between two screws, and even Brunner and Weber [33] used them. In particular, dorsal socket avulsions, which are frequently caused by dashboard injuries and falls onto a bent leg going up into the hip, which in turn posteriorly dislocates the head of the femur, can be firmly held together by cable stretched over the fragments.

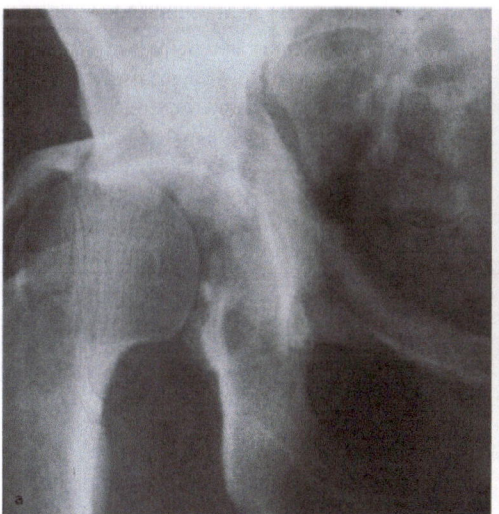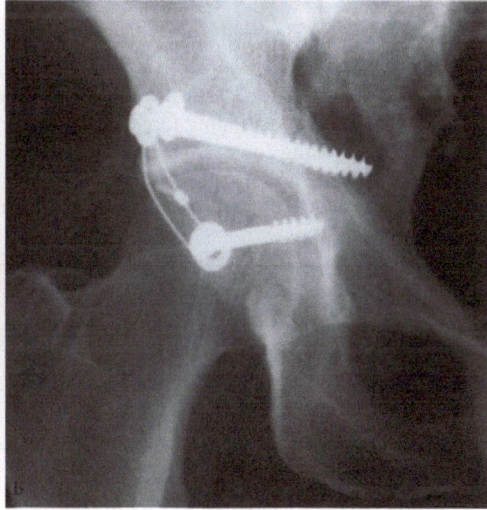

Fig. 110. Principle of operation. The posterior roof of the socket is held by cable tension banding, the proximal screws of which compress the column fracture at the same time

Principle of Operation

A cable is stretched around two or three cancellous screws, inserted divergently in the socket mass, in an O-shape or in the shape of a triangle, so that the repositioned fragment is firmly compressed. Washers will not do any harm as they become stuck to both cable and fragments.

Advantages and Disadvantages

- Stable osteosynthesis despite a small amount of material.
+ The disadvantages of plating – a lot of material, greater exposure, step formation due to inexact plate curvature, the danger of intra-articular screw entry – are reduced or do not apply.
- Post-traumatic and iatrogenic myositis ossificans caused by muscle tearing.

Indications and Contraindications

+ Dorsal socket avulsions with unstable joint management.
+ Letournel type A-E column fractures [154, 233, 433].
- Non-dislocated fractures.
- Narrow rim fractures without joint instability.
- Complex column fractures require plates.

Positioning

- Side position turned ventrally maintained by two supports. Large drape in the groin, the leg is covered from knee to foot and is freely movable.

Instruments

- In addition to the special cable instruments on the table there should be an electric drill together with accessories, large cortical and cancellous screws, pointed repositioning forceps and Jungbluth repositioning forceps, as well as pointed and blunt Hohmann retractors.

Operation Technique

- Posterior southerly access. This starts approximately 3 cm in front of the dorsal superior iliac spine and runs over the hip in an arc until just beneath the greater trochanter. Fascia lata and gluteus maximus are separated in the direction of the fibers. In strong internal rotation the short lateral rotators are held with holding threads without endangering the N. ischiadicus and detached from the trochanter. Gluteus medius and minimus are held anteriorly away so that the posterior capsule of the hip joint is exposed to view.

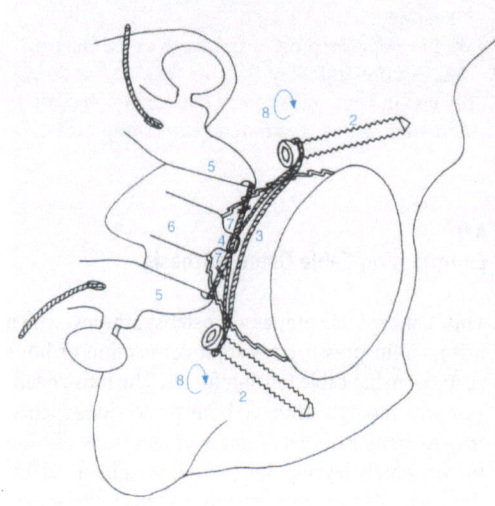

Fig. 111. Operation technique

If it is not torn, it is incised in a T-shape in order to make the inside of the joint and the fracture visible (Fig. 111).

- The posterior socket fragment is repositioned with pointed repositioning forceps without detaching it from the soft tissue.
- Screw canals (2) are drilled so that they do not enter the joint. The proximal screw is held securely in the roof of the acetabulum, whilst the one holding the fragment must end in front of the joint.
- Cable cut from the roll of an approximate length of 25 cm (3) is fitted in a crimp (4), stretched between the heads of the screws (5), and squeezed (6). Excess cable is cut off (7) and finally the screws (8) are tightened in order to provide further tension.
- Then the short lateral rotators are refixed, the fascia lata is adapted to enclose a subfascial Redon drain and the wound is closed.

Operative Peculiarities and Variations

- Trochanter osteotomy facilitates the overall view in complex fractures.

Complications, Mistakes, and Dangers

- The screws reach the joint.
- Convergently pre-drilled, the screw heads approach each other and on tightening cause reduction in cable tension.

- In determining the length of the screws the last turns after tightening the cable have to be taken into consideration. So that the joint is not perforated the screw holding the fragment is to be approximately 4 mm shorter than the length measured.
- Careless operating and drill dust left behind result in peri-articular ossifications, therefore rinse abundantly!
- Early weight-bearing endangers joint cartilage and osteosynthesis.
- Metal removal is ruled out because of the disproportionate nature of the operation.

Post-operative Treatment
- Electrical movement splints. Myositis prophylaxis with Indomethacin 4×25 mg/day for four weeks.
- Physiotherapy with strain relief for six weeks.

▶ **Results**
Up to the end of 1995, seven acetabulum fractures were stabilized with cable. They have healed in the right position, essentially without pain and so far without arthroses. In a polytrauma case with accompanying symphysis disruption, a painful peri-osseous calcification with reduction of hip mobility necessitated re-intervention; which showed a good result seven years later (Fig. 112).

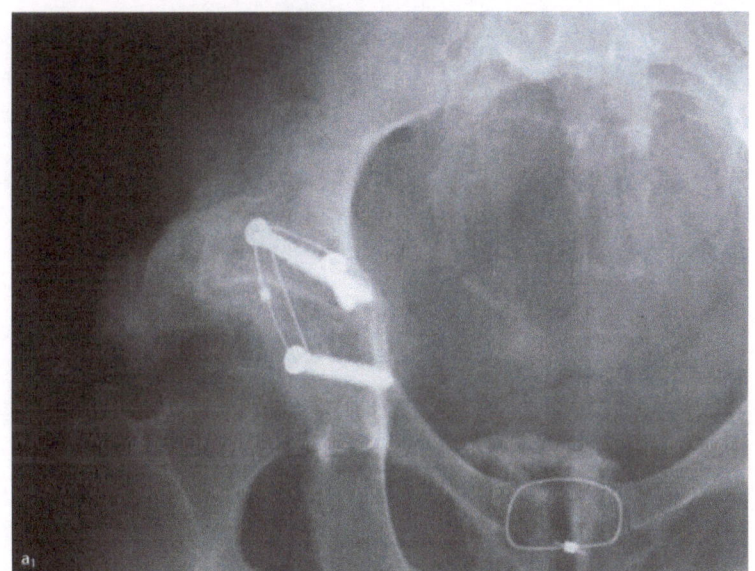

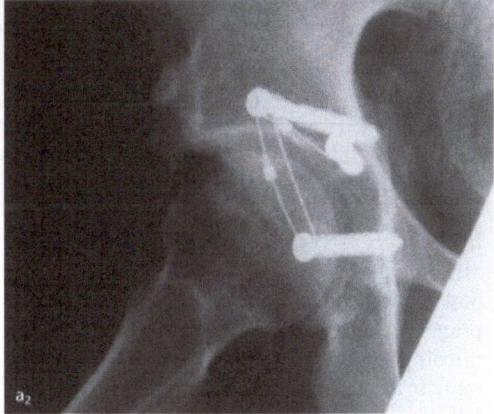

Fig. 112. Re-intervention due to hip calcification

Contemporary Alternatives and Conclusions
Cerclage wire should no longer be used; it does not compress.

Plates, which in experiments on cadavers resist higher destruction forces than screws [111], remain reserved for complex column fractures.

▶ It may be concluded that the cable osteosynthesis is a stable procedure for Letournel's "simple" column fractures and the dorsal rim break. It holds considerably better than cerclage wire.

4.9.2
Corrective Osteotomy in the Knee Joint Region

Straight legs with a physiologically neutral axis are a prerequisite for equal levels of strain on the knee joint. Axes out of true are corrected by realignment osteotomy. The resulting contact surfaces are pressed together so firmly by cable tension that plaster is not usually required for post-operative treatment. The most frequent indication is the varus position of the tibial head. Addition osteotomy is preferred in the less frequent supracondylar femur corrections – cf. Fig. 148.

meniscus was almost always removed. This procedure leads, after short-term improvement – because the meniscus, worn-down due to overloading makes the symptoms worse – to a rapid deterioration for two reasons:

1. The varus angle increases by 2° after removal of the wedge which the meniscus forms and holds the femur and tibia apart in the valgus position.
2. The overloaded medial compartment is robbed of its last buffer.

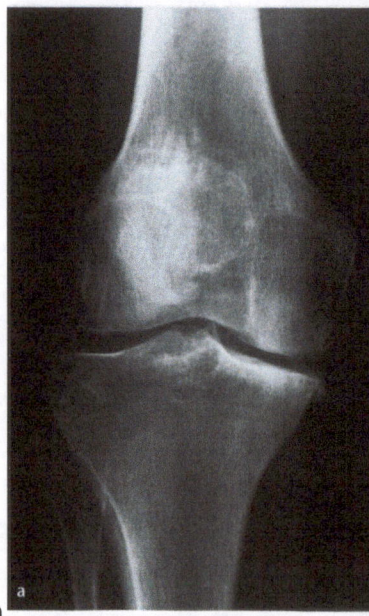
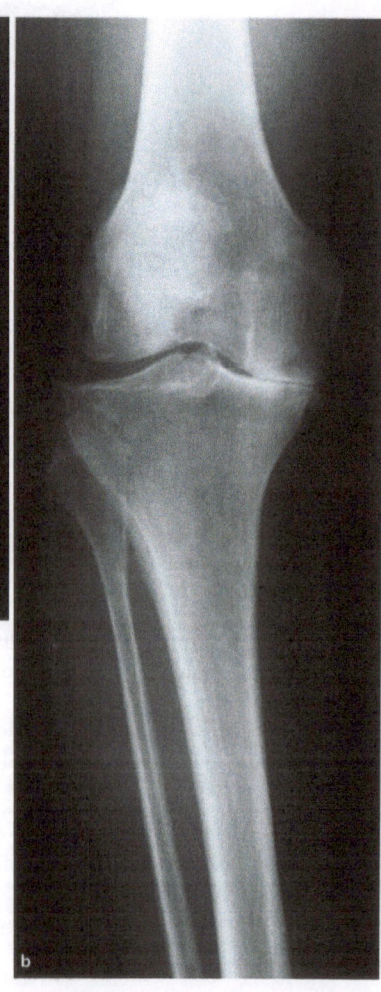

Fig. 113. Significance of the correct X-ray technique. The same knee X-rayed in lying down position (**a**) and whilst standing on the leg (**b**)

4.9.2.1
Cable Osteosynthesis to Compress Valgus Tibial Head Adjustment Osteotomy

In a primary axis error developing hemilateral gonarthrosis, tibial head adjustment osteotomy is the best biomechanical concept and the only one with a promising outlook [214, 393]. Because varus gonarthrosis goes together with medial meniscus symptoms, in former years (and, unfortunately still today following the fashion for arthroscopy), the medial

For this reason the meniscectomy becomes noticeable twice during each step, simultaneously in both peaks of the gait curve, as an impulsed "dynamic O-strain" of the medial compartment [212]. This increases the varus load also existing on the meniscus-intact knee joint [268], which the bent lever of the body weight causes. The joint cartilage is not up to long-term tolerance of this permanent over-loading when the meniscus is missing, especially when the other functions of the meniscus such as distribution of synovial fluid, nourishing massage of the cartilage, etc. [212, 352] fail. The medial over-loading of the joint after meniscectomy, which is gradually defined even to the point of becoming fixed can, surprisingly enough, remain persistently latent both clinically and radiologically, but unavoidably leads – in accordance with Hackenbroch's pre-arthrotic deformity – to medial compartment arthrosis.

In order to be able to assess the load conditions of the knee joint the usual X-ray films, taken on two layers lying down, are not sufficient. X-raying the axis of the leg whilst standing on one leg is part of biomechanical analysis, at least in the format 20 × 60 cm with the central beam directed on the joint gap (Fig. 113).

Principle of Operation

After wedge removal in accordance with the preoperative outline, the resulting osteotomy surfaces are pressed firmly onto one another using cable tension banding between two screws inserted proximally and distally to the osteotomy. The preserved narrow medial cortical bridge together with the periosteum and tractus iliotibialis remains as an effective natural opposing tension band (Fig. 114).

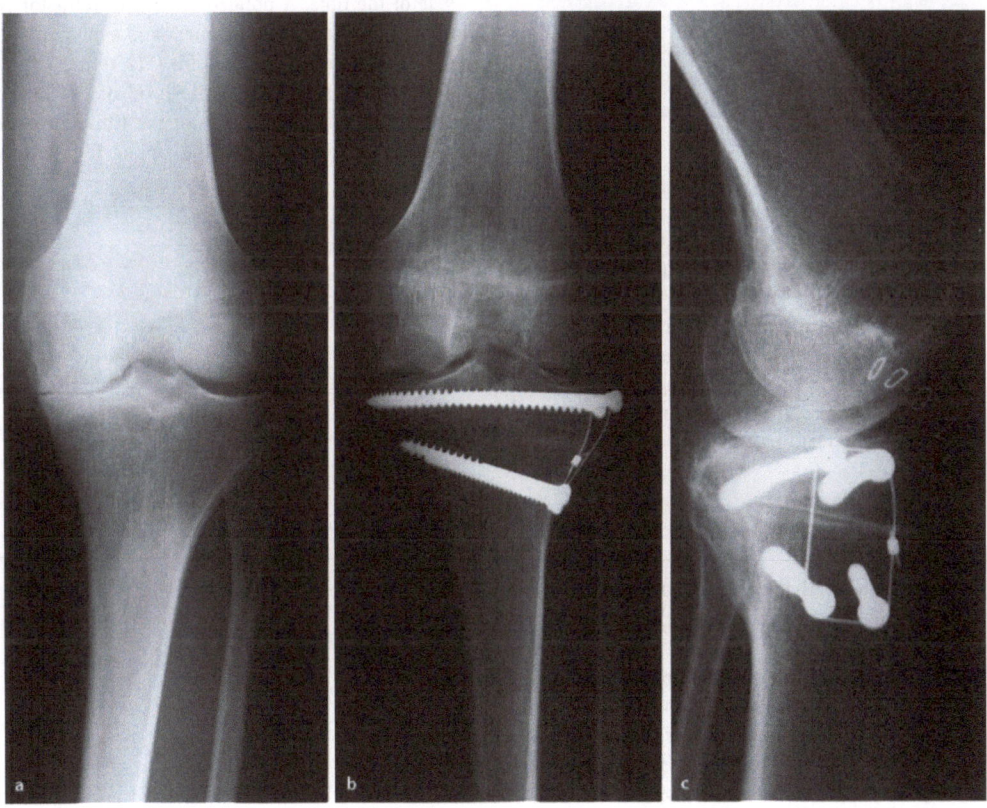

Fig. 114. Principle of operation. Note the bent screws as a sign of high cable tension, i.e. high interfragmentary compression

Advantages and Disadvantages

✚ High interfragmentary compression can be observed very well from the bent screws.

✚ The osteosynthesis is relatively simple to carry out; only a small amount of material is implanted. It is therefore comfortable for the patient; metal removal is usually superfluous.

✚ The flexible non-obstructive bond makes postoperative partial weight bearing possible immediately. Delayed healing and non-unions are hardly ever encountered.

− Subsequent correction of an already adjusted axis angle is not possible.
In the case of the osteosynthesis lacking rigidity the danger of spraining can occur if it is fully loaded too early.

Indications and Contraindications

✚ Medial compartment arthrosis, even in the elderly.

For them it is not medial meniscus "degeneration" – often falsely referred to – which is to blame but the faulty position of the axis. The term "degeneration" highlights an awkward biomechanical misunderstanding. It is not a question of regression but of *over-loading* that first affects the medial meniscus and then the whole medial compartment.

✚ In a large cartilage-deprived zone in young knees we have occasionally added a medial corium-interposition-plasty according to Lexer and E. Rehn [179]. For some time we have simultaneously been padding the cartilage defect with cartilage-bone cylinders that are transplanted press-fit using a Draenert diamond reamer [78]; primary healing [102].

− Panarthrosis.

− Compartment destruction after abnormal healing of a tibial head fracture.

Positioning

• Thermal mat, supine position, right and left side supports.

• Foam roll beneath the affected knee. Slight lowering of the opposite leg allows the surgeon freedom of movement.

• Cover in a similar way to the hip operation using a drape leaving exposed the spina iliaca ventralis. The lower leg is wrapped in sterile cloth to 15 cm below the tibial tuberosity. That facilitates axis control which is brought about by a 1.5-m wire cable fixed as a guidance cord from the spina to the first interdigital space.

Instruments

• In addition to the special cable instruments there should be on the table a bone tray with saws, chisels, and raspatories. Furthermore, an electric drill, drill sleeves, large cancellous and cortical screws together with thread cutters, a linear measuring device, and screwdrivers.

Operation Technique

• The hockey stick incision begins on the lateral side of the knee joint, two fingerbreadths beneath the tibial tuberosities on the anterior edge of the shin bone and curves to the posterior edge of the lateral joint space. Going immediately through the tractus iliotibialis to the periosteum, the muscles are pushed away from the tibia with a large curved raspatory. After freeing the posterior edge of the tibia the head of the fibula can be successfully loosened somewhat so that it can be moved higher more easily.

• The tractus is separated in the direction of the fibers and the musculature loosened as far as the posterior side of the tibia. A pointed Hohmann retractor is held under the patellar ligament and a blunt one at the posterior surface of the tibia (Fig. 115).

• Transverse osteotomy at the level of the lower edge of the lateral condyle of the tibia. Enough material is retained for the upper foundation screw.

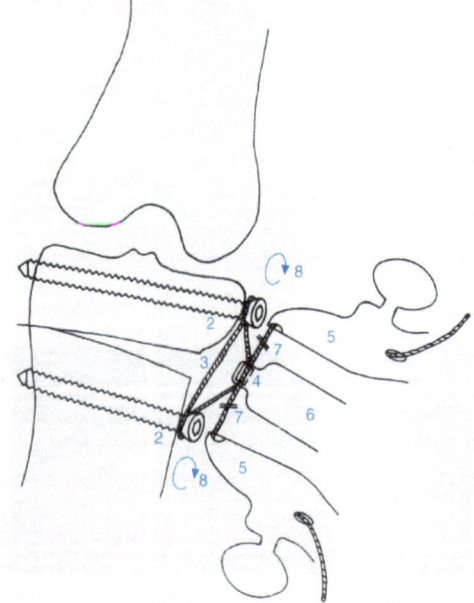

Fig. 115. Operation technique

- The base of the wedge is measured according to the pre-operative outline, both the angle and in millimeters. That increases precision.
- A narrow medial cortical sickle together with periosteum and pes anserinus tendons are left intact as natural opposing tension band.
- Passing transversely through the tibia two cancellous screws are inserted proximally (2), two cortical screws distally (2) until their heads just touch the bone.
- Then a cable (3) of 25 cm in length is placed around the heads of the screws, a crimp (4) is slipped over, and the cable is fixed in the cable tensioner.
- The first assistant takes the crimp pliers (6), the second assistant twists the lower leg to a valgus position until the bone surfaces make good contact. The surgeon tightens the cable and cuts off the excess with the cable scissors (7).
- The cancellous bone gained from the wedge is installed medially to the osteotomy.
- Finally all four foundation screws (8) are tightened in order to gain additional tension.
- Deep Redon drain, atraumatic layered wound closure. Compression bandage. No plaster. Positioning of the leg on a foam splint.

Operative Peculiarities and Variations
- A higher valgisation angle requires slanting subcapital osteotomy of the fibula so that it does not close up.
- If too much valgus threatens to develop, the wedge, correspondingly narrowed on its cortical base, is re-implanted as an interposition and then tension is applied. In each case the extracted cancellous bone is medially installed.

Complications, Mistakes, and Dangers
- If the osteotomy does not reach far enough into the medial cortical bone it can result in a chisel fracture in the middle of the head of the tibia on valgization. The resulting tent-shaped deformation of the tibial plateau causes incomplete correction (Fig. 116).
- The erroneous severing of the opposite cortical bone, periosteum, and pes anserinus results in instability. In this case cable tension banding (with two short screws) must also be applied medially and a plaster cast is fitted for four weeks.

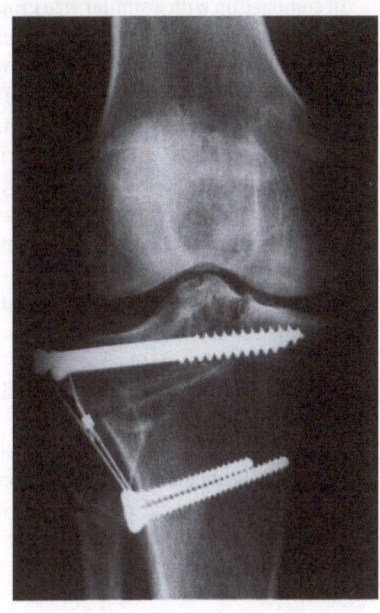

Fig. 116. Two-third osteotomy resulting in a chisel fracture

Post-operative Treatment
- Early mobilization is the best thrombosis prophylaxis. Immediate post-operative electric movement splints. Only partial weight-bearing for six weeks so that the osteosynthesis does not become compressed.
- In insufficient correction or over-correction, assessed on post-operative X-ray of the axes, counteract with outer or inner edge shoe supports.

Results

▶ Up to the end of 1995 we performed 267 valgized tibial head adjustment osteotomies with flexible wire compression. The first 60 patients were followed-up as part of a dissertation [393]. All osteotomies healed with osseous formation. Nonunions and delayed healing were not encountered, nor any peroneal nerve or vessel damage. In five cases cables loosened due to compression of the osteotomy surfaces after premature weight bearing. With it came a certain amount of valgus as well as varus loss of correction which was compensated through raised shoe edges. In three cases wounds healed superficially by second intention. Out of all 267 cases, 2 knee arthrodeses were necessary because an uncontrollable deep infection had spread to the joint.

In comparison with a similar size group of medial meniscectomies, whose results are extremely unsatisfactory, 53 patients (88%) were happy with the axis straightening, 2/3 were free of pain, 21% had significantly less pain and only in 7 patients (12%) did the pain remain the same. This correlates with a lengthened stride, the involution of recidivist contusions and quadriceps hypotrophy, and a radiologically visible recovery of the medial compartments

Contemporary Alternatives and Conclusions

Flexible Blauth clamps [18] and others have a similar principle to that of cable tension bands. Their disadvantage may lie in too little compression and too great a rate of loosening.

Angle plates [347] seem to be obsolete. Their technique is costly and angle correction is difficult to adjust. They are rigid and provoke non-unions.

Bell plates are not supposed to have this disadvantage [106].

The external fixator is not very comfortable, often causes painful irritation and infection of the pin entry points, and tends to work loose.

The curved Coventry osteotomy [55] is held with plaster and is therefore no longer up-to-date.

A good but expensive possibility is the Orthofix which, using callotasis, makes possible a step-by-step post-operative dilatation until the desired axis position is achieved.

> ▶ It may be concluded that for knee joint axis correction osteotomy surfaces can be highly pressed against each other flexibly with cable osteosynthesis. The procedure is effective, comfortable, and very economical.

4.10
Cable Arthrodeses

The high tension force of cables has opened up further therapeutic possibilities. Joints can also be advantageously stiffened with it. Clinically relevant indications are the arthrodesis of the upper ankle joint and tibio-calcaneous stiffening in Pirogoff amputation [394]. On the other hand, the lower ankle joint is more easily stabilized with two screws. At the knee, ventral cable tension-banding can save patients from the particularly uncomfortable tent construction of the external fixator – cf. Fig. 151.

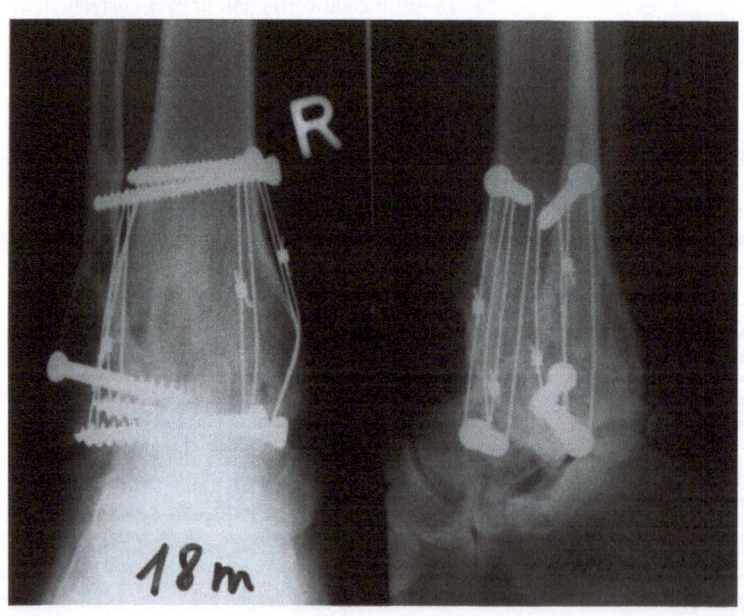

Fig. 117. Principle of operation. Even after 18 months cable tension is still high. Pre-arthrodetic state – cf. Fig. 119

4.10.1
Cable Arthrodesis of the Upper Ankle Joint

Principle of Operation
The principle corresponds to that of an internal frame fixator. Two pairs of wire cables, placed medially and laterally between the tibia and the talus on four screws forming the foundation, press the arranged de-cartilaged joint so firmly together that tibio-talar synostosis occurs without problems. The wire cables are placed around the heads and in the thread grooves of the corresponding pair of screws, which are proud of the opposite cortical layer, and are tightened (Fig. 117).

Advantages and Disadvantages
The construction that brings about the arthrodesis is very comfortable for the patient; he does not feel the small amount of metal lying predominantly in the bone.
+ The flexible compression construction does not gape. It therefore promotes bony reconstruction that rigid implants tend to prevent. The six weeks needed for consolidation is considerably shorter than with all other methods.

+ Hind foot and heel can be well-adjusted sagitally and frontally, pre-existing misalignments corrected and securely held. The bone surfaces are firmly pressed together using four tightened wire cable loops with a total of eight cross-sections. Their common resulting force runs through the center of the contact surfaces; shearing forces do not develop.
+ Cable arthrodesis fulfills the criteria of a biological process, the implants embedded do not impede problematic blood flow in this region lacking soft tissue, nor is there a possibility of external infection per continuitatem.
+ Metal removal is not necessary.
− No disadvantages observed.

Indications and Contraindications
+ Post-traumatic and iatrogenic arthrosis after pilon fractures and ankle joint and talus compression fractures (Figs. 118, 119).
+ Deforming osseous and neurological arthropathies such as Charcot's disease and primary chronic polyarthritis.
+ Stabilization of fallen foot and talipes equinus in peroneus paresis (3).
  Pain-free arthrosis, confinement to bed, old age.

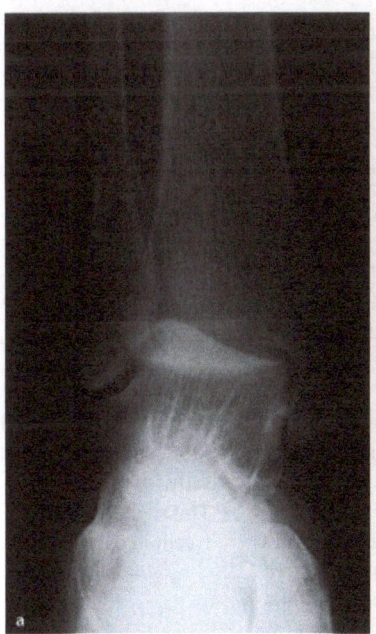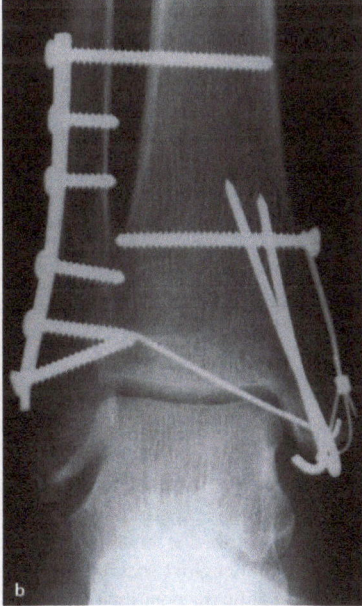

Fig. 118a–d. Indications. Arthrosis of the upper ankle joint after a fall from a height of 2 m. Probable primary cartilage damage: **a** trauma; **b** 10 days postoperative

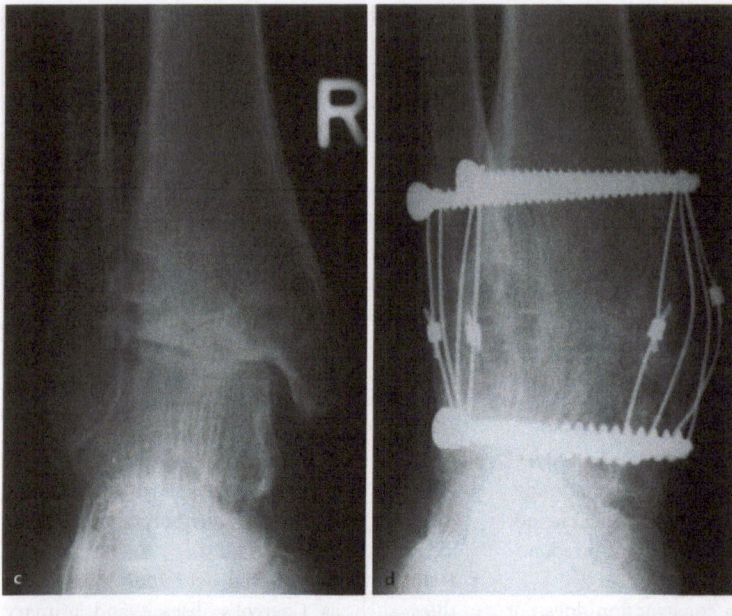

Fig. 118c, painful arthrosis 18 months later; **d** recovery under correction of the X-heel 14 months later

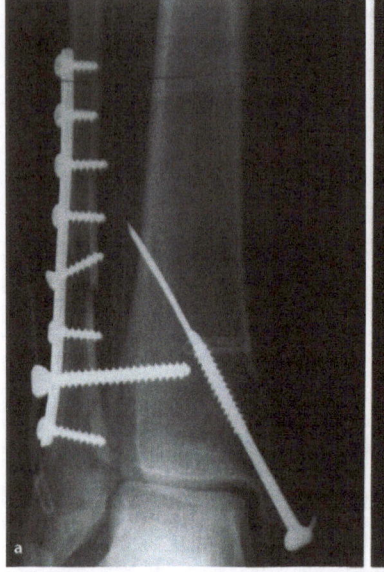
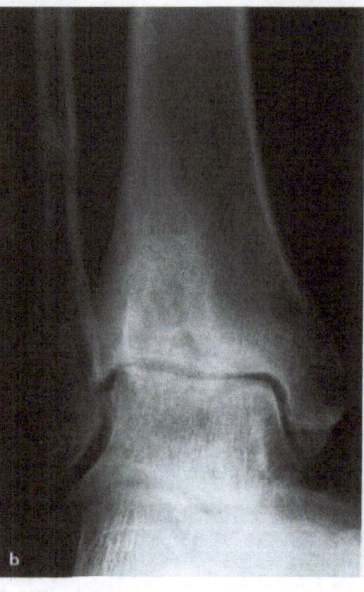

Fig. 119. Indications. Iatrogenically partially caused arthrosis of the upper ankle joint; **a** syndesmosis not correctly treated; probably also small outward rotation of the external malleus. The incomplete mortise recess results in cartilage-destroying shearing movements; **b** painful arthrosis 2.5 years afterwards. Stiffened in 15° talipes equinus. Healing – cf. Fig. 117. Unfortunately similarly incorrect upper ankle joint osteosyntheses are frequently seen – cf. Fig. 96

Positioning

- Thermal mat, supine position, right and left side supports.
- Wash the legs from the toes to above the knee.
- Cover with a large drape with a hole to a hand's breadth above the knee, the forefoot is covered with a rubber glove secured with tape. This is best for assessing the position of the foot in all planes.

- Foam roll under the distal lower leg, so that the foot can be freely manipulated, particularly dorsally.
- The slight lowering of the opposite leg results in freedom of movement for the surgeon.

Instruments

- In addition to the special cable instruments there should be on the table a bone tray, saws, chisels, raspatories, Hohmann retractors, Langenbeck hooks, an electric drill, 3.5-mm bits, drill sleeves, screw-measuring devices, thread cutters, cortical and cancellous screws, and screwdrivers.

Operation Technique

- Access to the joint is reached by straight-oblique 8 cm long cuts from the lateral and medial malleolus to the talus; it can be held wide open with Langenbeck hooks and Hohmann retractors and clearly exposed. Cartilage remains and sclerotic bone areas can now be easily removed.
- Tibia and talus are sawn even, sparingly. That produces two congruent surfaces on which the foot can be well adjusted dorsally. The lever of the forefoot is thus shortened, facilitating walking; leg shortening is slight (Fig. 120).

- slipped on, tightened (5), secured (6), and the excess cable cut off (7).
- The foot may now be turned gently in the varus or valgus direction – depending on the initial starting point. This is compensated with additional pressure gained from contra-lateral tension.
- On the opposite side a wire cable is carefully looped around two of the corresponding screw thread grooves lying directly against the bone and dealt with as described above. When positioning is correct in all planes, all screws (8) are finally tightened up. If it is not satisfactory or if there is even the slightest doubt about stability, tension bandings have to be renewed on one or both sides, whilst there is still time for correction.
- For details see Fig. 121.

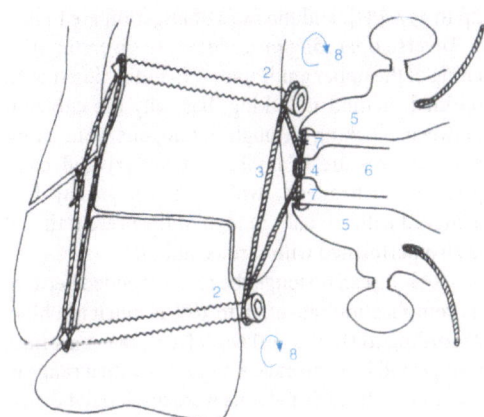

Fig. 120. Operation technique

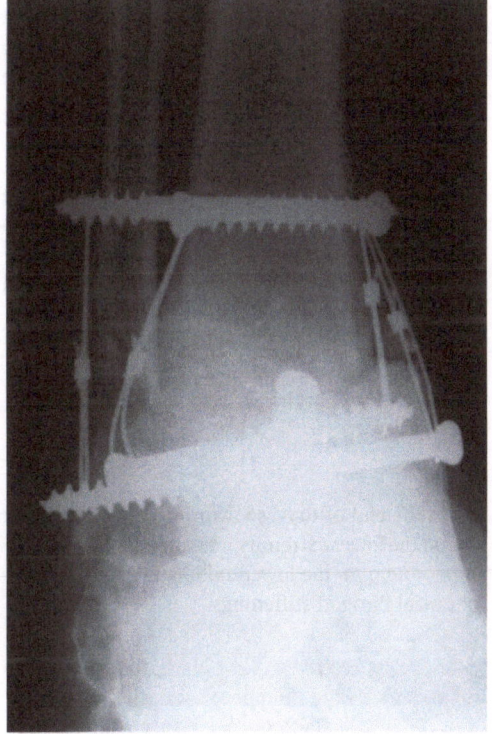

Fig. 121. Three operative details which contribute to optimal bone contact and higher interfragmentary compression: the lower posterior screw holds the osteotomy of the lateral malleolus; the cables lie well bedded in the screw thread grooves; the crimps optimally in free space

- Two cortical screws (2) are inserted into the side surfaces of the tibia, the first close to the anterior edge, the second right at the back. The length of the screws is chosen so that they perforate the opposite side before the heads touch. The first screw thread groove that appears of each screw will eventually take a wire cable.
- Two cancellous screws (2) are inserted in the same way through the neck and body of the talus.
- One after the other cable loops (3) are placed between the corresponding anterior and posterior screw heads – it is best to begin on this side – the position of the foot is checked, a crimp (4) is

Operative Peculiarities and Variations

- The bone material gained at arthroplasty is used in all cases; it is pressed in with a spatula.
- The osteotomized lateral malleolus can be fastened separately with a screw or caught in the posterior cable loop.
- The functional long-term result depends essentially on the adjustment of the foot. Shortening of the forefoot is crucial as is neutrality in the frontal plane (thus avoidance of an X- or O-heel).
- For men, the suitable neutral position is up to 5° talipes calcaneous, for women up to 5° talipes equinus.
- It is irrelevant whether the screws are inserted from a tibial or fibular direction.

Complications, Mistakes, and Dangers

- Wire cables must never lie over the ridge of the screw thread (danger of cutting!); they are well placed in a screw thread groove in an O-formation around the screws.
  Atraumatic surgery with loose cutaneous-subcutaneous sutures, skin clamps or Medi-Zip wound closure prevent problems relating to blood flow and infection, which easily occur in this area due to small skin-edge and soft tissue necrosis.

Post-operative Treatment

- Gradual weight-bearing with Aircast splints, in some cases with a brace with the foot in a well-made shoe.
- Patients for whom strain relief and partial weight-bearing is difficult, or where it is foreseeable that rules will not be observed during follow-up treatment, should be supplied with a below-the-knee support bandage for six weeks as a safety measure.

Results

Up to the end of 1995, 59 arthrodeses were carried out on the lower extremity, 16 on the knee, 25 on the upper and 9 on the lower ankle joints, and 9 tibio-calcaneal Pirogoff stiffenings.

▶ 21 cable arthrodeses were performed on the upper ankle joint (20 post-traumatic cases, one due to Morbus Charcot), the external fixator was only used 4 times. The post-traumatic cable arthrodeses were complete within six to eight weeks without any problems. The patients are pain-free and wear normal shoes with a

walking aid inserted. Imperfections in their gait are almost unnoticeable and their stride is not restricted. The single failure concerned the case of Morbus Charcot, which together with grotesque deformities of the skeleton of the foot results in gradual loss of sensation. No consideration was given to the patient having no feeling in the control of his weight bearing, which was allowed too early. Thus misalignment resulted with the formation of a large pressure sore. Using a fixator and a long period of strain relief the arthrodesis was finally successful.

Contemporary Alternatives and Conclusions

"To the experienced surgeon the problems occurring in a relatively high percentage of interventions on the upper ankle joint are well-known" says Niehaus in 1990 [278]. In fact the consolidation time often amounts to months, the non-union rate is set at up to 35% [85], and the rates of infection are high.

Diverse operating procedures are given for stiffening of the upper ankle joint – an indication that an optimal method is lacking. Basically the choice is between blocking through autologous bone chips without pressure (Campbell 1929) [57] and compression arthrodesis, which Charnley [48] first achieved with a fixator in 1951. At the present time it is also performed with screws and plates.

Blocking can no longer be recommended because its complication rate of up to 30% is much too high. According to Giolito and Grob [107], the consolidation period is on average 4.5 months with a range of 2.5–10 months. His patients were discharged on average after 7.5 months.

The fixator with variously shaped fittings is probably still the most frequently used procedure [19, 21, 50, 85, 122, 134, 152]. Infection rates from just 20% up to 80% in extreme cases [28], the fear of loosening of the pin, and the disability of the patient do not make it an ideal implant.

Muhr et al. [28] noted only 23% of patients as pain free after 4 months and 15 days, Jockheck noted only 37% pain free after 14 weeks. Cheng et al. [50] recorded wearing the fixator for up to 10 months (on average 5.6 months). According to Muhr, this is therefore only to be recommended for patients with severe soft tissue damage or complications of infection, an opinion with which we unreservedly concur.

Cancellous screws are said not to bring about such high compression as a well-placed fixator

[401]. They require, as they are not flexion stable, a below-knee walking cast for at least 8 weeks; after 10 weeks the arthrodesis should be complete, but the rate of loosening is 13%, amounting to 3 out of 24 cases; in 20% the screws broke; in osteoporotic bones they do not hold at all [134]. Niehaus and Staudte [278] claimed "56% serious complications with screw arthrodesis." On these grounds and because only 58% were free of pain – surprisingly, cited as a very good result [28] – we reject the screw arthrodesis. Even the recommended use of three (instead of two) screws [131], which record a higher compression in trials on cadavers [285], is biomechanically unconvincing.

Plates are rigid, compromising the thin soft tissue layer and have a rate of loosening of 30% [34]. According to Braly et al. [25] the arthrodeses were not complete until after 18 weeks. Nevertheless they were favored after stability tests on cadavers [74] (which do not reflect conditions in the living – cf. pages 46 and 64).

Information about arthroscopic stiffening techniques in ten cases is disillusioning: 30–80% nonunions, 50% recurrence of infections, and excessively long operating times [67, 131].

Konieczny [180] tried to by-pass talocrural arthrodeses from the start, instead keeping the joint able to function with a corium-interposition-plasty according to Lexer and Rehn; the Endo-clinic in Hamburg uses endoprostheses [358] under defined conditions.

An alternative could be the compression nail with which we have no personal experience however.

> It may be concluded that cable arthrodesis of the upper ankle joint is an elegant flexible procedure that, thanks to high interfragmentary compression by means of four cable tension bandings, shows an excellent rate of bony healing within a short time. It does not close (like rigid implants), does not encourage infection (like the fixator), and is extremely comfortable. Therefore, normal shoes may be worn shortly after the operation.

4.10.2
Pirogoff Amputation with Tibio-Calcaneal Cable Arthrodesis

Pirogoff, a Russian who studied in Berlin and Göttingen, presented an amputation through the tarsus in "Osteoplastische Verlängerung der Unterschenkelknochen bei der Exarticulatio des Fußes" (Leipzig, 1854). After removal of the talus it is performed as tibio-calcaneal arthrodesis. In our hospital it is performed almost exclusively on (diabetic) gangrene of the forefoot. This beneficial measure seems to have extensively disappeared today from surgical thinking.

Principle of Operation
A cable stretched *ventrally* between two screws together with the natural tension banding of the Achilles tendon extended by rotation of the calcaneus in the contact zone between tibia and calcaneus creates such high interfragmentary compression that the bony reconstruction can take partial weight-bearing after six weeks, provided that infection is successfully controlled (Fig. 122).

Advantages and Disadvantages
+ The greatest benefit of the technique described here lies in the projecting tread surface of the heel in the *unshortened* leg. With other techniques it becomes shorter [114, 406].

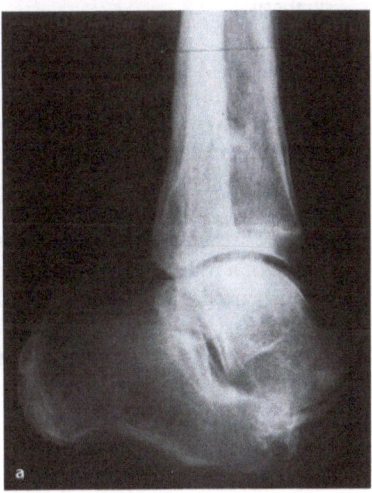

Fig. 122a–c. Principle of operation: **a** primary open Chopart operation in prevailing micro-angiopathy

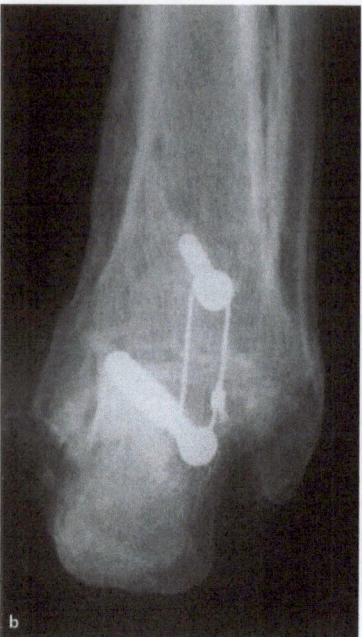
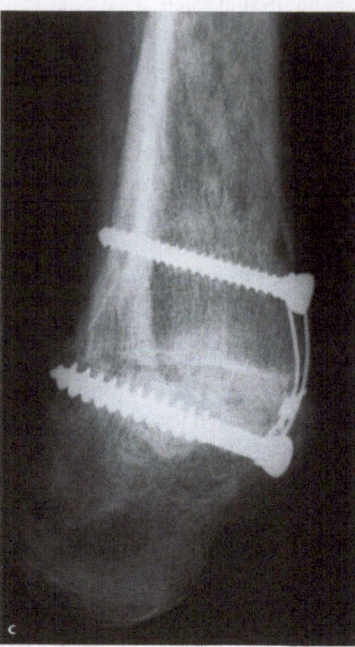

Fig. 122.b after infection control Pirogoff amputation; a.p. view; **c** lateral view

+ The optimal biological procedure as regards volume of material, which does not put additional strain on the precarious blood supply of a gangrenous foot.
+ Very comfortable, as the implant is not noticed.
+ Extremely cost-effective.
  There are no disadvantages as regards the osteosynthesis.

Indications and Contraindications

+ For the trauma-experienced general surgeon almost exclusively in the diabetic foot [114]. The micro-angiopathy presented here with open arcus profundus affects above all the peripheral third of the foot. Contrary to generalized arteriosclerotic ischemia this often allows peripheral amputation while preserving the tread surface of the heel, provided that one has decided on action at an early stage.
+ Reconstruction after traumatic midfoot amputation.
+ The neuropathic foot [406].
  Pirogoff's procedure is no longer successful if gangrene in the forefoot has spread as phlegmon to the hindfoot. Even in combined micro-macroangiopathy Pirogoff is not always successful.

Positioning

• Thermal mat, supine position, right and left side supports. Wash the leg from above the knee to the toes; cover to the middle of the lower leg.
• Foam rolls under the knee of the relevant side; the slight lowering of the opposite leg provides freedom of movement for the surgeon.

Instruments

• In addition to the cable instruments there should be on the table an electric drill, drill sleeves, thread cutters, screw measuring device, large cortical and cancellous screws, two pointed repositioning forceps, saws, chisel, and Hohmann retractors.

Operation Technique

• Usually a two-stage procedure: carry out border zone amputation in the region of the mid- or hindfoot with sufficient safety distance from the gangrene. The wound is rinsed several times daily with tap water. If the infection is controlled a Pirogoff intervention is carried out, otherwise the lower leg has to be amputated.
• Fish-mouth shaped incision which should preserve much of the heel and sole of the foot. It is

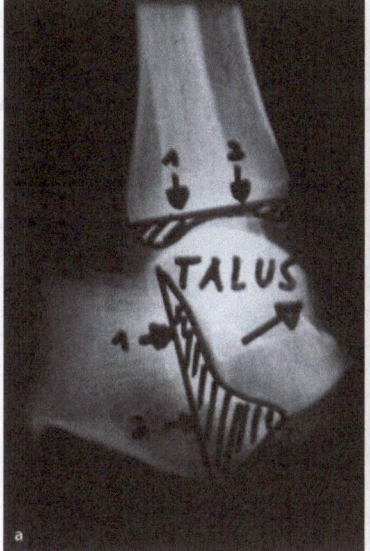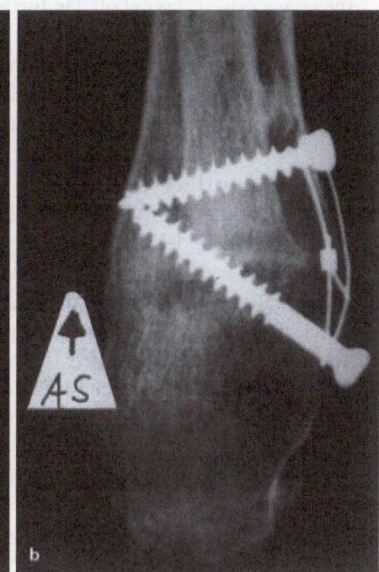

Fig. 123. (from [215]) **a** After removal of the talus and rotation of the previously sawn calcaneus, the bones fit together. **b** Ventral cable tension banding and the natural Achilles tendon tension banding produce relatively even compression in the osteotomy plane (first case, 1985)

made in one stroke as far as the periosteum. The longer flexor tendons are forcefully pulled out, cleanly cut through far above with a knife, and the cut ends of vessels and nerves are expertly dealt with. Deep preparation with the scalpel loosens the talus and separates it from the calcaneus (Fig. 123).

- After removal of the talus, the anterior soft tissue flap is pushed 3 cm over the tibia without lifting away the periosteum.
- The joint surface of the tibia is trimmed horizontally very sparingly with a saw.
- The calcaneus is prepared for arthrodesis by sawing the anterior joint-carrying portion of its neck at an angle of 20° to the vertical diagonally posteriorly upwards.
- The freshly prepared contact surface of the calcaneus is placed under the tibia using bone-gripping forceps laterally. This demands a certain force because on doing so the Achilles tendon is stretched at the same time. If correctly sawn the calcaneus is now positioned like the Leaning Tower of Pisa, inclined anteriorly at 20° to the vertical. This position creates a favorable heel appearance.
- A screw (2) is inserted approximately two finger-breadths above the tibial osteotomy transversely, or better still slightly diagonally upwards into the tibia and a further screw (2) at the same distance

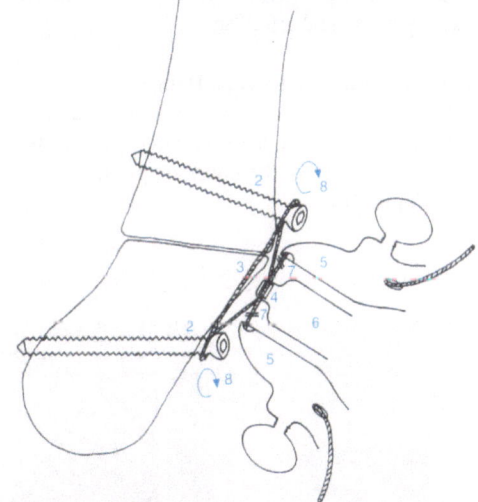

Fig. 123.c Operation technique

parallel to the sawn surface into the calcaneus. Both screws must perforate the opposite layer of cortical bone in order to give a better hold. After the bone surfaces have been positioned on top of each other, the screws lie horizontally or slightly divergently one above the other.

- One cable of suitable length (3) is looped around both screw heads, the crimp (4) is slipped over, and the cable tightened (5) until the arthrodesis has an absolutely firm hold. After squeezing (6)

the excess cable (7) is cut off. On further tightening of the screws (8) more tension is achieved.
- Bipolar point hemostasis, easy-flow drainage, small amount of loosely adapting dermal-subdermal sutures as far as the periosteum.

Operative Peculiarities
- There are no variations; one should keep strictly to this proven model. After the forefoot amputation patients feel better, local and general signs of inflammation recede, and the diabetes can be adjusted. But the infection is not always controllable. If it flares up again further surgery is immediately undertaken; in some cases the treatment according to Pirogoff may not have been in vain. Cable tension banding contributes by firmly pressing together the bone surfaces thus hindering infection.
- The skin incision is carefully planned so that the soft tissue flap remains well perfused and can be closed without stretching. Therefore, the incision must be deep right from the start.
- The single stage operation is only successful with a very peripheral infection.

Complications, Mistakes, and Dangers
- If too much is sawn off the calcaneus and/or the tibia, the Achilles tendon remains slack so that the surfaces of the osteotomy are put under only slight pressure.

- A calcaneus adjusted too flat or too steeply is less favorable for the prospective heel tread than the 20° angle.

Post-operative Treatment
- Slightly raised positioning in flat foam splints is suitable for venous drainage without hindering the arterial supply.
- Early stepping exercises without weight-bearing improve the circulation of the heel. If they are well tolerated, mobilization can soon be initiated with full weight-bearing from the sixth week. A stump shoe can be fitted relatively early. Later, if desired, a normal-looking fashion shoe can be ordered.

▶ Results
Of the total 48 amputations of the foot performed up to the end of 1995 (border zone, toes, Adelmann, midfoot), 9 were performed according to Pirogoff's technique. Five (55%) had complete bone healing, one case with secondary healing. These patients were very pleased that the leg had not been shortened; they can apply pressure painlessly and walk well. In fashion shoes the disablement is almost unnoticeable (Fig. 124). Four patients had to be operated on again with an amputation at a higher level.

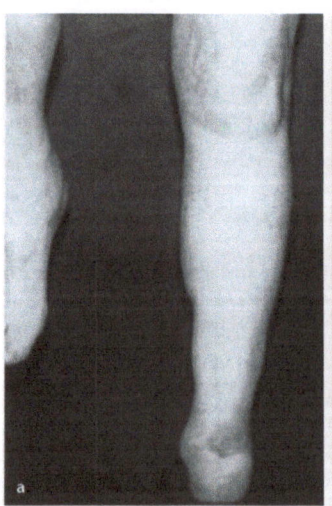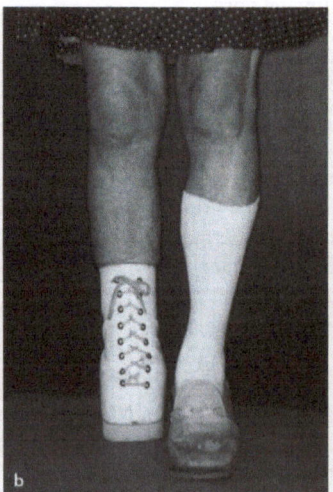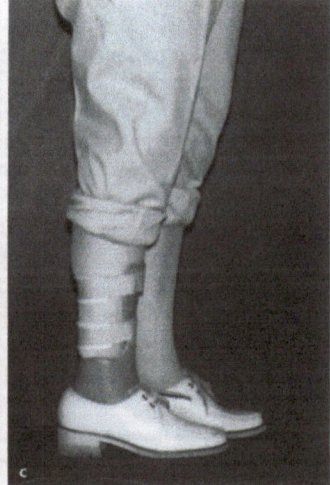

Fig. 124. (from [215]) Ideal result

Contemporary Alternatives and Conclusions

Pirogoff's procedure seems to be a forgotten method of reconstruction. There is hardly any current literature on the subject [406]. Amputations through the midfoot according to Lisfranc and Chopart or of the whole foot according to Syme are apparently rated more highly, or proximal amputation is primarily recommended [357].

▶ It may be concluded that Pirogoff's amputation with tibio-calcaneal cable arthrodesis is a resilient load-bearing amputation giving a very good tread surface to the heel. In some cases it spares the patient below-the-knee amputation. Standing on one leg as well as hopping on the stump is possible. The high compression of the contact surfaces due to the cable restraint increases the chances of successfully warding off infection and the low-volume implant does not impair blood flow.

4.11
Cable Cerclages

Historically, cerclage follows the first bone sutures. For more than a century this concept dating back to Berger [14] has been synonymous with loops placed around bones. In the years to follow, cerclage was used so frequently that it lent its name to the round wire used medically – cerclage wire. Before this there were many names that were in use for a long time: silver wire, aluminum-bronze wire, tempered iron wire, Vienna wire cable, piano-tuning wire, and Krupp wire [64, 223, 388, 395].

Vienna wire cable seems to have been used in a wire connection similar to "wire plate suture of the abdominal wall. The twisted Vienna wire is just about the worst bone material in existence" meant Kirschner in 1925 [167]. It was never accepted.

Nowadays cerclage is only used in exceptional cases. It is no longer an independent procedure but is effective in femur shaft repair during the fitting of a hip endoprosthesis or during prosthesis exchange [261].

Simple wire cerclage provides a fracture with only inadequate and usually not even adjustable support [44]. More can be achieved with tension cables. Wire cable cerclages can be used well as a restraint, provided the cables are squeezed together in free space.

In our clinic tension wire cerclages are used exclusively as emergency measures in hip endoprosthesis surgery.

4.11.1
Shattering of Femur Shaft Following Total Endoprosthesis

The frequency with which a femur shatters on introduction of the prosthesis undoubtedly depends to a high degree on the method of insertion. Anyone who drives the shaft of the prosthesis in with a hammer, whether it is a cement-free pressfit insertion or one using bone cement, will see this complication repeatedly. Since we have been accurately implanting CTS-prostheses with diamond precision reamers using Draenert and coworkers' [78] vacuum cement technique, this problem no longer arises. In prostheses exchange, the removal of the loose prosthesis only still held by friction, or of the cement casing via a sawn longitudinal gap or by reaming the femur, weakens the latter so much that it is necessary to strengthen it with wire cerclages.

The stable bone-implant connection is a conditio sine qua non for permanent anchorage of the prosthesis. Radial tension, which is encountered on implantation and during walking, is effortlessly absorbed by cerclage wires, so that partial weight-bearing is again permitted.

In addition to the special cable instruments one requires a renal peduncle crimp, a large Overholt clamp, or a hollow Dechamps, with which the cable can be directly fitted around the femur.

Principles and technique of operation are described in Chap. 4.2.

Operative Peculiarities
- The sawn out bone lamella is refitted.
- All cerclages are put on and squeezed tight prior to the implantation of the shaft. The cable tension selected is somewhat less than usual because the

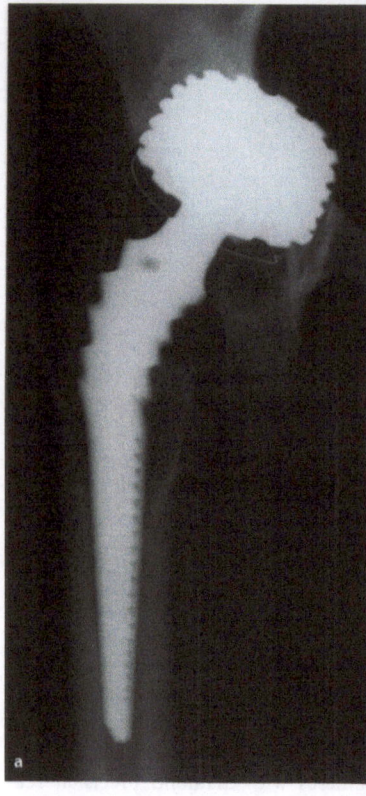

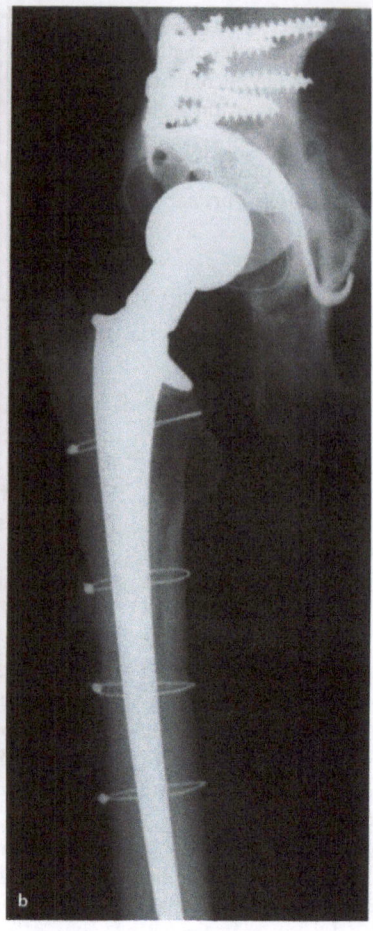

Fig. 125. Cable cerclage in prosthesis exchange

prosthesis shaft puts radial strain on the cerclages. Too much restraining tension could cause the
cable to break.

- All cerclages go around the bone at exactly 90 ° to
the longitudinal axis. This position corresponds
to the resulting forces. Placed on the diagonal in
an oval shape, they eventually adapt to this position and lose their tension.

- If after tightening a second cerclage the first becomes loose, it is renewed (Fig. 125).

▶ Results
Up to the end of 1995, 32 cable cerclages were
necessary during prosthesis exchange. The patients were urged not to undertake full weight-
bearing for the first four weeks. Cable breaks
and loosening of the shaft were not observed.

Contemporary Alternatives and Conclusions
As regards the stability of the femur after complications or in total endoprosthesis exchange, there is no
alternative to cerclage. It is most stable when performed with tension cables. Binding wires or metal
ribbons achieve only low radial strength. Iprenburg
(personal correspondence 1994) secured homologous cortical lamellae with cable cerclages on the femur with good results (Fig. 126).

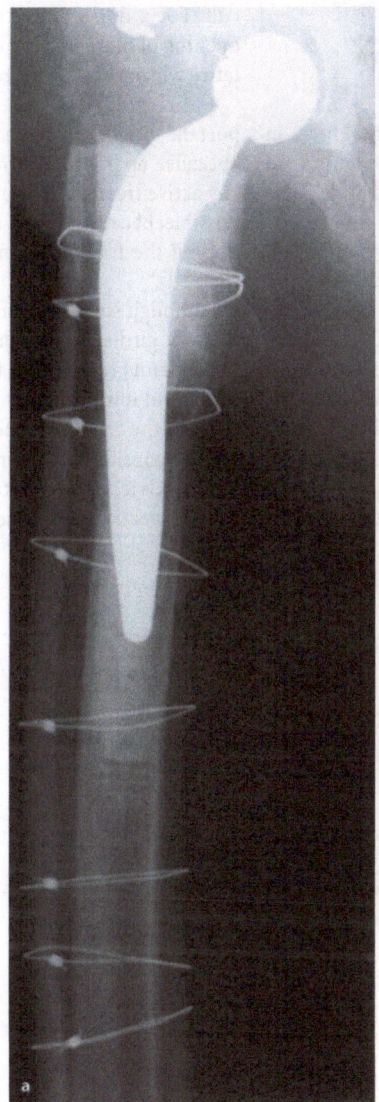
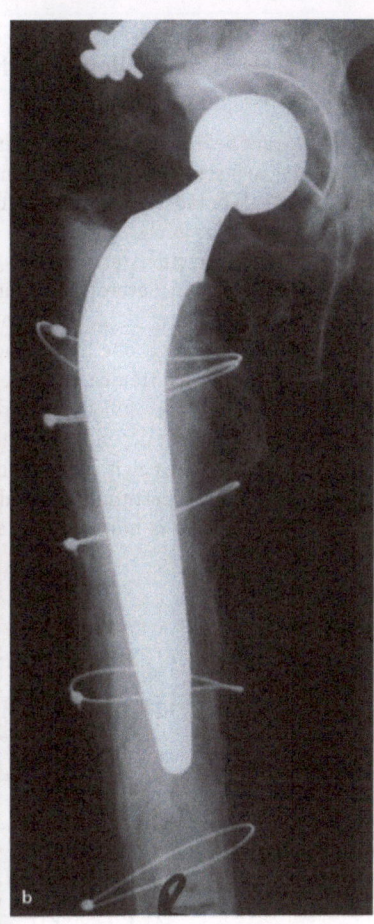

Fig. 126. Homologous strut grafts with prosthesis exchange and healing four years later. (Dr. Iprenburg, Assen NL, 1994)

Tangentially inserted screws are seldom practical and probably also less durable than cable cerclages. Plates, unsuitable proximally, are reserved for fractures in the distal third of the prosthesis.

According to Voorhoeve et al. [399] femur funnel nets prove successful in bone defects at the site of the prosthesis. Here even fragments can be well secured with cables.

▶ It may be concluded that cable cerclages are optimal for the stabilization of a weakened or fractured femur during endoprosthesis replacement. They keep it load-stable by means of high centripetal tension and give the prosthesis a secure hold.

4.12
Sleeve-Cable Banding of Unstable Pelvic Ring Injuries

When X-rays became routine procedure, Thiem in 1909 [378], in just under a year, "found no fewer than 8 detachments or loosenings of the symphysis pubis and the sacro-iliac joints."

Today pelvic fractures account for 3–8% of all those occurring [304]. Severe girdle injuries of types A-C according to Tile et al. [299] form a distinct minority of these, though one that is increasing because of speed-related trauma. All types can be unstable if the dorsal ring segment is severed on one or both sides. Nor does it depend on whether the rupture runs through the pelvic joints or the neighboring bony areas. The restitution of Malgaigne-type ligamentous injuries is however particularly diffi-

cult. For a dorsal break of continuity , symphysis opening of more than 2.5 cm has been shown, a distance which occurs arbitrarily.

For Leser [232] in Halle in 1904, it was still unimportant to have exact knowledge about the injury, "because apart from providing complete bed rest, any active treatment for pelvic girdle fracture is impossible; because there is no target point for repositioning the fragments and holding them in place correctly."

Although since then great steps have been made in pelvic girdle osteosynthesis, in 1996 Tscherne and Pohlemann [391] came to the conclusion: "Low incidence, but unsatisfactory results."

From the external fixator, which "could not fulfill expectations in the treatment of translationally unstable pelvic girdle fractures" [304], an acknowledged spectrum of osteosynthesis ranges from

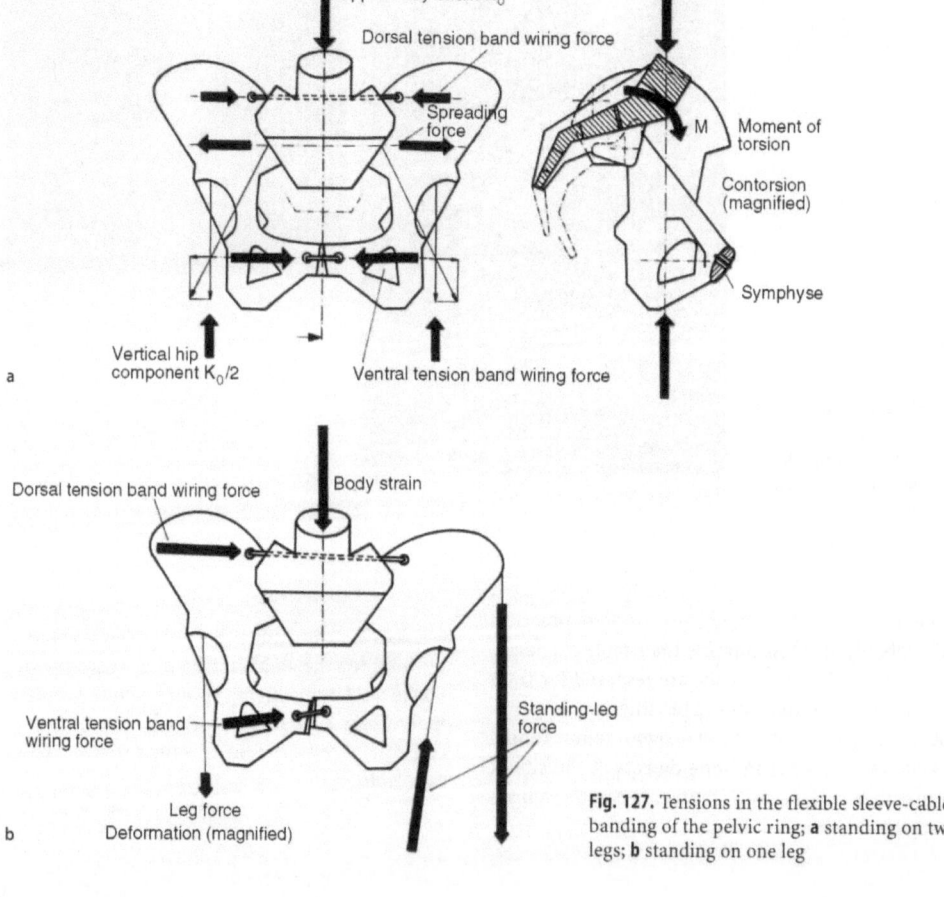

Fig. 127. Tensions in the flexible sleeve-cable banding of the pelvic ring; **a** standing on two legs; **b** standing on one leg

transarticular immobilization of the pelvic dorsum using screws through to plates or the internal fixator [88, 158, 269, 325, 346, 386] to wire banding or tying with PDS cords of the symphysis and sacro-iliac joints [82, 156]. In 1986, flexible sleeve-cable banding was introduced by the author [210].

The pelvis is a ring in three parts, which move three-dimensionally against each other under load [117]. The principle of functional unity of the lumbar spine, pelvis, and hip joints, referred to by the au-

thor because of its central significance in the kinetic chain of the human skeleton as the "central movement segment," stands for tension neutralization by means of controlled distortion [204]. It is fulfilled by a series of anatomical details:

1. The three-part form which exists thanks to an articulation of both ilia with the sacrum.
2. A useful adaptation of the sacrum that is operated on and held by strong ligaments and opposingly inclined joint surfaces, and *twist-*

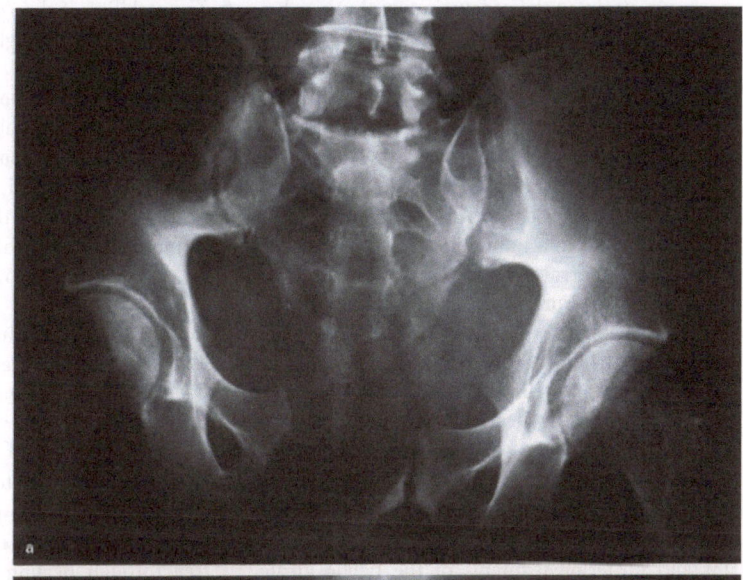

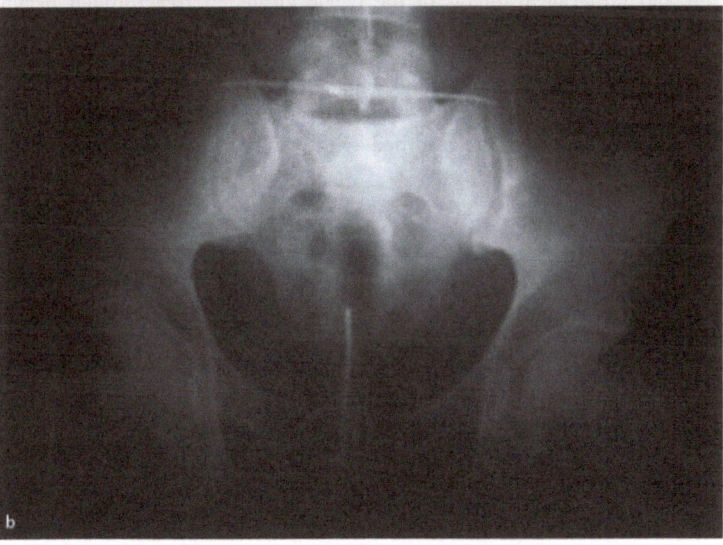

Fig. 128. Principle of operation. Open-book-lesion with ligamentous symphysis and sacro-iliac joint rupture

ed by means of the load provided by the trunk. It does therefore *not* function like the keystone of a Romanesque vault. Such an element pressed in place by weight would have no shock-absorption properties.

3. A number of ligaments and muscle groups working synergistically and antagonistically, which convert and divert the pressure exerted on the pelvis from the body weight and acceleration into tension.

Meißner et al. [253, 254] determined the resulting maximum strain on the cadaveric symphysis as being 398 N in the vertical direction and 148 N in the sagittal direction. These results are looked upon by the author as too low for the living.

The rupture of this ring connected by synchondrotic ligaments cancels out pelvic girdle tension and disrupts the kinetic forces. All therapeutic procedures which lead to a immobilization of the pelvic girdle have left themselves open to the biomechanical criticism on working against "the pelvis as a three-dimensional gearbox, a swing with the task of neutralizing the vibration" declares Teubner [373]. Flexible sleeve-cable banding is biologically as well as mechanically ideal because it avoids such stiffening.

The banding effect of cables for the symphysis and the sacro-iliac joints using the two dorsal iliac spines creates a flexible interplay between the anterior and posterior segments of the pelvic girdle [210]. This technique is very efficient in contrast to PDS-cords and other methods using wires [82, 254].

When standing on one leg and when walking, spread effects and vertical shifts, which arise due to the weight of the trunk, are absorbed by the cables (Fig. 127).

Principle of Operation

The sleeve-cable bandings of the symphysis and the sacro-iliac joints, performed in a single session, holds the pelvic girdle together *flexibly* and thereby preserves the physiological stimulus which promotes the healing of the torn capsule ligaments. The polyethylene sleeves are not X-ray opaque (Fig. 128).

Advantages and Disadvantages

✚ The operation is performed in one session of anesthesia, unlike in other procedures where often two sessions are required [88, 325, 386]. The trauma is very limited because it is the upper surface of the body which is worked on. Damage to nerves and vessels is – in contrast to transarticular screwing and plating – not observed.

✚ The operation can be carried out in an emergency. Temporary fixator is not advisable.

✚ Loosening and infections, which are a disadvantage of plates and fixators [88, 303, 373], do not occur.

✚ The stability of the "pelvisynthesis" is high, so that early partial weight-bearing using a walking frame is allowed.

✚ Material removal is not required.

✚ The dorsal wire cable running transversely through the back musculature does not cause pain. The procedure is, in contrast to the fixator, very comfortable for the patient, something that cannot be valued highly enough.

– No disadvantages known.

Indications and Contraindications

All unstable ruptures and fractures of types A – C, open-book-lesions, and isolated symphyseal ruptures with a gap below 2.5 cm. It does not always require ventro-dorsal stabilization, occasionally anterior or posterior tension is enough.

✚ The operation is also practicable when it comes to older cases, because walking can become pain free through healing of the torn ligamentous structures.

– There are no contraindications. The primary restoration of the pelvic girdle is vital because of the threatening danger of hemorrhaging (Fig. 129, 130).

Positioning

• At first a supine position for the treatment of intrapelvic abdominal injuries and symphysis rupture.

• After ventral treatment and sterile dressing, turn to pronate position. Shave, disinfect, and cover anew.

Instruments

• The special cable instruments are supplemented with self-tapping polyethylene sleeves 10 – 18 mm in length. Additionally there should be on the table an electric drill with 3.5-mm bits, drill sleeves, and a large-lumen venous catheter for threading the cables and passing them through the sleeves.

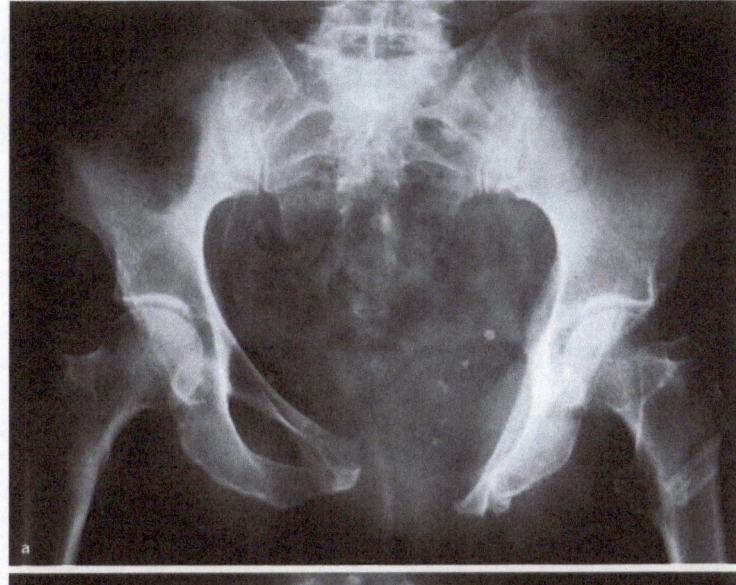

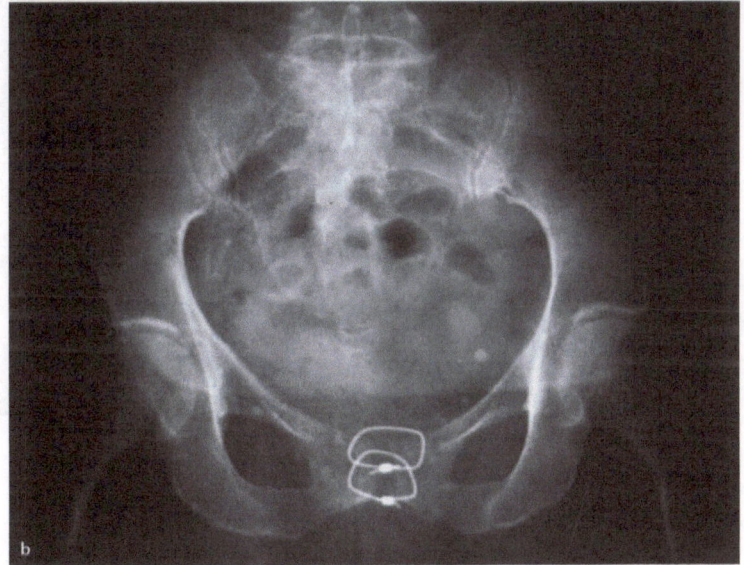

Fig. 129. Indications. Single symphysis banding: the posterior segment of the pelvis is not really unstable. Early weight-bearing and pain-free healing

Operation Technique

- Regarding the technical part – inserting the sleeves and threading the cables – see Chap. 4.2.3.

Symphysis

- Pfannenstiel's incision on the superior edge of both pubic bones. After separation of the subcutaneous fat tissue the opened symphysis lies free. It is cleared of coagulations and impacted tissue.

Now locate the pelvic bones and expose them up to approximately 3 cm.

- Two bore canals are drilled right and left, approximately in the middle of the symphysis and at a good distance from its edge, from the outside to the inside or the reverse with a 3.5-mm bit.
- After determining the length, a self-tapping sleeve is inserted in each one.

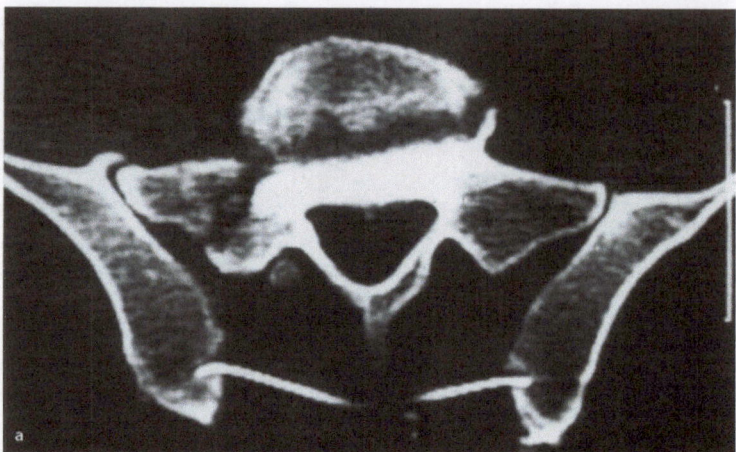

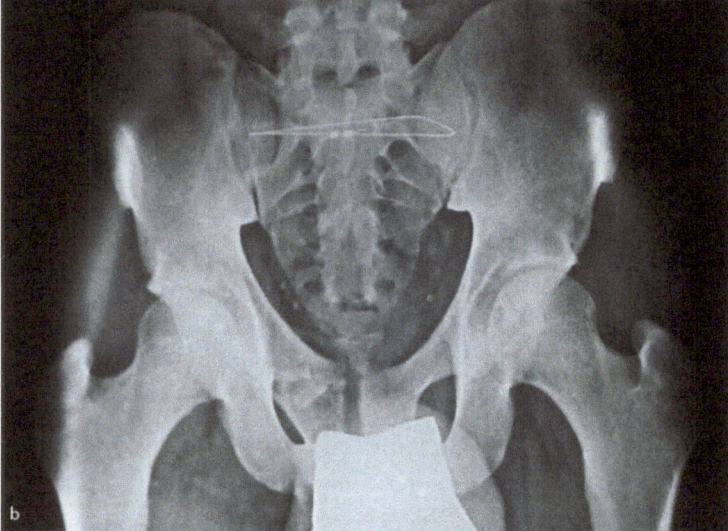

Fig. 130. Indications. Banding only of the posterior segment of the pelvis on post trauma day 17. From the sixth post-operative day "walking with full weight-bearing without the slightest pain."
(After primary treatment of a bladder rupture severe back pains were encountered on attempting mobilization, the cause of which could not be determined on X-rays. Only much higher resolution CT showed the injury (here already treated). Note the cable supported on a spiny process and anchored in both spinae by means of PE sleeves. (Prof. Dr. Scheuba, Wetzlar, 1986))

- A roughly 25 cm long wire cable is now threaded directly through one sleeve and a venous catheter through the other. Into the latter at a comfortable distance *in front of* the symphysis the cable is threaded and both are pulled from the inside to the outside through the second sleeve.
- The crimp is then slipped over, tightened until the symphysis cartilages touch, squeezed, and the excess cable cut off.
- The ligaments and periosteum are adjusted with sutures, one or two deep Redon drains are inserted, and the wound is closed. Compression dressing with Fixomull.

Sacro-iliac Joints
- The patient is turned pronate and the pelvis and upper thorax are padded with foam cushions so that breathing is made easier. The incision runs from one spine, following it downward for approximately 3 cm, transversely over the sacrum to the other spine and then upward. By means of this dish-shaped incision, which is similar to a very wide flat U, both iliac spines are well exposed. After reaching the periosteum, the musculature is pushed medially with a curved raspatory.
- Then, using a 3.5-mm bit, a bone canal is drilled straight through each spine laterally to medially,

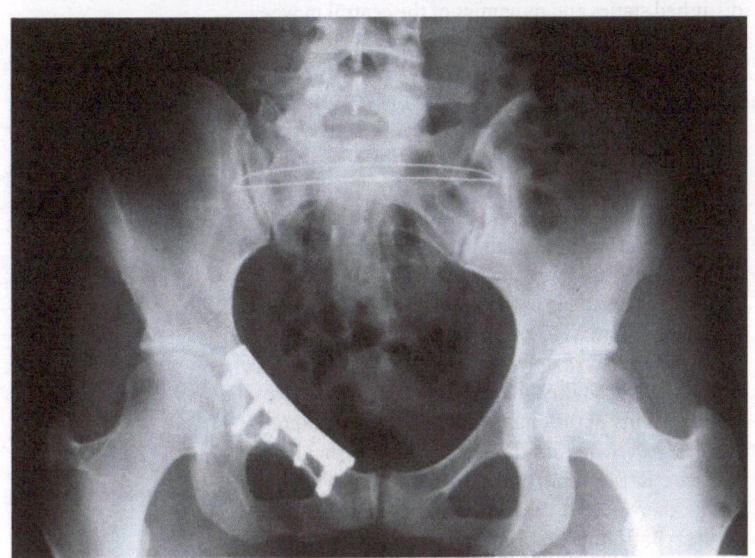

Fig. 131. Combined osteo-synthesis

the self-tapping sleeves are inserted, an approximately 30 cm long cable is threaded through one sleeve laterally to medially, guided with the straight awl parallel to the sacrum through the back extensors to the opposite side, and threaded, again with the help of the venous catheter – medially to laterally through the second sleeve. The rest is routine.

> Note: The dorsal stretch of cable lies without pressure on the fascia of the back extensors without irritating them, the internal one, crossing the muscle, rests on a spinous process – occasionally visible radiologically.

Operative Peculiarities and Variations
- Urethral, bladder, and intra-pelvic injuries as well as bleeding are immediately dealt with on opening the site. The closing of the open-book-lesion helps to staunch venous hemorrhaging by tamponade.
- Repositioning of the symphysis and sacro-iliac joint is made easier with two assistants working under the sterile cloths who push the pelvis together from the side. The prominent half of the pelvis is easily repositioned by forceful traction on the leg because the dislocation is still quite fresh.

- In mixed bone-ligament pelvic rupture sleeve-cable banding can be combined with a plate (Dr. Walter, Emmerich, 1987) (Fig. 131).

Complications, Mistakes, and Dangers
- So that the symphysis is held together evenly, the tension banding must encircle it in the middle as far as possible. If it is too far towards the upper edge of the pubic bone the symphysis opens in a reverse V-formation below. That makes its load-bearing healing difficult.

Post-operative Treatment
- Intensive care.
- As soon as possible, early partial weight-bearing in a walking frame, otherwise passive hip movements in bed.

Results
Up to the end of 1995, 22 Malgaigne injuries of the pelvis were treated with sleeve-cable banding. Some of the patients were operated with colleagues, Dres. Scheuba (Wetzlar), Schretzmair (Hamm), Walter (Emmerich), Kramer, Schneider-May, and Richter (Dortmund), to whom this procedure had been demonstrated.

The complex pattern of injury makes judging the results difficult. Some of the consequences cannot be attributed to the reconstructed pelvic girdle, others however can. This group includes the cases of disturbed statics and dynamics of the central movement segment, the most important connection between the trunk and the extremities. Chronic lumbago and symphysis pain are always due to instability and excessive movements between the three pelvic bones under strain. They are practically resistant to therapy. Therefore, the restoration of the flexible pelvic girdle is an essential aim of the treatment. With regard to determining what sleeve-cable banding achieved for post-operative load-bearing capacity, all contactable patients were further checked or consulted and all X-rays examined.

Six patients were polytraumatised. There were 15 cases of full instability and 7 cases presented particular instability of the anterior or posterior segment. Besides severe to life-threatening hemorrhaging, which occur as a result of the bursting of the venous plexus, there were 12 cases of damage to intra-pelvic organs. Both these conditions made immediate treatment obligatory.

▶ In 19 cases an anatomical adjustment had been primarily achieved, in which the distance between the symphysis bones did not exceed 0.5 cm. These patients have no complaints. In three cases it widened to a maximum of 1 cm which causes localized complaints and premature tir-ing after lengthy walking. Peri-symphysis calcification was encountered three times, severe in two cases – cf. Fig. 112 – without causing pain; in one case an infection, later healed, with osteomyelitis of the pubic bones contributed to bowel, urethral, and bladder rupture. The sleeve-cable banding had to be removed prematurely. The now 54-year-old farmer is able to continue in his job.

In the first patient, an obese 18-year-old motorcyclist, the symphysis cable had broken. He had been operated on in May 1982 with metal sleeves made for sternotomy closure. In one, the cable had worn through. This experience was what prompted the introduction of softer polyethylene sleeves. After having new tension cables and PE-sleeves inserted he recovered without pain (Fig. 132).

Contemporary Alternatives and Conclusions

Stabilization of the pelvic girdle with rigid osteosynthesis materials is still standard practice. However one should consider that transarticular plates immobilize the symphysis and sacro-iliac joints and temporarily stiffen the mobile pelvic girdle. When this happens not only is its shock absorbing func-

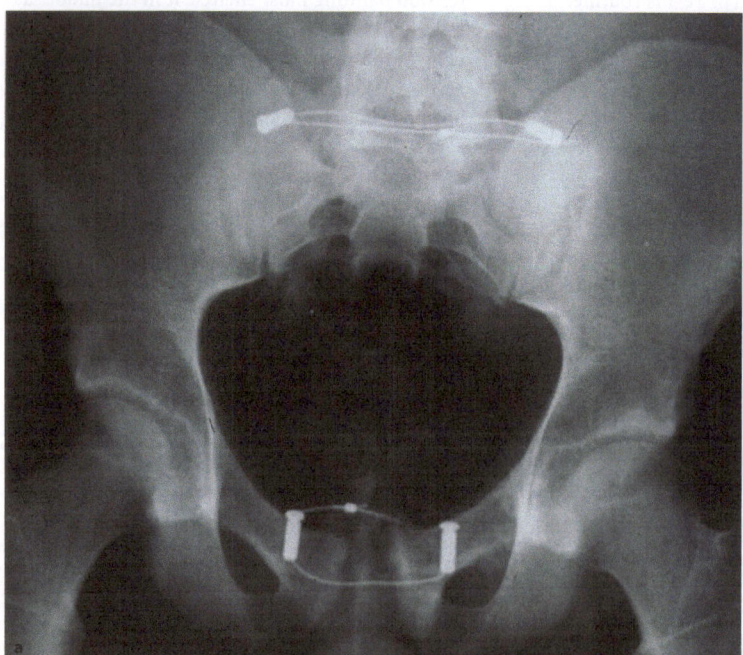

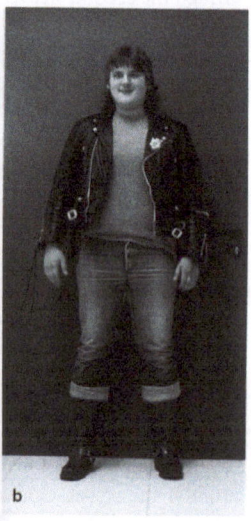

Fig. 132. Optimism after a full recovery

tion for the skeleton eliminated, but the healing of the ligaments is also delayed. This requires limited tension-loading as a physiological stress, which inflexible implants prevent [210, 373]. After metal removal, the remaining instability of the joints of the pelvic girdle therefore often leads to therapy resistant pain in the sacral region and symphysis [88, 299, 304, 325]. In addition, there is the fact that these osteosyntheses are not easy from a technical point of view; specific injury patterns for nerves and vessels are inherent.

Dorsal positioning of screws and plates for fixation of the sacro-iliac joints and "plate osteosynthesis of the superior pubic ramus requires time-consuming access with preparation of standard windows for separating the structures that run ventrally" writes Trentz [386]. The shearing and thrusting forces that occur can lead to loosening of the screws, as is clearly demonstrated on X-rays [354].

In order to eliminate stiffening of an osteosynthesis, special symphysis and sacro-iliac joint plates with tension banding effect have been developed [373].

Symphysis wire tension banding dates back to Jungbluth [156]. Ecke [82] bridged torn amphiarthroses with wire or PDS-cords. These procedures are, however, biomechanically advisable because they do not stiffen the pelvic girdle. Unfortunately the traction material used is not up to the job [438], so that the high surgical expenditure is not worthwhile.

In 1998 Meißner et al. [254] investigated the stability of the cadaveric symphysis in a dynamic walking simulator. Dynamic and reconstruction plates achieved primary stability of the symphysis only in non-osteoporotic bones, in other cases the screws came away. This led to a clear *surpassing of the physiological limitation of movement* of the symphysis. This condition also clinically observed as painful hypermobility is the expression of a *post-osteosynthetic* instability of the pelvic girdle, which is underestimated and positively assessed as *"approaching anatomical reconstruction"* [88].

Triple tension banding with a 1 mm thick wire around 4.5-mm cortical screws loosened according to Meißner due to breaks of one or more of the cerclage wires; with 2-mm PDS cords not even sufficient initial stability could be measured. Therefore he rejected this procedure.

The external fixator made popular by Slätis and Karaharju 20 years ago [359], should today only "be applied as a temporary therapeutic solution" [373]; it has been seen to be inadequate [303]. Despite that it is still used. "Type B injuries react well and can be stabilized best with a simple anterior fixator" [325].

Good results have been achieved using the internal fixator, in particular for vertical-shear-lesions [158].

The problematic nature of chronic pain after operative stabilization of the pelvis is clearly described in the following statement of Tscherne et al. [304]: "Out of 486 patients, 47% of type A injuries and 75% of type C had slight to severe pain with proportionally shorter stride length." We consider this as criteria for pelvic girdle stability only approximately restored. It also shows however that concepts of pelvic osteosynthesis must be further adapted to the physiology of pelvic girdle movements. Sleeve-cable banding may be a step in the right direction.

Continuing analyses – according to Tscherne – are necessary to clarify "whether possible causes of pain and disability can be surgically influenced."

> ▶ It may be concluded that the ventro-dorsal sleeve-cable banding of Malgaigne's ligament rupture and comparable unstable bony injuries is a convincing flexible "pelvisynthesis" which does not stiffen the pelvic girdle, but stimulates healing of the ligaments via quasi-physiological movements. It safely absorbs the strain that the symphysis has to withstand during weight-bearing whilst standing on one leg and during walking [403]. Partial weight-bearing exercises are therefore possible very early on, provided that other aspects of the injury allow it.

4.13
Sleeve-Cable Osteosynthesis of Longitudinal Sternotomy

Longitudinal medial sternotomy makes possible the opening of the thorax via the mediastinum. The prime reason is open-heart surgery; the thoracic surgeon reaches mediastinal tumors and the general surgeon is occasionally forced by an oversized intrathoracic growing goiter to perform at least an upper sternotomy. Whilst the longitudinal incision of the sternum with the Codman saw presents no difficulties, osteosynthesis of each of the two halves of the sternum is laden with different problems. These result on the one hand from the cancellous structure, which is particularly weak in elderly and osteoporotic patients, and on the other hand from the strains accompanying breathing and the distraction of the osteotomy, which arise at each inspiration and with every cough or are initiated by artificial ventilation. The cancellous bone, surrounded only by a delicate layer of cortical bone, offers hardly any resistance to the rigid osteosynthesis material (Fig. 133).

These well-known complications are still reported [281]. At least 15 operative procedures have become established which are very similar to each other and are mostly variations of cerclage [208, 209].

What begins initially as a split can lead, via increasingly separating softening of both halves of the sternum, to a deep infection and in the worst situation to mediastinitis. How often a successfully completed heart operation ends in complications or even death is difficult to ascertain statistically because a cardiac patient is sent back to his local hospital within a few days of the operation.

At the start of the 1980s sleeve-cable closure of the sternum was used together with Reidemeister in the Cardiac clinic Essen, at first for infected dehiscence, but later became routine. Despite the safety of the method, it has not been widely accepted, possibly because cardiac surgeons rarely see the above-mentioned complications or because they do not like working with electric drills and screwdrivers.

> Both halves of the sternum are compressed evenly by means of three to four transosseous pairs of cable guided through sleeves (Fig. 134).

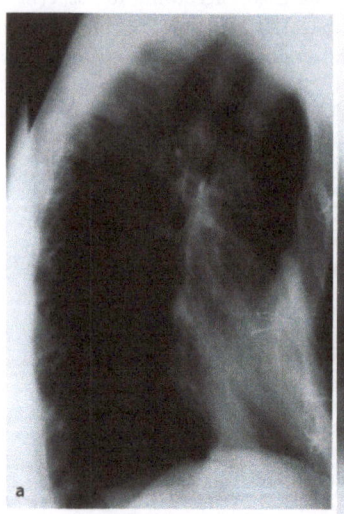
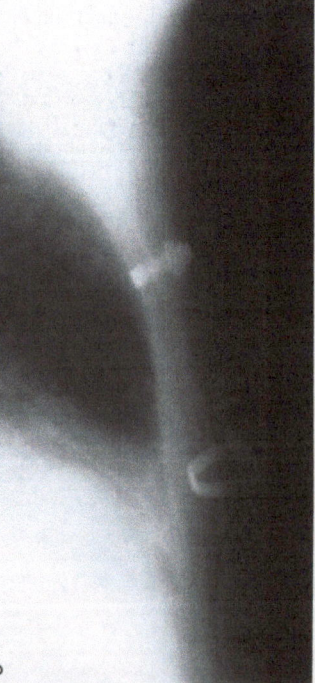
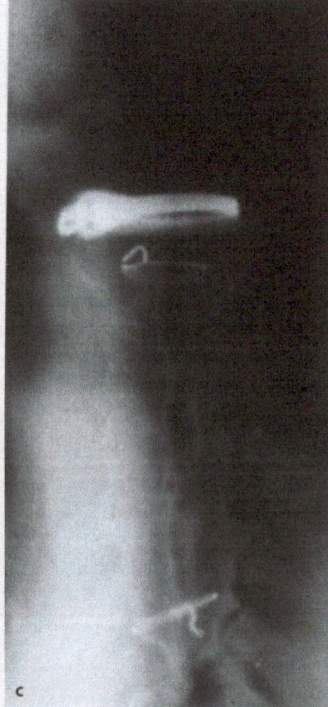

Fig. 133a–c Complications following conventional closure. Three different cases (**c** with mediastinitis)

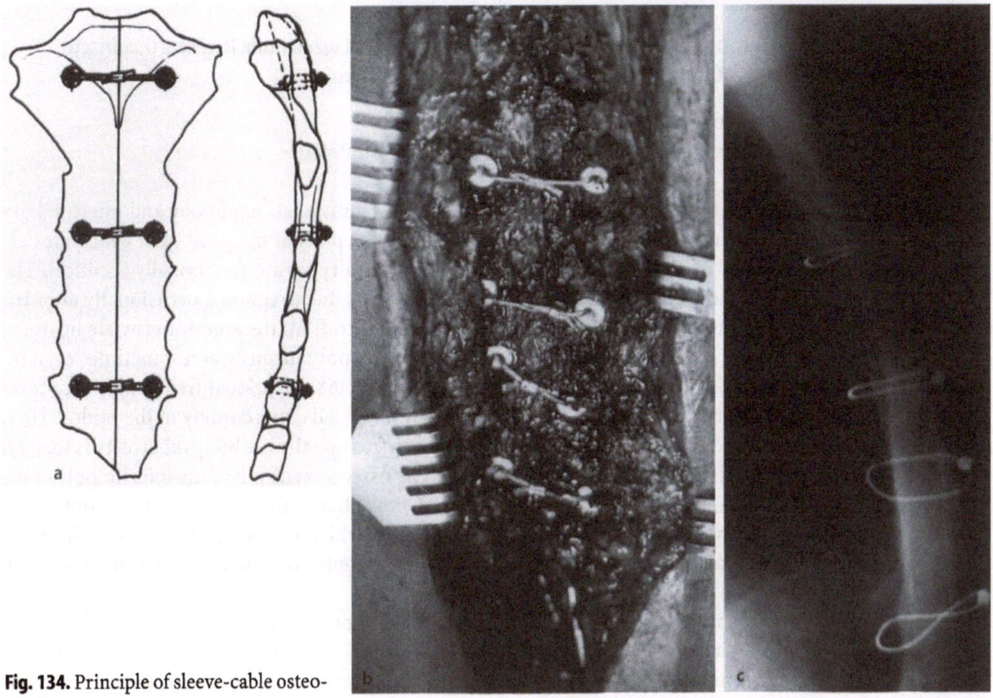

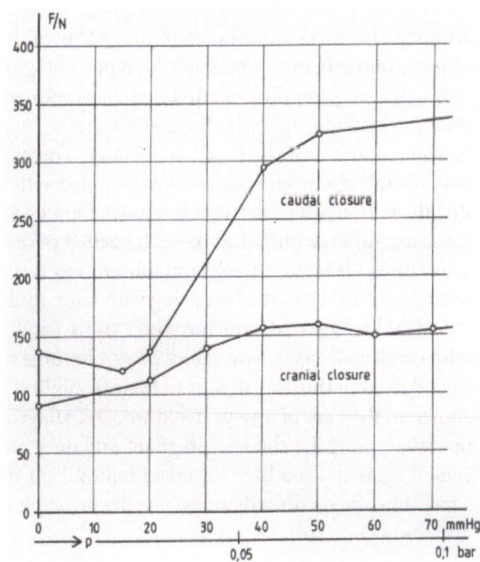

Fig. 134. Principle of sleeve-cable osteosynthesis

Fig. 135. Distraction forces on the osteotomized sternum of a cadaver dependent on the force of artificial ventilation

The V4 A cylinder sleeves used in the beginning were soon replaced with self-tapping polyethylene thread sleeves which are not radio-opaque. Their external diameter is 5 mm. They are screwed into 3.5-mm bore canals as near as possible to the lateral edge of both sternum halves. So that the drill cannot pierce too deeply, it has a cut-off mechanism which acts as a stopper.

Together with Witzel in 1986, dehiscence tension forces were measured using stretch measuring strips on the sternum of an artificially ventilated cadaver. Up to 330 N was recorded, particularly distally. Coughing leads to peak loading, which can result in tearing off the sleeves if the bone is porotic. Therefore the individual sleeve-cable units should only be put under enough tension to establish easily visible contact along the whole length of the osteotomy. This is recognized at the point when no more blood exudes from the gap (Fig. 135).

▶ Over 50 patients were treated at that time by this method, of whom one-third had infected dehiscence after wire and steel band cerclage [208]. The procedure would be worth re-establishing with simplified instruments.

4.14
Soft Tissue Trauma – Temporary Protection of Ligament Sutures Using a Cable

A tear of the quadriceps tendon, the patellar ligament, the cruciate ligaments, and the Achilles tendon still produces problems, as can be verified from numerous experiences, for which up to now no ideal solution has been found. Thus variations of a standard procedure consisting of suturing the torn structures and providing additional protection are common. Besides still commonly used plaster casts, special movement-limiting splints have become popular. They are expensive and relatively uncomfortable. The ligamentous and tendon structures that lie around the knee are not well treated with splints as no rigid flexion axis exists here, but rather one which passes through a hyperbolic-wandering hinge movement [268]. For some ligament tears internal protection is favored, achieved with a wire cable. To be optimal it has to be firmly anchored in soft tissue and if possible be absorbable so that a second intervention – however posing few problems under local anesthetic – can be omitted.

In securing the ruptured patellar ligament and in tears of the inferior pole of the patella there is no better procedure than securing with cable [328]. The high tensile strength cable protects the suture admirably, is not disruptive, and allows plaster free follow-up treatment. The characteristic fatigue breaking of conventional wiring is not observed with correct use.

For quadriceps and Achilles tendon ruptures, conditions are not so favorable because the fixation of the proximal end of the cable in soft tissue cannot be as firm as in bone.

Even temporary protection of the cruciate ligament with cable is physiologically favorable. It protects from stretching of the graft during the recovery phase [24] and prevents subsequent arthroses.

4.14.1
Rupture of the Ligamentum Patellae, Quadriceps, and Achilles Tendon

4.14.1.1
Ligamentum Patellae

Indications for operation of bony and intermediary rupture of the patellar ligament exist widely; for assessment both types are functionally identical. The ligament tears due to trauma, occasionally after the removal of a graft for the anterior cruciate ligament [404], rarely spontaneously and sometimes even bilaterally [187, 368, 385]. Most frequently it ruptures beneath the patella, more rarely in the middle [194] and very occasionally the bony tuberosity is torn off [30]. The osseous avulsion of the inferior pole of the patella is probably the most frequent continuous break [194], which is actually not included here but under the patella fracture and is treated by osteosynthesis.

Different non-absorbable and absorbable sutures are described including reinforcement with the Leeds-Keio-Band and PDS cords, usually with the protection of wire loops and immobilizing bandages [99, 186, 187], as well as assistance with autologous tendons [225] and even an external patello-tibial transfixation with a rotating fixator [110]. Securing with wire however has the disadvantage of breaking almost routinely in an extremely high percentage of cases. Träger [385] documented a vivid example of double-sided multiple wire breakage. Cerclage wire is rigid and becomes fatigued through constant small bending movements beyond the range of flexible distortion after relatively few movement cycles [104, 300] often within the six-week healing period. Therefore at least four weeks immobilization is recommended in the case of securing with wire. Rudig et al. [328] secures the suturing with a trans-patellar wire cerclage. Tensile wire cables do not become fatigued used in this way thanks to their flexibility, as shown in the case of a 32-year-old woman, who was operated on whilst she was pregnant and only presented again 4 years later for metal removal. At the same time the pictures demonstrate the principle of operation (Fig. 136).

> **Principle of Operation**
> The distance between the patella and the tibial tuberosity is maintained by a peri-patellar cable that is attached to two screws on the tibial head and which does not cross over the ligament. The

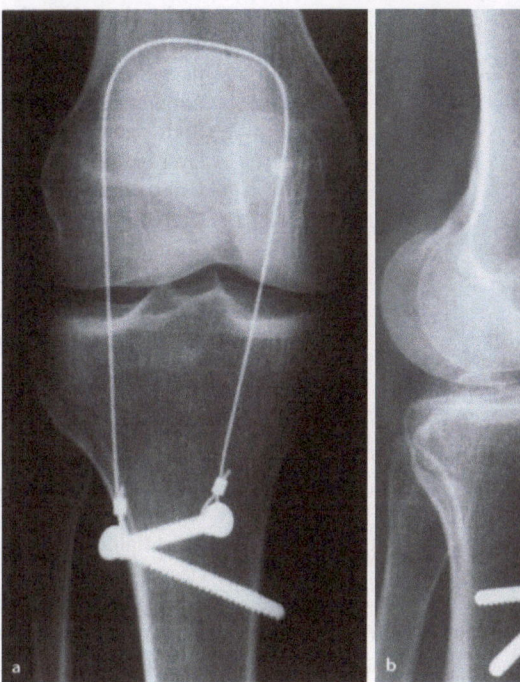

Fig. 136. Principle of operation. Cable modification of McLaughlin's technique. No cable break 4 years postoperative

screw fixation of the wire on the head of the tibia dates back to McLaughlin and Francis [251]. We treat the bony rupture in the form of a tear of the inferior pole with distally-crossed bilateral patellar tension banding, which holds the fragments together well, and with additional cable tension banding.

Advantages and Disadvantages

+ Safe protection of the suturing with free flexion to 90°, no immobilizing bandages or splints.
+ The cable running parallel to the ligamentum patellae interferes with neither the latter's sutures nor with its blood flow.
+ Correctly placed cables do not break.
+ Metal removal can be performed under local anesthesia above the two screw heads or under an epidural if desired.
− There are no disadvantages regarding this procedure.

Indications and Contraindications

+ Every rupture, bony and ligamentous, has to be treated surgically; there are no contraindications.

Positioning

As for patella fractures – see Chap. 4.5.

Instruments

• In addition to the special cable instruments there should be on the table an electric drill and cortical screws. For this indication 50 cm long cables with an end loop are supplied, which one could also prepare oneself.

Operation Technique

• A straight incision from the tuberosity to just above the superior edge of the patella next to or above the ligament exposes the site of the tear. Normally the injury is not limited to the ligament. The torn anterior joint capsule is sutured first. Then the cable is put on and the ligament treated (Fig. 137).
• A cortical screw (2) is first of all inserted through the cable loop and then screwed downwards slightly obliquely next to the tuberosity into the head of the tibia so that its head just touches.
• The cable (3) is guided with the curved awl through the middle of the quadriceps tendon directly around the upper circumference of the pa-

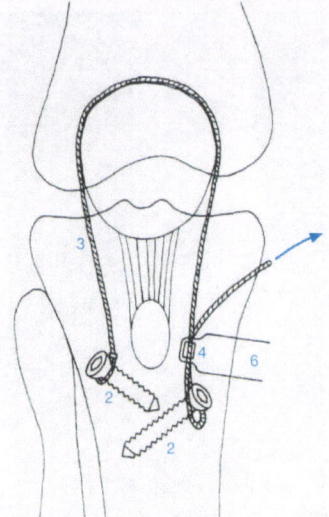

Fig. 137. Operation technique

tella and on both sides of the tendon as far as the tibial tuberosity.

- On the other side another cortical screw (2) is inserted next to the tuberosity.
- The ligament is sutured with the lower leg in the extended position.
- With the free cable end, a loop is formed using a crimp (4) and put around the head of the second screw. Now the crimp is gently gripped with the crimp pliers (6) and guided up to the head of the screw, still without squeezing it. The free cable end is pulled by hand – the cable tensioner is not applied – and tightened just so far that the suturing remains without strain up to 90° knee flexion. This is tested by repeated extensions and flexions between 0° and 90°.
- Only now is the crimp squeezed directly next to the head of the second screw and the excess cable cut off. Finally both foundation screws are firmly tightened.

Operative Peculiarities and Variations

- With simple ligament ruptures the joint does not need to be opened.
- The bony polar avulsion is first treated with bilateral tension band, where the cables cross over beneath the pole – cf. Fig. 73, and is additionally secured in the way described with a cable. Schretzmair also anchored cables to a patella transverse screw (personal correspondence, 1987), as did Rudig et al. [328].

Complications, Mistakes, and Dangers

- The superior pole of the patella should be encompassed around the middle so that the patella is not unnecessarily tilted.
- Both screws must include the opposite cortical layer of the tibia; a short one would come away.
- Using one straight screw, a cable loop was anchored in one of the thread grooves. It loosened during post-operative treatment. Since then we have been using two screws.
- The second loop pulled through by hand has to be narrow so that it does not come off the head of the screw. Washers are not favored as they could wear through the cable.
- The cable must not, under any circumstances, cross the tibial head in a bore canal; it would cut into the bone and become loose.
- A crossed cable damages the ligament.
- "Post tightening" was once tried using a thin cerclage wire after a cable was found to be somewhat loose. After three months it naturally wore through; the ligament had healed. The inferior very narrow polar avulsion had been refixed using atypical cable tension banding (Fig. 138).

Post-operative Treatment

- Positioning on flat foam splint. Electrical movement splint from day two. Sitting up to 90° knee flexion and early walking with two crutches is permitted from the second week with increasing weight-bearing. Climbing stairs and squatting remain forbidden for six weeks.

4.14.1.2
Quadriceps Tendon

Typically the quadriceps tendon tears slightly above or directly at the edge of the patella. Often it also partially involves the secondary extensor apparatus. Trans-osseous suturing, also augmented with PDS cords or a Leeds-Keio polyester band, is usually protected for six weeks with immobilizing bandages or movement-limiting orthotics. This is considered necessary on the one hand because the suturing has only slight hold in the fibrous tissue and because extension of the lower leg requires considerable expenditure of strain. We try to relieve the strain on it with a cable which is pulled transversely through the patella and proximally guided on the inside of the quadriceps in a pear-drop shape. There it is held in the extended position under gentle tension directly on the tendon reflector over a stopper with a crimp.

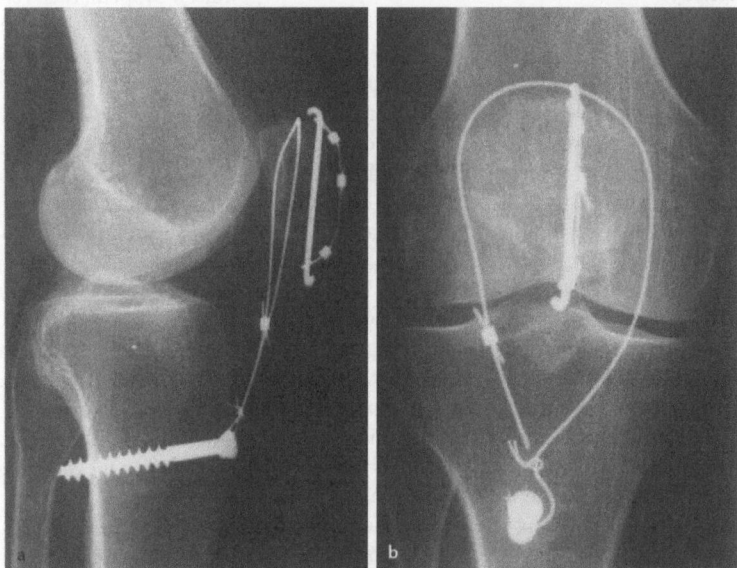

Fig. 138. Cerclage wire notch effect caused cable breaking

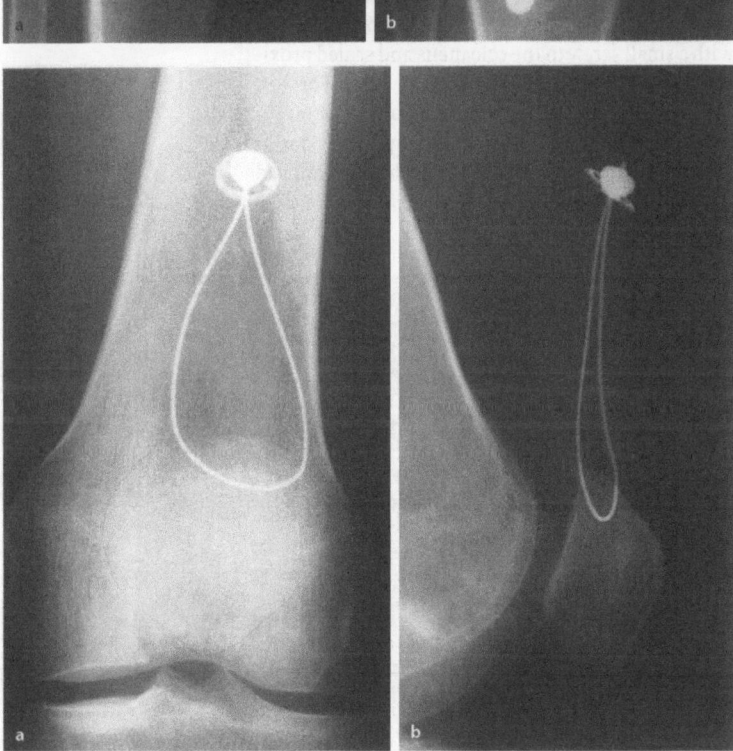

Fig. 139. Quadriceps tendon rupture in an amateur footballer in whom both Achilles tendons were also torn a few months earlier and who had been treated with cable augmentation

For this purpose at present we use a plastic washer for the large cancellous screw in which we put a grooved screw head which the sealed-in cable cannot slip out of. An improvement is being worked on.

For three weeks a split plaster cast is worn, during which time electrical splints are used to practise flexion between 0° and 60°. Re-mobilization with voluntary weight-bearing (Fig. 139).

4.14.1.3
Achilles Tendon

A sign of the worldwide enjoyment of sport, Achilles tendon rupture is encountered more and more frequently. Correspondingly, many methods of treatment are in use. Different suture techniques [47, 229], strengthening with the patients own plantar tendon, PDS-weaving [98, 374], and plastic therapy with reversal of the tendon reflector [424], with autologous corium [372] and the flexor hallucis longus tendon [405] are now in competition with the long favored conventional functional therapy of Anglo-American and Scandinavian specialists [236, 376]. Our own operating team is able to choose freely the type of treatment which allows us to compare these various methods objectively. Irrespective of the individual suture technique – if available, the plantar tendon is woven in and stuck with Fibrin – a cable may also be introduced to make a core, fastened with a small screw to the calcaneus and sealed proximally over the tendon reflector on a washer. For this, the cut off grip of the piston of a 20-ml plastic syringe is used. Until wound healing, apply dorsal splint in the pointed foot position, which is removed for movement exercises. After that the heel is raised by 4 cm, then reduced to 2 cm in the fourth week and after a further month is completely removed. Temporary partial strain relief by means of crutches until the gait is sure again. Orthotics are not prescribed in cable augmentation (Fig. 140).

Results

Up to the end of 1995, 26 ruptures of the knee extensors and 54 Achilles tendons were treated surgically. At the knee, the patellar ligament was affected 19 times and the quadriceps tendon 7 times. In 4 cases the ligament had intermediate tears, 7 cases directly at the inferior pole of the patella, and 8 cases with bony involvement (as a distal pole fracture); the quadriceps tendon was always torn immediately at the superior pole. The Achilles tendon usually tears just above its insertion on the calcaneus and is usually very frayed.

4.14.1.4
Ligamentum Patellae

▶ The 11 purely ligamentary tears healed after securing with cable without loss of function or decrease in the circumference of the quadriceps. The results of the eight distal fractures of the patella were included in Chap. 4.5.

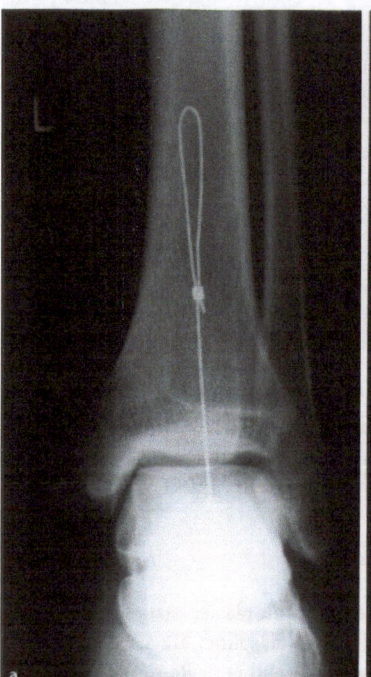
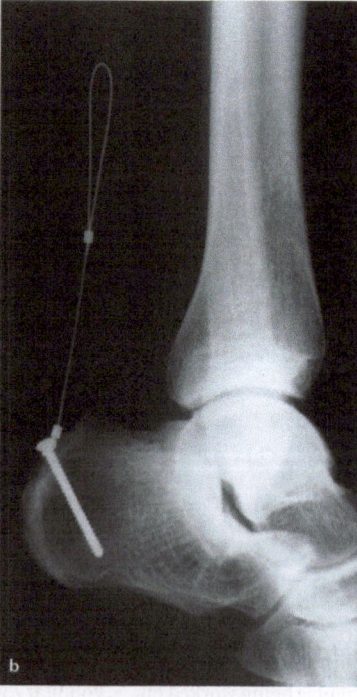

Fig. 140. Temporary protection of the Achilles tendon with a doubly anchored wire cable

4.14.1.5
Quadriceps Tendon

▶ Six quadriceps ruptures healed without problem, without functional loss, and without lasting reduction of the muscle girth. In one case a flexion deficiency in wasted thigh muscles required extensive outpatient physiotherapy.

4.14.1.6
Achilles Tendon

▶ Out of 54 Achilles tendon tears, 36 were augmented with cable that was removed again after 3 months via 2 minimal access points; 28 cases were operated on without using cable and treated for 8 weeks with pointed foot orthotics.

The results of both groups are equally good; obstructive functional loss was not found. The cables however are felt to be especially pleasing because uncomfortable external aids become dispensable; metal removal (under local anesthesia) is not a deterrent. The procedure is very economical and is especially suitable for the young and active patient.

Contemporary Alternatives and Conclusions

The suturing of the ligamentum patellae is generally acknowledged as unavoidable as is its temporary protection by some means of additional strain absorption [251, 328]. Rigid cerclage wires break [385], prolonged resting periods result in immobility-induced illness, and are no longer standard practice. The bridging joint fixator [110]or other minifixators [226] may relieve the strain on the sutures but have all the disadvantages of fixators; they are uncomfortable and expensive. Securing with cable, which can be fastened to two bones – the patella and the head of the tibia – produces an optimal procedure. It makes an early start to post-operative treatment possible without danger. Cable breakage is not observed even in excessively long-lasting implantation; in one case over four years, the single exception was caused by surgical error.

Clearly, in quadriceps and Achilles tendon tears unfavorable conditions are present. Unfortunately there is only the possibility here of anchoring the augmenting strain absorber osseously on one side. In the region of the tendon one tries to strengthen by means of weaving techniques using PDS cords or fine wires [229] or to protect the suturing by six weeks' immobilization [311]. We lock the proximal end of the cable on an artificial stopper directly on the tendon reflector. Results show that the cable is acceptable to patients owing to comfortable, early functional post-operative treatment, which is free of plaster and orthotics. Here load-bearing, soluble material – mass produced – would be an ideal implant.

Achilles tendon tears can also be treated without internal augmentation as the results of work using suturing and orthotics and conventional concepts [236, 375] show. These procedures are however less comfortable and very expensive.

▶ It may be concluded
1. that the McLaughlin augmentation of a ruptured patella ligament with a cable is without competition. The cable resists fatigue fractures for a long time
2. that in quadriceps and Achilles tendon ruptures cables are a compromise. They could better be substituted by resorbable strings like PDS-cords.

4.14.2
Rupture of the Anterior Cruciate Ligament: Treatment According to Weigand

In 1990, Weigand [414] performed "temporary post-operative securing of the anterior cruciate ligament using a trans-articular wire cable". This is his answer to the unresolved problem of protecting the reconstructed cruciate ligament from stretching and lengthening during the recovery period by unrestrained thrust and rotation forces. During this time the loadability of the transplant proportional to the reduction in circumference of the newly-formed collagen fibers is reduced by 40% [24]. Extension of the cruciate ligament during healing is the starting point on a slowly developing vicious circle, which results in secondary damage as a consequence of disintegration of the rolling-gliding movements in the joint [268]. The immensely important transmission function of the cruciate ligaments cannot be taken over by other ligament structures of the joint capsule. The over-taxed dorsal parts of the meniscus tear, and the shearing movements lead to cartilage damage and end in a late arthrosis. A cable parallel to the anterior cruciate ligament running trans-articularly over the top and fixed to the femur and tibia prevents the elongation of the cruciate ligaments

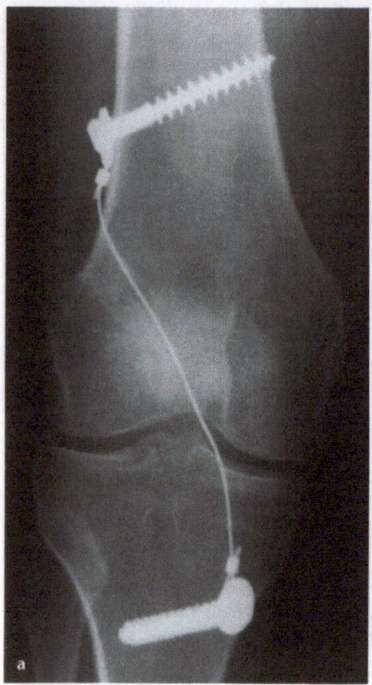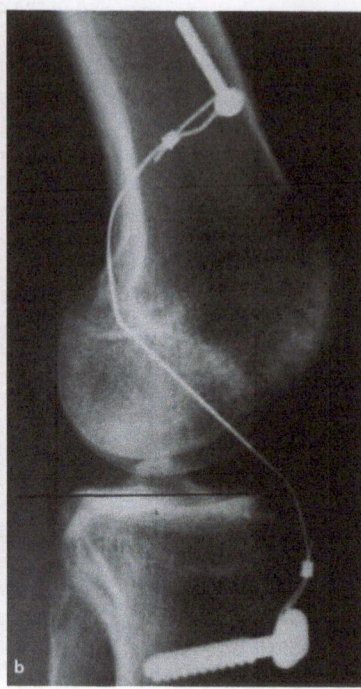

Fig. 141. Weigands' cable augemntation for the reconstructed anterior cruciate ligament (b from [414])

during healing and permits early functional postoperative treatment without negative effects on the graft. The pre-operatively positive Lachmann test becomes negative when using a cable, as shown in Fig. 141. Weigand considers it important that the cable does not go through the bone, "but is placed in the region of the lateral femoral condyle as well as on the tibia, exclusively on the upper surface of the bone. In this way the cable is prevented from becoming too long in relative terms, as a consequence of resorption processes in the bone, thus losing its protective effect."

The distal insertion of the anterior cruciate ligament lies some 10–15 mm posterior to the cable fixation point on the anterior side of the tibial head. In a legal argument the author was reproached that because of this the biomechanics of the cruciate ligament had been disturbed. A simple model proves that this is not the case: the hinge movement of the knee joint guided by means of the wire cable does not lengthen the distance in any position between the origin and insertion of the cruciate ligament. Weigand also clinically refuted such an assertion: of 144 patients operated on in this way he carried out a follow-up on

50. According to the Lysholm Score 37 patients were classified as very good, 8 as good (90%), 3 as satisfactory, and 2 as poor. The radiologically measured Lachmann test which showed an average pre-operative measurement of 12 mm, had been normalized to 5 mm after removal of the cable.

Ihara et al. [144] explained that this could also be achieved conventionally with the Kyuro knee brace because "it minimizes abnormal sagital deviation between the femur and the tibia."

▶ In 86 patients operated on in our clinic according to Weigand's proposal similarly good results were obtained, which are also confirmed by Sellmann and Walter (personal correspondence 1992 and 1996).

However in 1993 the trend towards arthroscopic intervention forced the abandonment of his method. In the meantime, however, we have rejected unprotected reconstruction because cruciate ligament elongation was observed during the recovery phase. An arthroscopic version of the procedure, an improvement of which we are working on, seems to be clinically as successful as the open technique.

4.15
Special Indications

Here examples of applications for cables will be demonstrated which are not found in the daily routine of orthopedic trauma surgery, but which have been performed approximately 100 times. In some cases the cable is the icing on the cake (for example in axis correction), occasionally it helps to master a surprisingly unusual situation (for example in the thorax and knee joint or temporarily in osteosyntheses). From time to time it is the final resort in tumor surgery.

Colleagues with other operative spectra have provided further indications for cables. Kluger (personal correspondence 1992, [173]) straightens the spinal column and stabilizes non-unions of the odontoid peg; Blömer, Walter, and Weigert (personal correspondence 1985 and 1997) wire up acromio-clavicular joint dislocations with different techniques [351]. Baumgart et al. [11] and other authors [310, 331] lengthen limbs; Iprenburg stabilizes the femur with homologous cortical lamellae – cf. Fig. 126; Hertel et al. [438] refix the tuberculum majus with our cables to shoulder prostheses. Weigand et al. [414] have demonstrated cruciate ligament protection.

Some procedures have been abandoned again because they did not prove reliable or because they have become obsolete due to improved techniques. Secondary collapse of a straightened vertebral compression fracture using dorsal sleeve-cable banding could not be prevented. Here the internal fixator has proved to be most successful. Only two out of four knee-joint cable arthrodeses recover free of complications and we have returned to the external fixator. But the ventral compression of cable tension banding is still preferred to the tent construction. The interlocking nail has made open procedure with cable cerclage of oblique fractures and flexion wedges superfluous, but there are exceptions. Very frequently acromio-clavicular joint dislocation is repaired with cable using the AO procedure. In our clinic it has been replaced by Hahn's process plate, which is undoubtedly best [260] (Figs. 142–155).

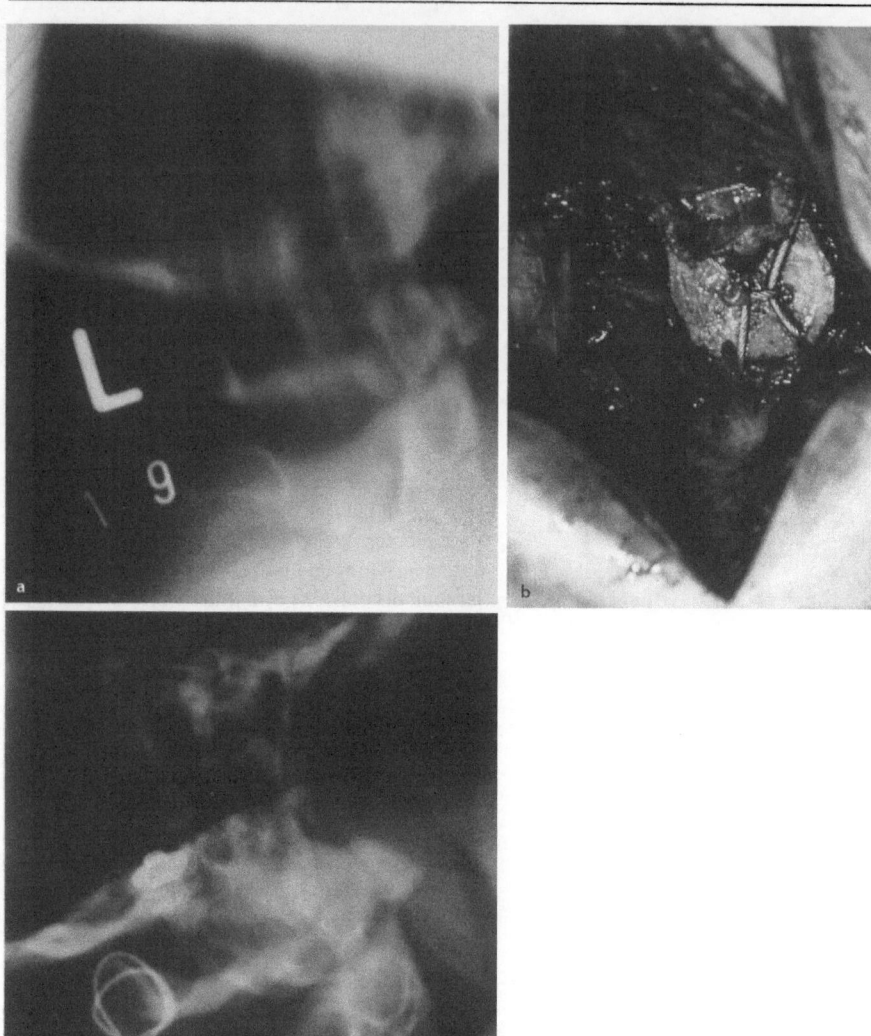

Fig. 142. Non-union of the odontoid peg: dorsal fusion with a fitted cancellous block and cable tension according to Brooks-Gallie (Dr. Kluger, Ulm)

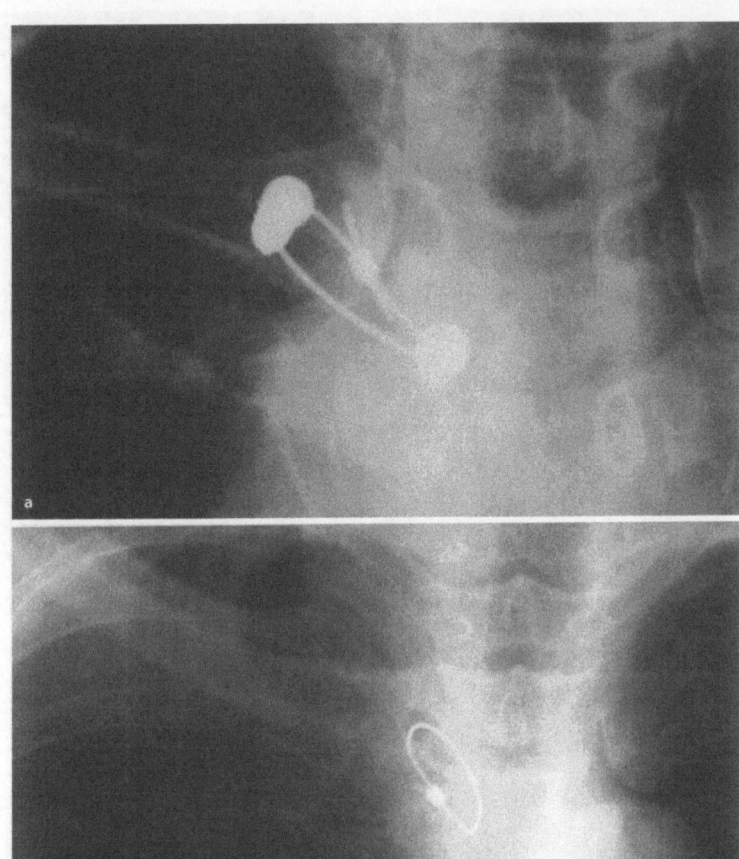

Fig. 143. Rupture of the sterno-clavicular joint. Sutured and secured with cable tension banding using: **a** two screws; **b** non radio-opaque polyethylene sleeve-cable tension in the clavicle and sternum. Implant removal not required

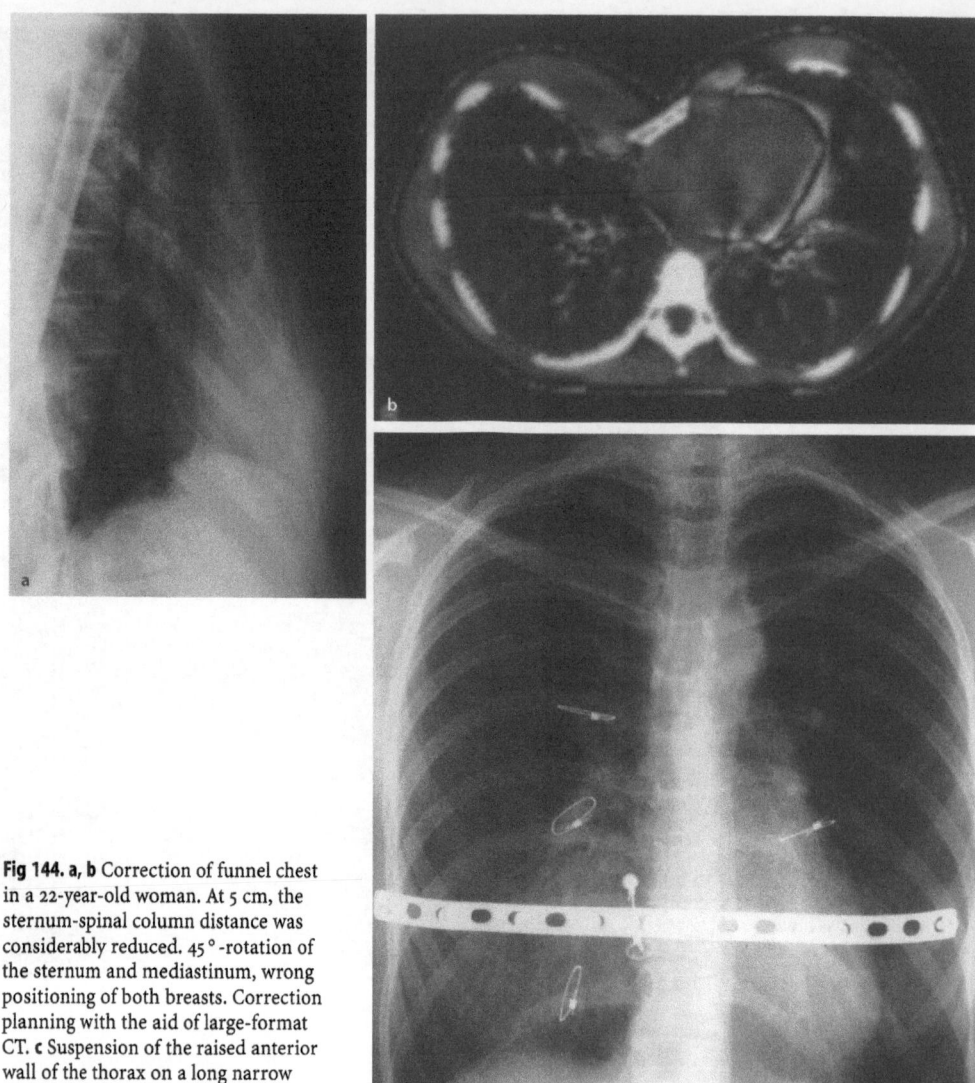

Fig 144. a, b Correction of funnel chest in a 22-year-old woman. At 5 cm, the sternum-spinal column distance was considerably reduced. 45 ° -rotation of the sternum and mediastinum, wrong positioning of both breasts. Correction planning with the aid of large-format CT. **c** Suspension of the raised anterior wall of the thorax on a long narrow plate. Some osteotomized ribs were held together with polyethylene sleeve-cable osteosyntheses; the sleeves form a firm foundation for the cable in the soft rib cartilage

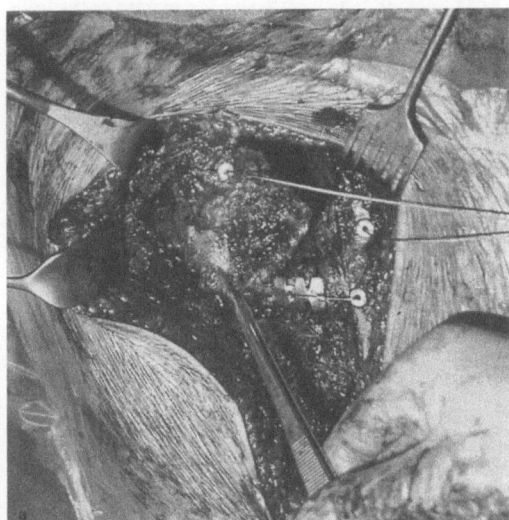

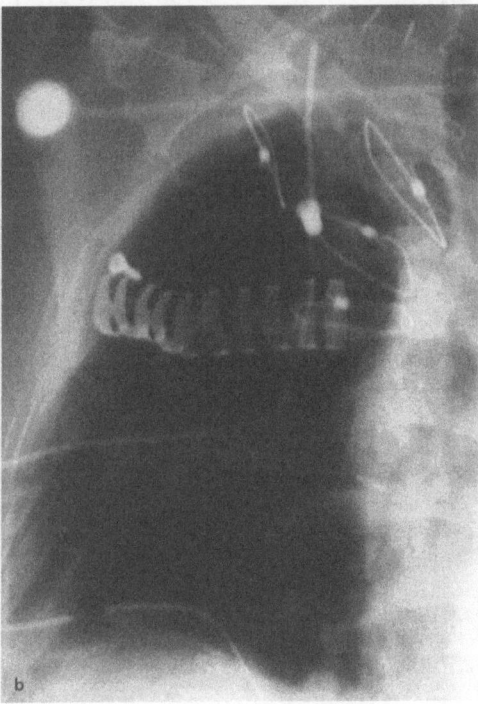

Fig. 145. Thorax trauma with rupture of the entire sterno-clavicular joint and the first rib; rupture of the first and second sterno-costal joints, fractured second to fourth ribs. Readjustment of the sterno-clavicular joint which is maintained by means of sleeve cable tension as are the first two ruptured rib joints (a metal sleeve lies at the chondral end of the second rib, the polyethylene sleeves are only indirectly recognizable from the straight course of the cable). Stabilization of the fracture of the second rib with flexible rib clamp [201]

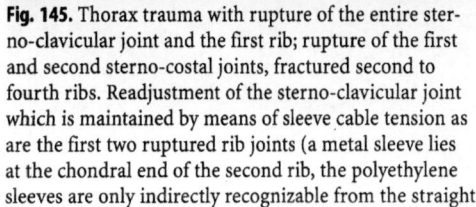

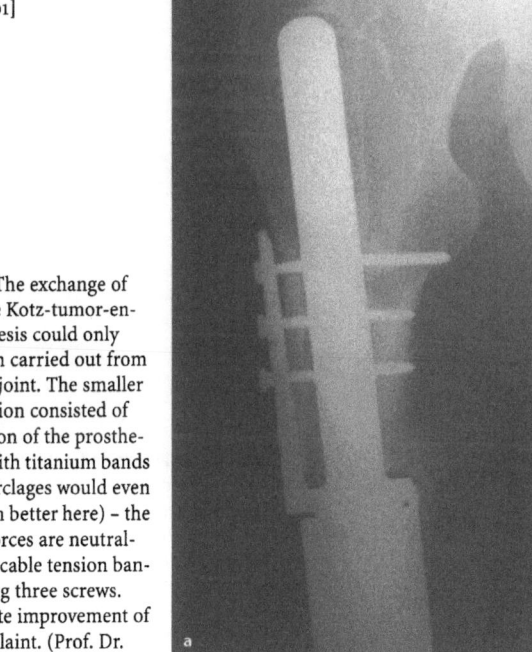

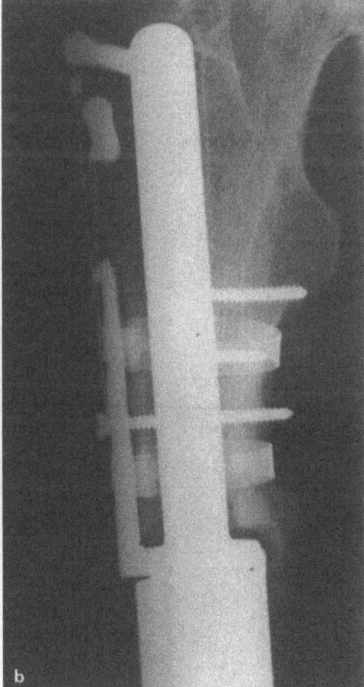

Fig. 146. The exchange of this loose Kotz-tumor-endoprosthesis could only have been carried out from the knee joint. The smaller intervention consisted of the fixation of the prosthesis flap with titanium bands (cable cerclages would even have been better here) – the flexion forces are neutralized by a cable tension banding using three screws. Immediate improvement of the complaint. (Prof. Dr. Becker, Volmarstein)

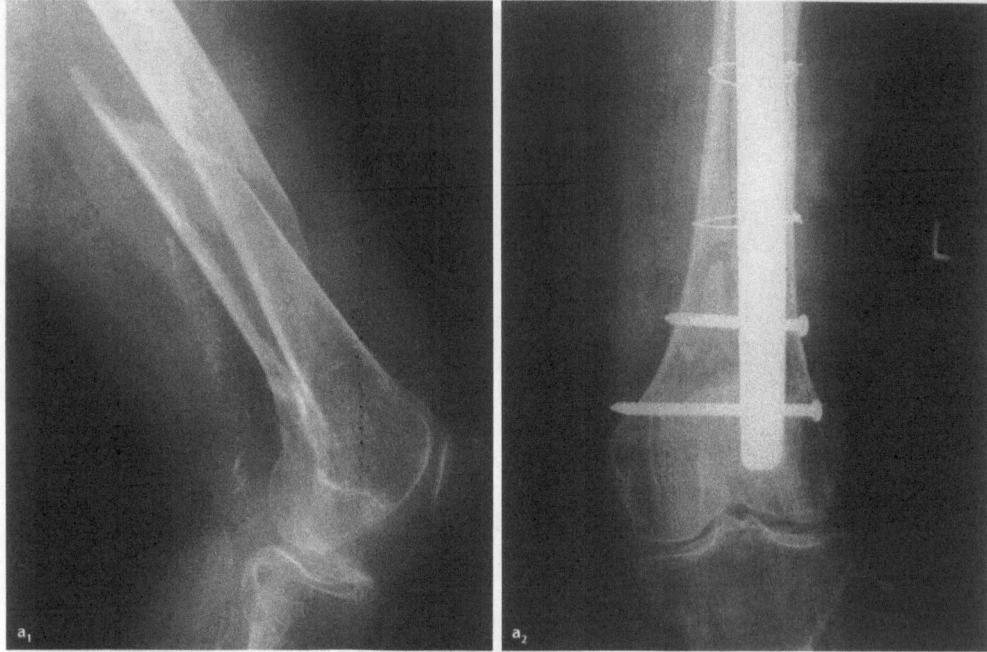

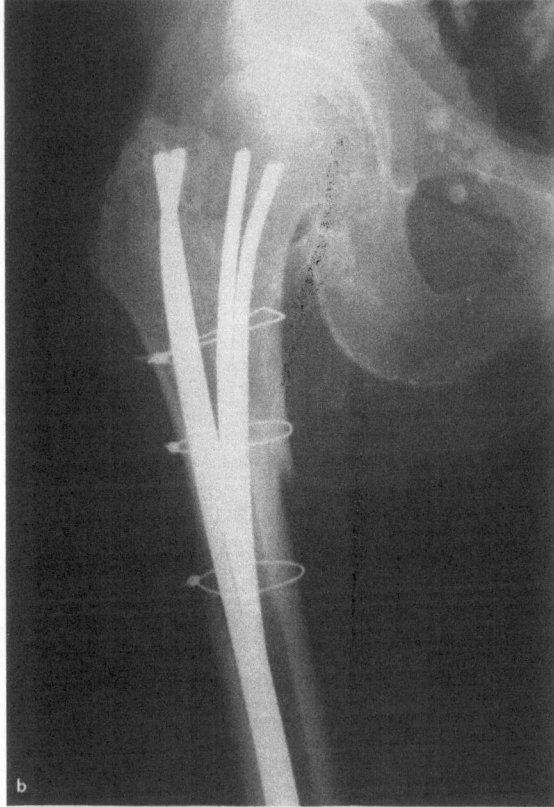

Fig. 147. a Long distal torsion fracture of the femur in a 94-year-old woman that extends into the intercondylar region. The interlocking nail is not inserted until after adjustment of the fracture with two cable cerclages. **b** Per- and subtrochanteric fracture of the femur in a 83-year-old man. Despite the advance of the gamma nail, Ender's nails and cable cerclages are still a worthwhile procedure permitting early re-mobilization

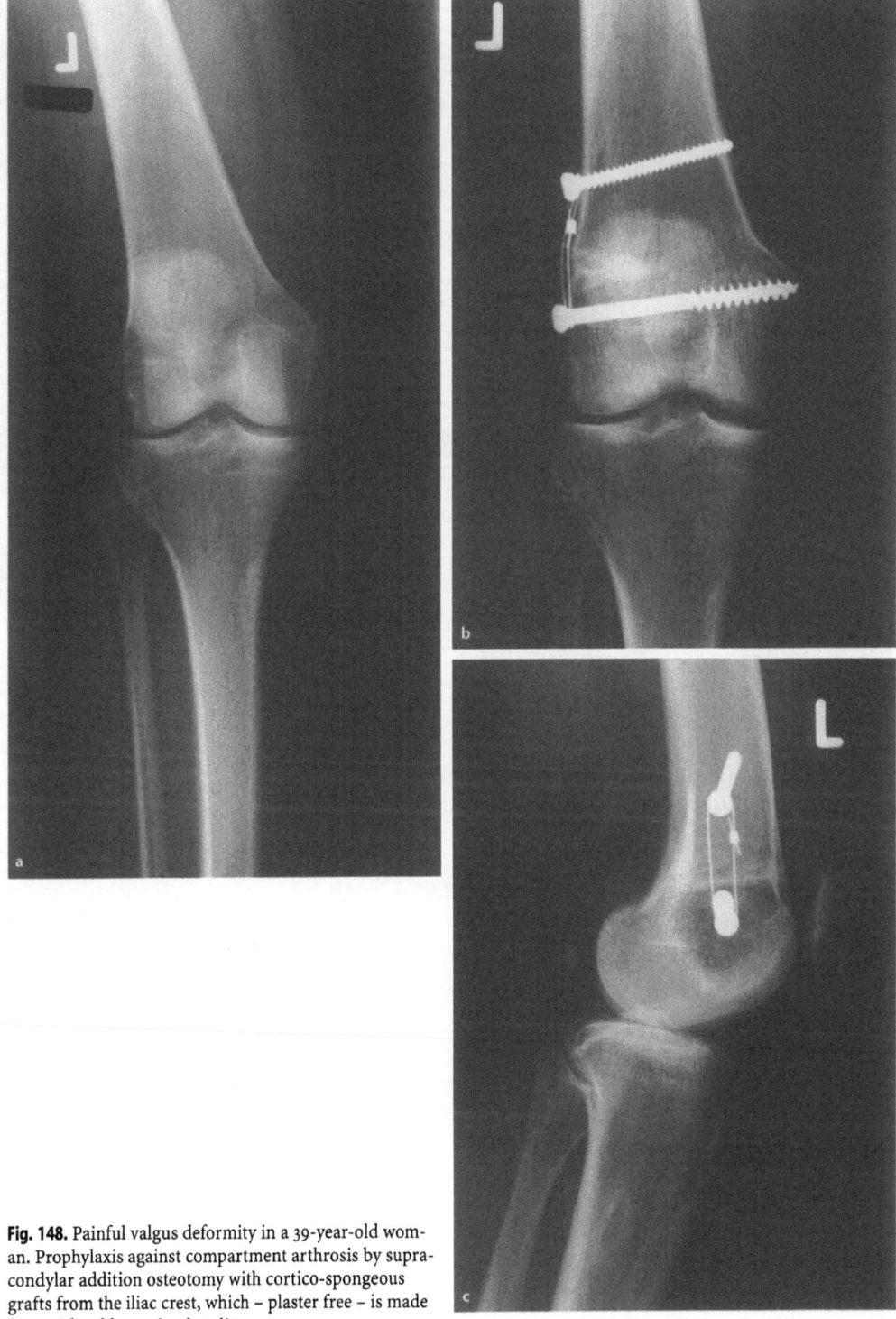

Fig. 148. Painful valgus deformity in a 39-year-old woman. Prophylaxis against compartment arthrosis by supracondylar addition osteotomy with cortico-spongeous grafts from the iliac crest, which – plaster free – is made firm with cable tension banding

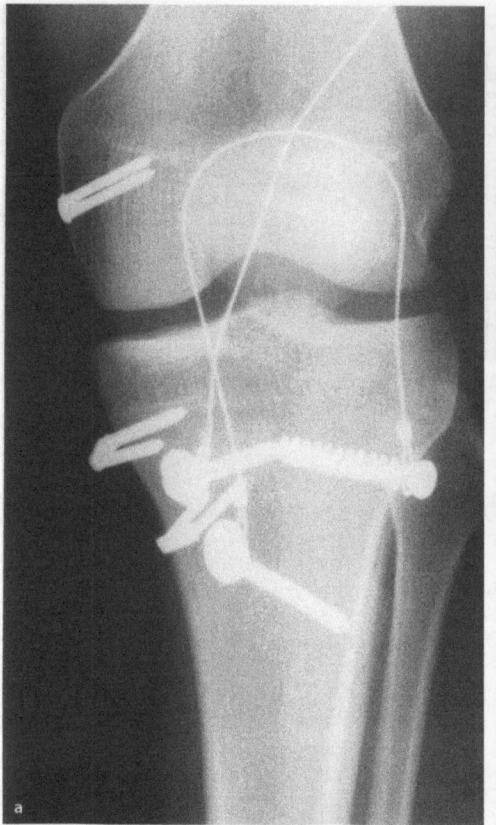

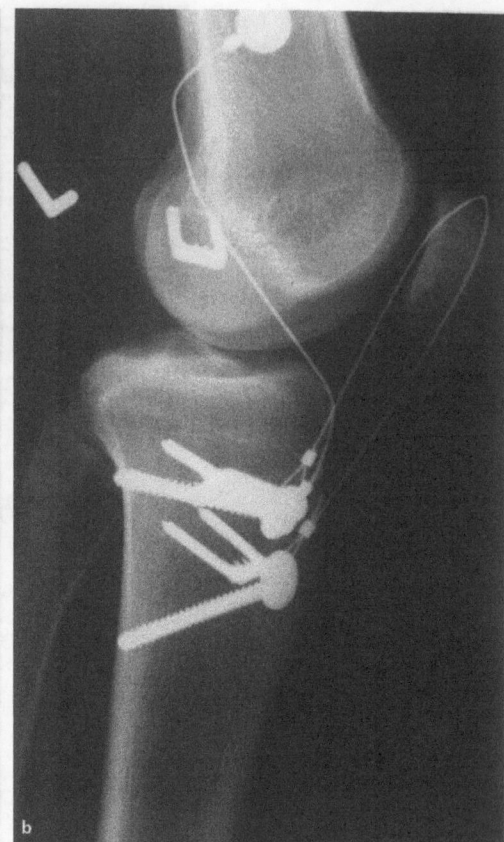

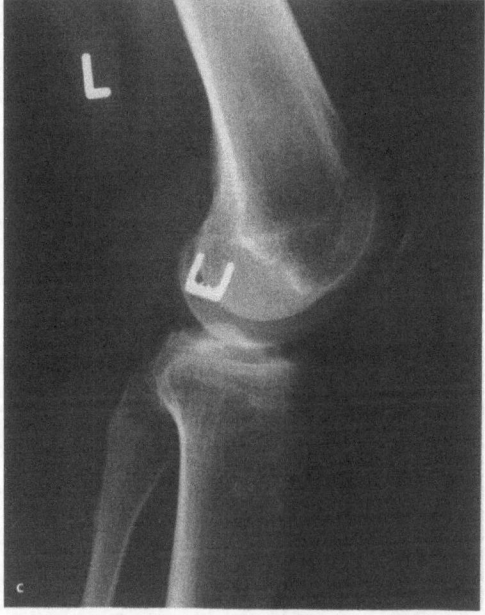

Fig. 149. Complex first grade open injury of the knee joint of a motorcyclist with rupture of both cruciate ligaments, the medial collateral ligament and the pes anserinus, the patella ligament and the anterior joint capsule, avulsion of both posterior horns of the menisci, extensive cartilaginous contusions with cartilage-bone flakes: **a,b** suturing and reconstruction of all ligaments, temporary augmentation with wire cables, no plaster, immediate movement splints; **c** healing after five years with slight shortening of the patella ligament, flexion deficit of 30°, reduction of the thigh musculature by 2 cm. Few difficulties, full functional ability

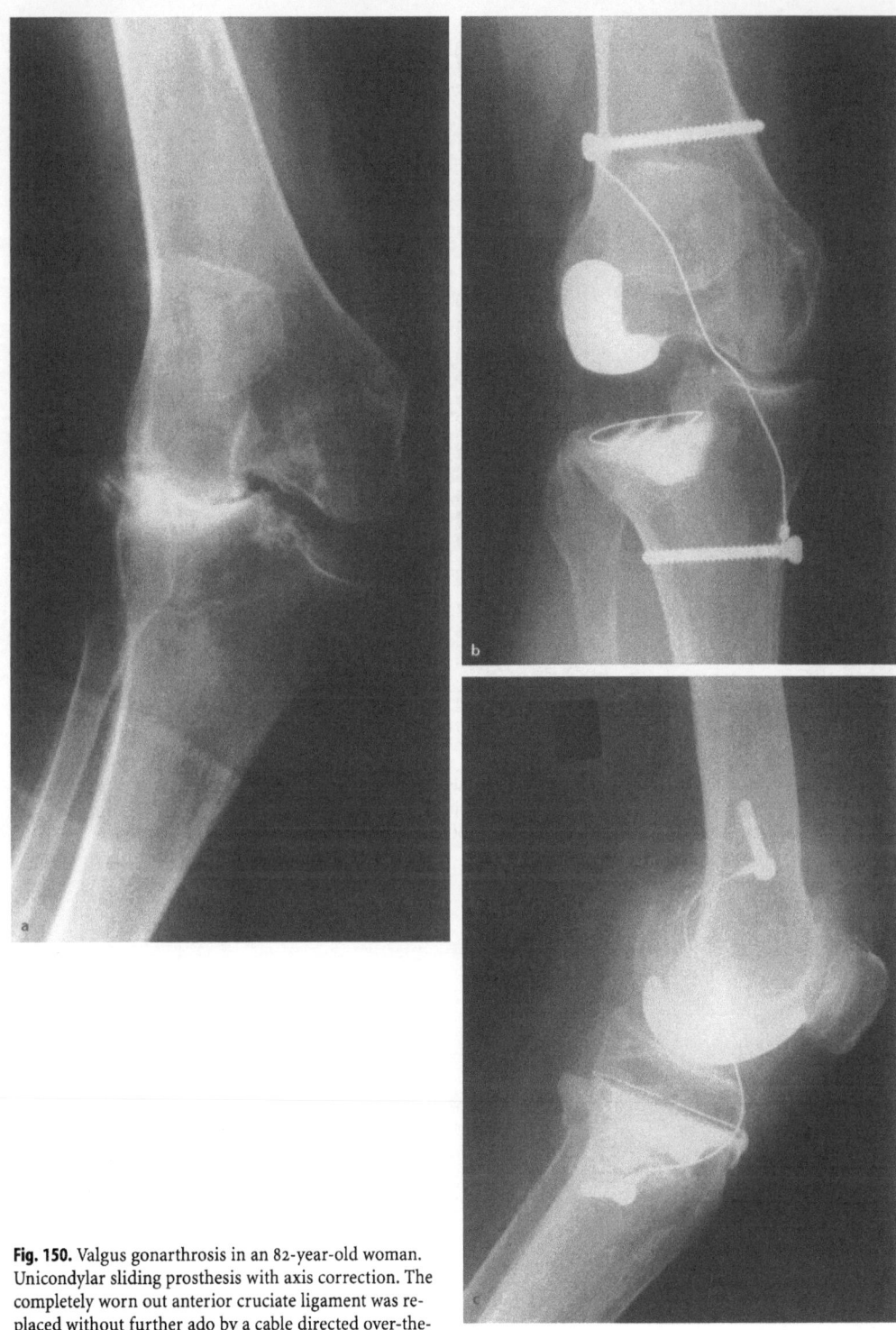

Fig. 150. Valgus gonarthrosis in an 82-year-old woman. Unicondylar sliding prosthesis with axis correction. The completely worn out anterior cruciate ligament was replaced without further ado by a cable directed over-the-top. Five years post-operatively it is still problem free and has not broken

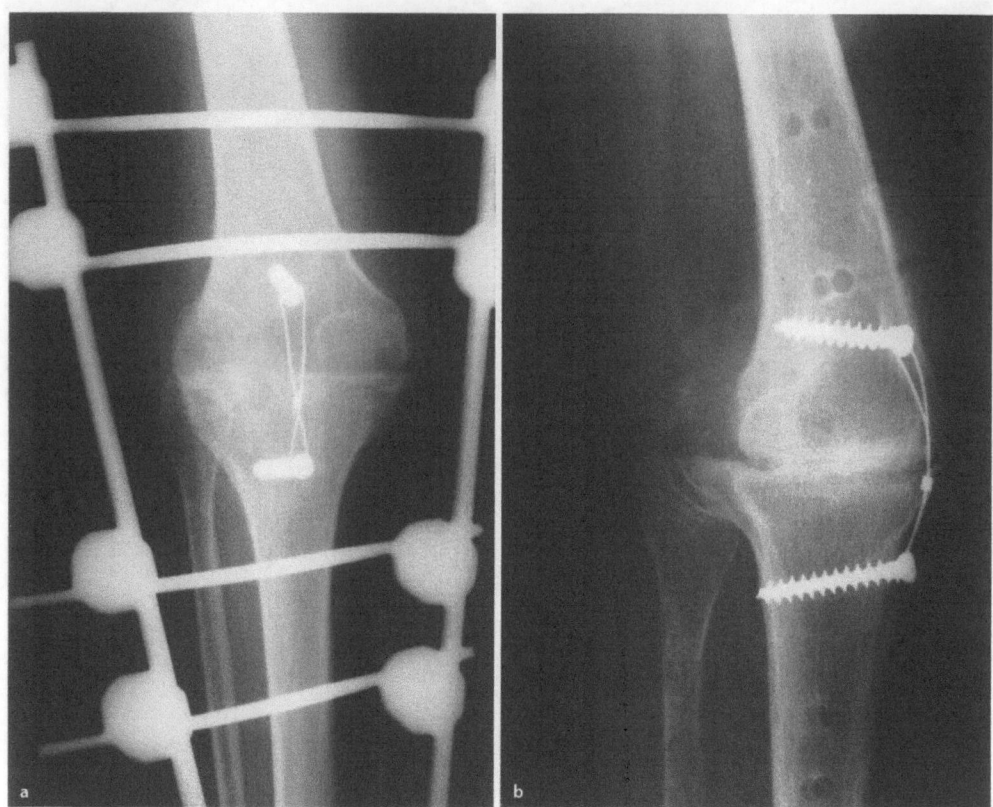

Fig. 151. Frame fixator for six weeks and extensor-side cable tension banding to the knee-joint arthrodesis. Bending forces whilst walking are transferred flexibly through tension banding into the bone contact zones. (Shortening of the quadriceps made it impossible to pull the patella in front of the arthrodesis gap)

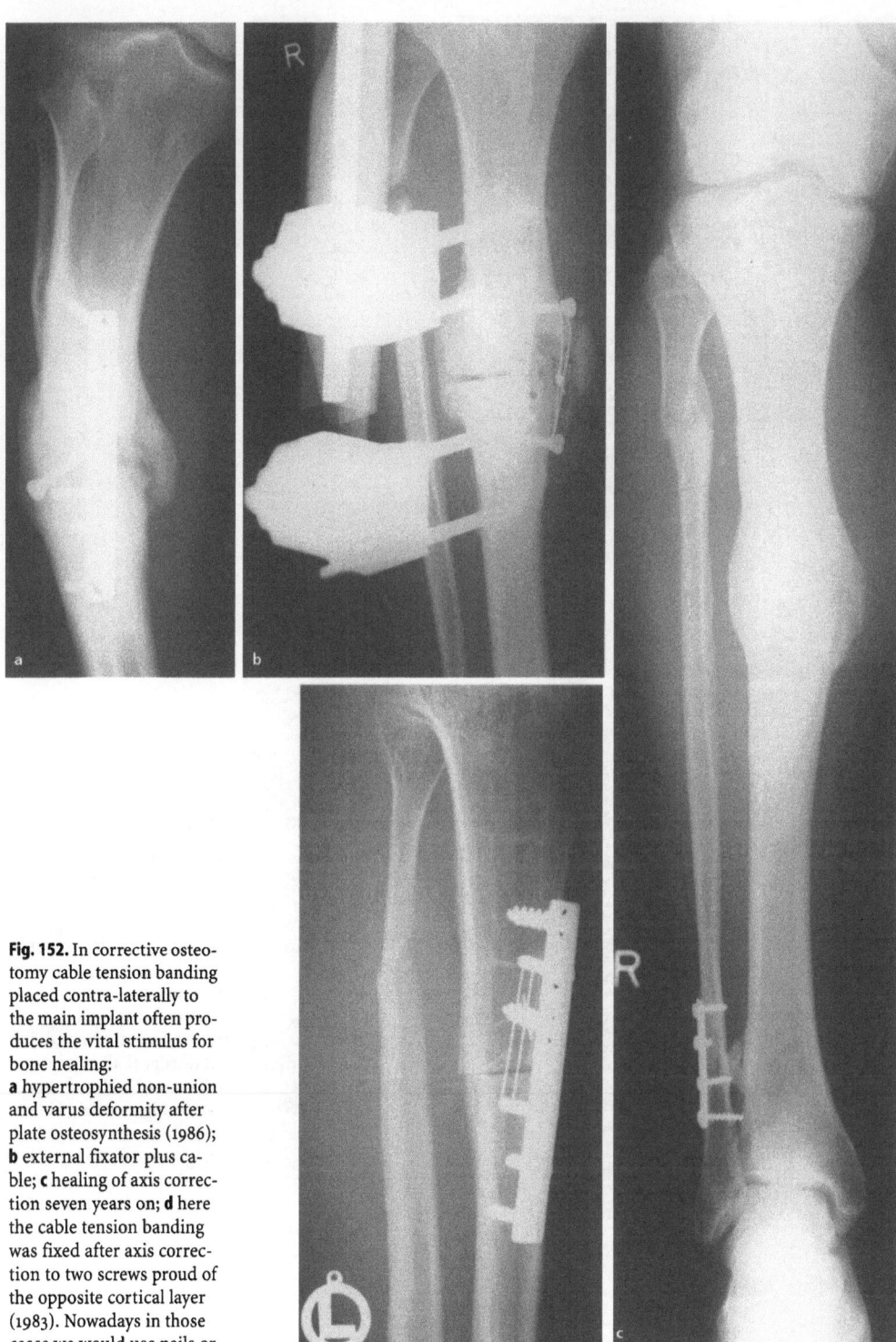

Fig. 152. In corrective osteotomy cable tension banding
placed contra-laterally to
the main implant often produces the vital stimulus for
bone healing:
a hypertrophied non-union
and varus deformity after
plate osteosynthesis (1986);
b external fixator plus cable; **c** healing of axis correction seven years on; **d** here
the cable tension banding
was fixed after axis correction to two screws proud of
the opposite cortical layer
(1983). Nowadays in those
cases we would use nails or
a fortified EndoHelix

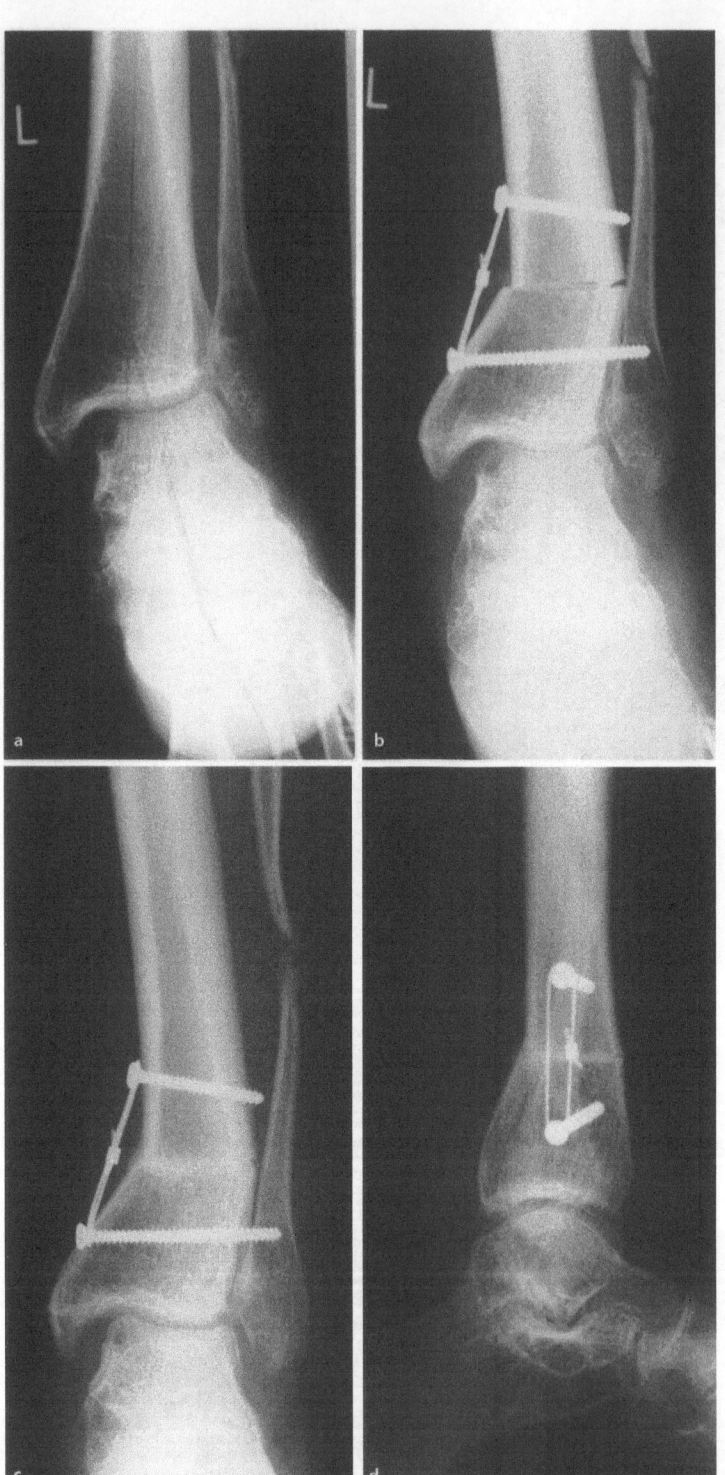

Fig. 153. Corrective osteotomy of a valgus deformity of the distal tibia of 15° after a childhood injury by wedge removal and medial cable tension banding with preservation of the lateral periosteal membrane as a naturally effective counter-tension band. The cable protruding from the bone did not disrupt at all as it was well covered with soft tissue. Note its high tension, identifiable by the absolutely straight course. Spongiosa apposition from the wedge. For the low blood flow and soft tissue covering of the distal tibia cable is ideal. Completely plaster free postoperative treatment with increasing load-bearing. Fully healed. Metal removal after seven months

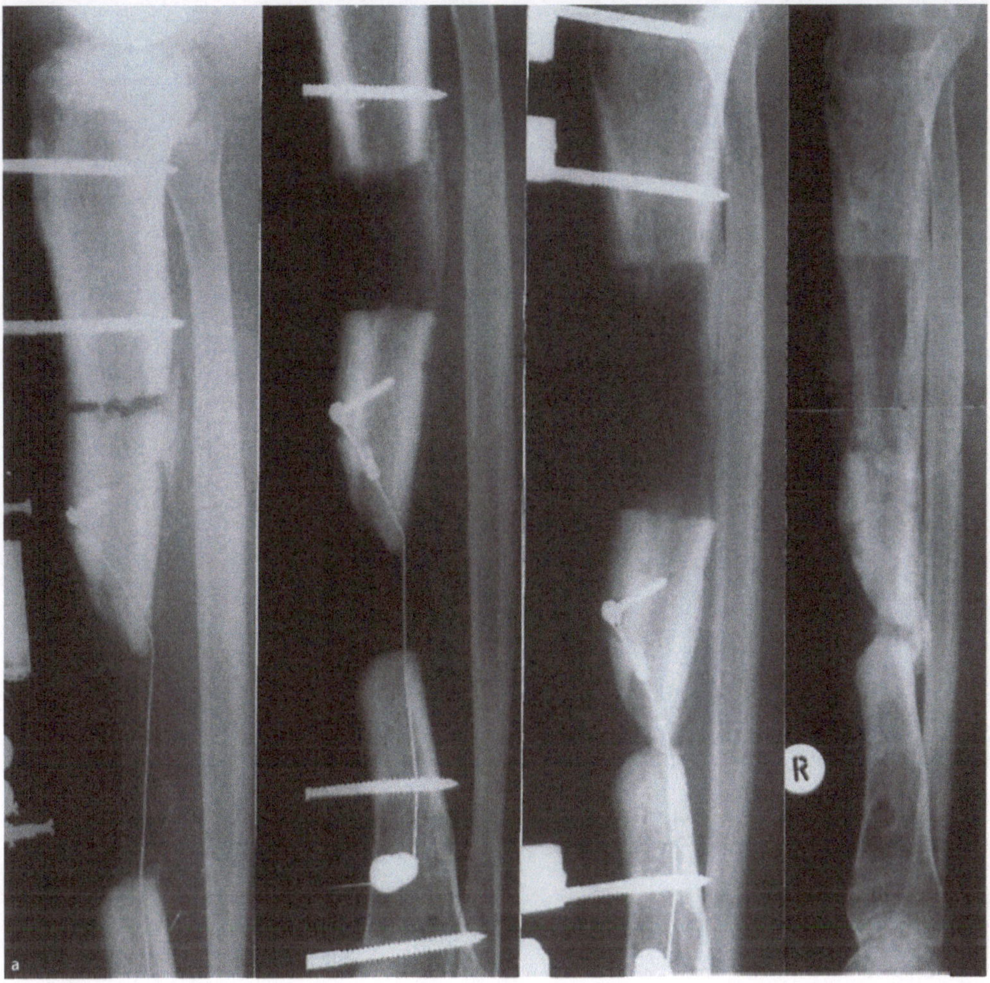

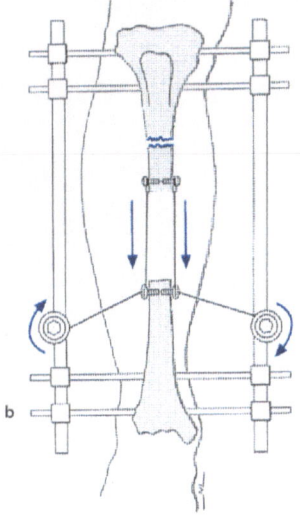

Fig. 154. Callus distraction with cables: **a** "central cable band system" according to Baumgart (from [11]); **b** Rüter's procedure (from [331])

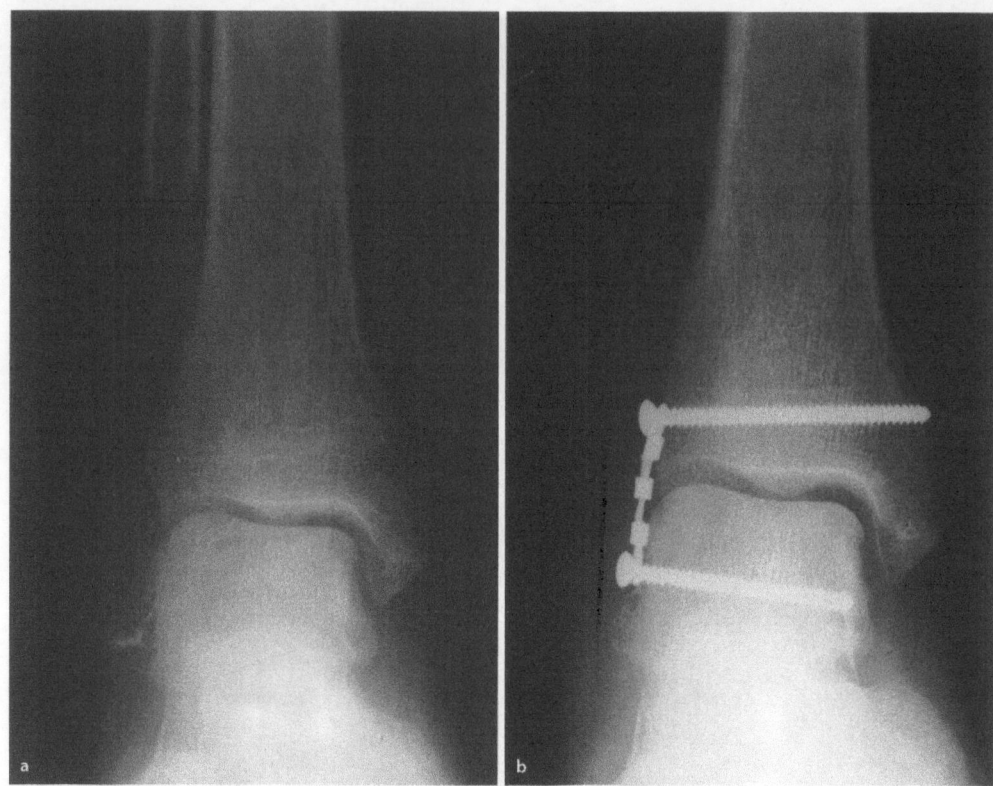

Fig. 155. Destructive fibular sarcoma in an 84-year-old man. After resection the lateral ligament stability of the ankle joint which was lacking was successfully restored with cable tension banding (Prof. Dr. Becker, Volmarstein)

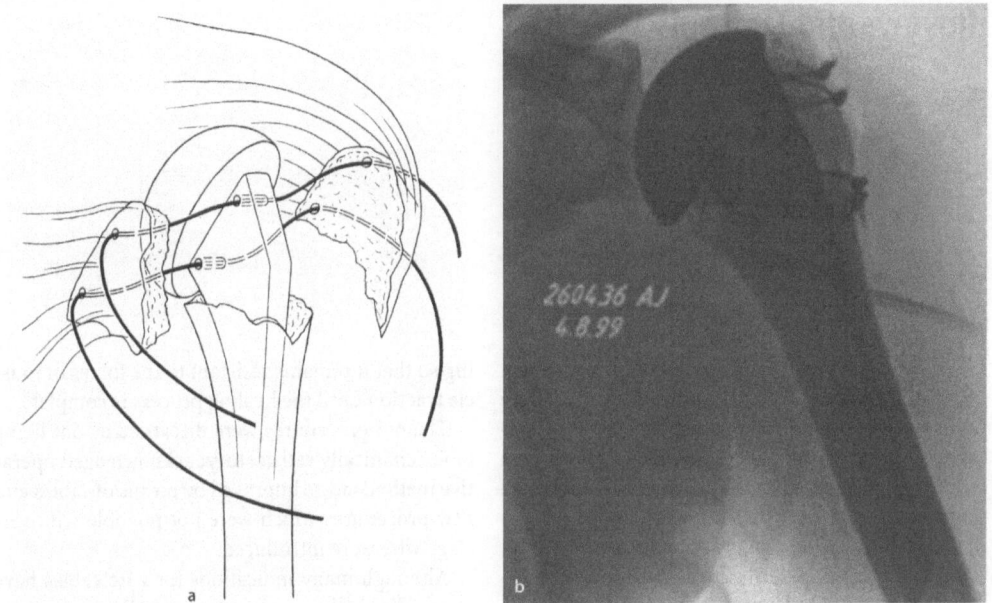

Fig. 156. Refixation of the greater Tuberculum with two special laser-finished cables (provided by ABAmed Express – cf. page 2) around the shoulder endoprosthesis [438] (PD Dr. A. Hertel, Bern CH)

CHAPTER 5

Review and Outlook

This work has discussed the historical development of rigid wire, the medical term of which is cerclage wire, and has highlighted the many different application possibilities of wire cables. Basic information relating to mechanics and engineering was provided in order to deepen the understanding of the cable as a means of traction. The practical value of wire cables in surgery is underlined by overwhelming experimental data and superior clinical results. It is the rational alternative to "florist's wire," as the Americans aptly call cerclage wire.

The biomechanics of tension banding had to be revised because the "eccentric-dynamic" model has too many disadvantages for bone healing. Tension bands, irrespective of whether used by engineers or surgeons, are a static principle. The entire fracture has to be compressed by means of cable pre-tension-

ing so that it remains resistant to the forces of muscle traction until the healing process is complete.

The old procedures were discarded as not being biomechanically satisfactory; acknowledged operative methods were improved by means of cables and new procedures which were not possible with cerclage wire were introduced.

Although many indications for wire cables have materialized, they may only symbolize an interim stage on the development scale. Kevlar threads achieve a 10- to 15-fold higher stability than steel wires. A carcinogous softener however prohibits its use in humans. It seems likely that one day materials with such qualities and the advantage of gradual reabsorption in the body will be available. Until then, the wire cable remains the most superior choice.

References

1. Ackerknecht E (1992) Geschichte der Medizin. Enke, Stuttgart
2. Albert W (1835) Die Anfertigung von Treibseilen aus geflochtenem Eisendrath. Arch Mineral Geognosie Bergbau Hüttenkd 8:418–428
3. Alvarez R, Barbour T, Perkins T (1994) Tibiocalcaneal arthrodesis for nonbracable neuropathic ankle deformity. Foot Ankle 15:354–359
4. Anderson W (1892) Treatment of fracture of the patella with an account of a new method. Lancet Juli 2:10–11
5. Ansorge D (1978) Die Anwendungsmöglichkeiten der Zuggurtungsosteosynthese (Drahtzuggurtung) in der operativen Knochenbruchbehandlung. Zentralbl Chir 103:420–431
6. Armstutz H, Mai L, Schmidt I (1984) Results of interlocking wire trochanteric reattachment and technique refinements to prevent complications following total hiparthroplasty. Clin Orthop 183:82–87
7. Bassett C (1962) Current concepts of bone formation. JBJS 44A:1217–1244
8. Bassett C, Becker R (1962) Generation of electric potentials by bone in response to mechanical stress. Science 137:1063–1064
9. Bastian L, Blauth M, Thermann H (1995) Verschiedene Therapiekonzepte bei schweren Frakturen des Pilon tibiale (Typ C-Verletzungen). Unfallchirurg 98:551–558
10. Bauer G, Zenkl M, Schierle M (1993) Störung der Gangfunktion nach Metatarsale-5-Basisfrakturen. Unfallchirurg 96:483–487
11. Baumgart R, Betz A, Schweiberer L (1994) Möglichkeiten der Rekonstruktion von Knochendefekten. Orthopäde 23:396–403
12. Baumgartel F (1964) Das Kniegelenk. Springer, Berlin Göttingen Heidelberg New York
13. Benjamin J, Bried J, Dohm M (1987) Biomechanical evaluation of various forms of fixation of transverse patellar fractures. J Orthop Trauma 1:219–222
14. Berger P (1892) Suture de la rotule par un procede nouveau (cerclage de la rotule). Bull Soc Chir Paris 18:523–527
15. Bernard A, Brooks S (1987) The role of trochanteric wire revision after total hip replacement. JBJS 69B:352–354
16. Blank H (1972) Osteosynthese bei Olecranonfrakturen. AO Bulletin
17. Blatter G, Jackson R, Bayne O (1987) Patelektomie als eine "Salvage Operation." Orthopäde 16:310–316
18. Blauth W (1984) Zur Technik der valgisierenden kniegelenksnahen Tibiakopfosteotomie. Unfallheilkunde 87:397–404
19. Blömer W, Ungethüm M, Stuhler T (1994) Vergleichende mechanische Untersuchungen verschiedener Fixateur-externe-Montagen bei Sprunggelenksarthrodesen. In: Stuhler T (ed) Arthrodesen. Thieme, Stuttgart, pp 228–236
20. Böhler L (1937) Technik der Knochenbruchbehandlung, vols 1 and 2, 5th edn. Maudrich, Wien
21. Böhmer G, Böhm H, Settner M (1995) Die Arthrodeseoperation am oberen Sprunggelenk mit minimiertem Ringfixateur. Aktuel Traumatol 25:191–196
22. Börner O, Contzen H (1983) Indikation und Technik der Eingriffe am Sprunggelenk. BG-UMed 50:165–174
23. Boldt H (1989) Meilensteine der Bergtechnik. Glückauf 125, Nr 23/24
24. Bosch U, Kasperczyk W, Tscherne H (1994) Biology of the posterior cruciate ligament healing. Sports Med Arthrosc Rev 2:88–99
25. Braly W, Baker J, Tullos H (1994) Arthrodesis of the ankle with lateral plating. Foot Ankle 15:594–653
26. Braun W, Wiedemann M, Rüter A (1993) Indications and results of nonoperative treatment of patellar fractures. Clin Orthop 289:197–201
27. Braune C, Fischer O (1895) Über den Schwerpunkt des menschlichen Körpers. Der Gang des Menschen, 1. Teil. Teubner, Leibzig
28. Breitfuß H, Muhr G, Mönning B (1989) Fixateur oder Schraube bei Arthrodesen am oberen Sprunggelenk. Unfallchirurg 92:245–253
29. Brill W, Hopf T (1987) Biomechanische Untersuchung verschiedener Osteosyntheseverfahren bei Patella-Querfrakturen. Unfallchirurg 90:162–172
30. Brulhart K, Sartoretti C, Roggo A (1993) Ausriß des Ligamentum patellae an der Tuberositas tibiae als Komplikation nach Kreuzbandersatzplastik. Unfallchirurg 96:387–389
31. Brunn v M (1906) Über das Schicksal des Silberdrahtes bei der Naht der gebrochenen Patella. Brun's Beitr Klin Chir 50:83–117
32. Brunner A, Henschen C, Heusser H (eds) (1950) Lehrbuch der Chirurgie, vol II. Schwabe, Basel

33. Brunner C, Weber B (1981) Besondere Osteosynthese-techniken. Springer, Berlin Heidelberg New York

34. Brunner C, Hoffmann R (1983) Arthrodesen nach Verletzungen des oberen und unteren Sprunggelenkes. BG-UMed 50:193–198

35. Brutscher R (1991) Frakturen und Luxationen des Mittel- und Vorfußes. Orthopäde 20:67–75

36. Bühren V, Trentz O, Hennerberger G (1989) Die operative Behandlung der Patellafraktur. Chirurg 60:723–731

37. Bürgel (1993) Carl Hansmann (1852–1917) – die Plattenosteosynthese als neue Technik der operativen Frakturbehandlung. Dissertation, Hamburg

38. Bürger K, Hennert D (1978) Die Methode der Zuggurtungsosteosynthese bei der operativen Behandlung der Olecranonfracturen. Monatsschr Unfallheilkd 70: 528–534

39. Burri C, Lob G (1982) Operative Therapie der distalen Humerusfrakturen. Hefte Unfallheilkd 155:35–49

40. Burri C, Lob G, Rüter A (1983) Frakturen im Breich des Ellenbogengelenkes. 15. Freiburger Chirurgengespräch 18.3.1983. Gödecke, Berlin

41. Burri C, Rüter A, Spier W (eds) (1975) Knochenverletzungen im Kniebereich. Hefte Unfallheilkd 120. Springer, Berlin Heidelberg New York

42. Burvant J, Thomas K, Alexander R (1994) Evaluation of methods of internal fixation of transverse patella fractures: a biomechanical study. J Orthop Trauma 8:147–153

43. Busch W (1857) Lehrbuch der Chirurgie, vol. 1 Hirschwald, Berlin

44. Buzzi R, Aglietti P, Gandenzi A (1989) Frattura transversali di rotula: valutazione sperimentale del metodo di fissazione interna di Lotke e Ecker. Arch Putti Chir Organi Mov (Italy) 37:283–291

45. Cassady S (1986) Spanning the gate. Squarebooks, Santa Rosa

46. Ceci A (1886) Eine neue Operation der Patellarfractur. Subcutane Metallnaht der Kniescheibe. Dtsch Z Chir 23:285–290

47. Cetti R, Henriksen L, Jacobsen K (1994) A new treatment of ruptured Achilles tendons. A prospective randomized study. Clin Orthop 308:155–165

48. Charnley J (1951) Compression arthrodesis of the ankle and shoulder. JBJS 33B:180–191

49. Charnley J, de Ferreira A (1964) Transplantation of the greater trochanter in arthroplasty of the hip. JBJS 46B:191–198

50. Cheng Y, Lin S, Tien Y (1993) Ankle arthrodesis. Kao Hsiung 9:524–531

51. Chissel H, Jones J (1995) The influence of a diastasis screw on the outcome of Weber type-C ankle fractures. JBJS 77/3B:435–438

52. Clarke R, Shea W, Bierbaum B (1979) Trochanteric osteotomy: analysis of pattern of wire fixation failure and complications. Clin Orthop 141:102–110

53. Colton C (1973) Fractures of the olecranon in adults. Classification and management. Injury 5:121–124

54. Cornell C, Levine D, Pagnani M (1994) Initial fixation of proximal humerus fractures using the screw-tension band technique. J Orthop Trauma 8:23–27

55. Coventry M (1965) Osteotomy of the upper portion of the tibia for degenerative arthritis of the knee. JBJS 47A:984–990

56. Crawford R (1973) A history of the treatment of nonunion of fractures in the 19th century in the United States. JBJS 55A/8:1685–1697

57. Crenshaw A (ed) (1971) Campbell's operative orthopaedics, vol 1 and 2. Mosby, St Louis

58. Dall D, Miles A (1983) Re-attachment of the greater trochanter. JBJS 65B:55–59

59. Damanakis K, Schaal O, Mann J (1996) Ein modifiziertes Behandlungskonzept bei Humeruskopffrakturen des älteren Menschen. Unfallchirurg 99:561–568

60. Danziger M, Healy W (1992) Operative treatment of olecranon non-union. J Orthop Trauma (US) 6/3: 290–293

61. Darder A, Gastaldi E, Gomar F, Sandris V (1993) Fourpart displaced proximal humeral fractures: operative treatment using Kirschner wires and a tension band. J Orthop Trauma 7:497–505

62. Deliyannis S (1973) Comminuted fractures of the olecranon treated by the Weber-Vasey technique. Injury 5:19–24

63. Demel R (1925) Zur Technik der Knochennaht. Zentralbl Chir 52/2:71–76

64. Demel R (1926) Operative Frakturenbehandlung. Springer, Wien

65. Dennert H (1986) Bergbau und Hüttenwesen im Harz vom 16.–19. Jh, dargestellt in Lebensbildern führender Persönlichkeiten. Pieper'sche Verlagsanstalt, Clausthal-Zellerfeld

66. Dennert H (1986) Oberbergrat Wilhelm August Julius Albert, der Erfinder des Drahtseiles – ein Lebensbild. Schriftenreihe der GDMB Gesellschaft Deutscher Metallhütten- und Bergleute 46:31–41

67. De Vries L, Dereymaeker G, Fabry G (1994) Arthroscopic ankle arthrodesis. Preliminary report. Acta Orthop Belg 60:389–392

68. Dexel M, Stuflesser H (1977) Ergebisse der Patellektomie bei schwerem posttraumatischen Knorpelschaden im Femoropatellargelenk. Hefte Unfallheilkd 129: 378–381

69. Dickmann H (1962) Neue Beiträge zur Geschichte des Drahtseiles. Stahl und Eisen 82:166–169

70. Diehl K (1974) Biomechanische Berechnungen und Untersuchungen zur Notwendigkeit der Hohlbiegung bei der Plattenosteosynthese. Arch Orthop Unfall Chir 80:247–256

71. Dieterich G (1908) Die Erfindung der Drahtseilbahnen. Zieger, Leipzig

72. Dittrich V, Stedtfeld H (1992) Manual der Frakturklassifikation. Deutscher Ärzte-Verlag, Köln

73. Doebbelin D (1898) Zur Behandlung der frischen Kniescheibenbrüche. Dtsch Z Chir 49:461–478

74. Dohm M, Benjamin J, Harrison J (1994) A biomechanical evaluation of three forms of internal fixation used in ankle arthrodesis. Foot Ankle 15/6:297–300

75. Doursounian L, Prevot O, Touzard R (1994) L'osteosynthèse par hanbanage de fractures deplacees de l'olecrane. Ann Chir 48:169–177

76. Draenert K, Draenert Y (1984) Der Knochen als hydraulisches System. Information of the Institute of lightweight structure (IL), University of Stuttgart. IL 36:108–109

77. Draenert K, Draenert Y (1987/III) Ein neues Verfahren für die Knochenbiopsie und die Knorpel-Knochen-Transplantation. Sandorama 62:5–12

78. Draenert Y, Garde U, Ulrich C (1999) Manual of cementing technique. Springer, Berlin Heidelberg New York

79. Dwyer A, Newton N, Sherwood A (1969) An anterior approach to scoliosis. Clin Orthop 62:192–202

80. Dwyer A (1973) Experience of anterior correction of scoliosis. Clin Orthop 93:191–206

81. Ecke H (1977) Prinzipien der Zuggurtung. Hefte Unfallheilkd 129:64–65

82. Ecke H, Hofmann D, Patzak H (1990) Die Rupturen der Amphiarthrosen am Beckenring. Unfallchirurgie 16:311–321

83. Edwards B, Johnell O, Redhund I (1989) Patellar fractures. A 30-year follow-up. Acta Orthop Scand 60:712–714

84. Egyed B, Kazar G (1977) Die Rolle einzelner biomechanischer Faktoren bei der Heilung der dislozierten Patellafraktur. Beitr Orthop Traumatol 24:29–37

85. Eingartner C, Winter E, Volkmann R (1995) Zur Rearthrodese des oberen Spunggelenkes. Aktuel Traumatol 25:217–223

86. Eitel F, Schweiberer L (1983) Olecranonfrakturen. Retrospektive multizentrische Therapiestudie an 175 Fällen. Hefte Unfallheilkd 86:143–151

87. Eriksson E, Sahlin O, Sandahl U (1957) Late results of conservative and surgical treatment of fracture of the olecranon. Acta Chir Scand 113:153–166

88. Felenda M, Dittel K (1993) Instabile Beckenringverletzungen. Klassifikation – Behandlungsstrategie. Aktuel Traumatol 23:263–271

89. Fick R (1911) Handbuch der Anatomie und Mechanik der Gelenke Dritter Teil: Spezielle Gelenk- und Muskelmechanik. Fischer, Jena

90. Fischer A, Gohrbandt E, Sauerbruch F (1958) Bier-Braun-Kümmell – Chirurgische Operationslehre. Barth, Leipzig

91. Flinchum D (1966) Patellectomy when why and how. South Med J 59:897–902

92. Fourati M, Essadam H, Hassine H (1987) Resultats longtains du traitement de fractures de la rotule. Rev Chir Orthop 73:361–364

93. Frank M (1849) Systematisches Lehrbuch der gesamten Chirugie. 1. Bändchen, 2. Abtheilung. Enke, Erlangen

94. Frank E, Zitter H (1971) Metallische Implantate in der Knochenchirurgie. Springer, Wien New York

95. Franke D, Glatz R, Henning K (1981) Theoretische Grundlagen und tierexperimentelle Untersuchungen mit einer neuen stabilitätsverbessernden Methode der Drahtcerclage durch ablenkungsfreie Drahtführung. Hefte Unfallheilkd 84:338–344

96. Franke D (1985) Die stabile, ablenkungsfreie Drahtcerclage. Chirurg 56:408–410

97. Freuler F, Brunner C, Rüter A (1974) Spätresultate bei operierten Patellafrakturen. Hefte Unfallheilkd 120:68–75

98. Frisch W, Machens K (1995) Die frühfunktionelle Behandlung der operativ behandelten Achillessehnenruptur – ein neues Behandlungskonzept. Aktuel Traumatol 25:56–58

99. Fujikawa K, Oktani T, Matsumoto H (1994) Reconstruction of the extensor-apparatus of the knee with the Leeds-Keio ligament. JBJS 76B:200–203

100. Fürmaier A (1953) Beitrag zur Mechanik der Patella und des Gesamtkniegelenkes. Arch Orthop Unfall Chir 46:78–90

101. Ganz R (1989) Die Trochanterversorgung bei adduzierender (varisierender) intertrochanterer Osteotomie. Operat Orthop Traumatol 1:211–218

102. Garde U Histomorphologie der primären Knochenheilung bei Osteochondralfrakturen. Habilitationsschrift, Witten-Herdecke (in Vorbereitung)

103. Geller F (1847) De resectione pseudarthroseos e femoris fracturae ortae. Inaugural-Dissertation, Bonn

104. Georgette F, Sander T, Oh J (1984) The fatigue resistance of orthopaedic wire and cable systems. Biomaterials 7:146

105. Gersdorf v H (1967) Feldbuch der Wundarznei (Nachdruck). Wissenschaftliche Buchgesellschaft, Darmstadt

106. Giebel G, Tscherne H, Daiber M (1983) Die Tibiakopfosteotomie zur Behandlung der Gonarthrose. Orthopäde 14:144–153

107. Giolito A, Grob C (1994) Verriegelungsarthrodese des oberen Sprunggelenkes. In: Stuhler T (ed) Arthrodesen. Thieme, Stuttgart, pp 252–253,

108. Goetze O (1933) Subcutane Drahtnaht bei Tibiaschrägfrakturen. Arch Klin Chir 177:445–449

109. Gotzen L, Hütter J (1976) Experimentelle Untersuchungen zur Plattenvorbiegung – ein Beitrag zur Biomechanik der Plattenosteosynthese. Arch Orthop Unfall Chir 85:129–138

110. Gotzen L, Ishaque B, Morgenthal F (1997) Die externe patellotibiale Transfixation. Unfallchirurg 100:24–28

111. Goulet J, Rouleau J, Mason D (1994) Comminuted fractures of the posterior wall of the acetabulum. JBJS 76A:1457–1463

112. Goymann V (1975) Umlenkung und Flächenpressung im femoropatellaren Gelenk, eine biomechanische und klinische Studie. Habilitationsschrift, Essen

113. Goymann V, Haasters J, Heller W (1974) Neuere Untersuchungen zur Biomechanik der Patella. Z Orthop 112:623–625

114. Greitemann B (1998) Der diabetische Fuß. Chir Prax 54:279–296

115. Griffith A (1920) The phenomena of rupture and flow in solids. Philos Trans R Soc Lond A 221:163–198

116. Gurlt E (1862) Handbuch der Lehre von den Knochenbrüchen, Bd 1. Grote'sche Buchhandlung, Hamm

117. Gutmann G, Biedermann H (1992) Funktionelle Röntgenanalyse der Lenden-Becken-Hüftregion. Fischer, Stuttgart

118. Hachez-Leblanc M (1958) Osteosynthese de rotule et cerclage fonctionelle. Acta Orthop Belg 24:107–113

119. Hackenbruch P (1894) Zur Behandlung der queren

Kniescheibenbrüche durch die Knochennaht. Beitr Klin Chir 12/1:409–438

120. Hansmann C (1886) Eine neue Methode der Fixirung der Fragmente bei complicirten Fracturen. Verh Dtsch Ges Chir 15:134–137

121. Hasselbach v C, Witzel U (1987/1988) Die Schenkelhalszuggurtungsplatte. Chir Prax 38:235–260

122. Hawkins B, Langermann R, Anger D (1994) The Ilizarov technique in ankle fusion. Clin Orthop 303:217–225

123. Heide M, Hohndorf H (1990) Therapeutisches Konzept für Frakturen des Trochanter major bei der Hüftgelenksalloarthroplastik. Beitr Orthop Traumatol 37:52–57

124. Heinrich W, Nixdorf J (1972) Grundlagen zur Berechnung der mechanischen Eigenschaften von Faserverbundwerkstoffen. VDJ-Zeitung 114:1

125. Heister L (1763) Chirurgie. Raspe, Nürnberg

126. Helferich H (1897) Atlas und Grundriß der traumatischen Frakturen und Luxationen. Lehmann, München

127. Helm H, Hornby R, Miller S (1987) The complications of surgical treatment of displaced fractures of the olecranon. Injury (England) 18/1:48–50

128. Hendrich V, Siewecke W (1993) Offene Gelenkfrakturen am distalen Unterschenkel. Unfallchirurg 96:253–258

129. Hoffa A (1891) Lehrbuch der Fracturen und Luxationen für Ärzte u. Studierende. Stahel'scher Verlag, Würzburg

130. Hoffmann A (1908) Zur Technik der Patellarnaht. Dtsch Z Chir 91:623–627

131. Hofmeister M, Hempfling H (1997) Die arhroskopisch kontrollierte Schraubenarthrodes des oberen Sprunggelenkes. Chir Prax 52:267–276

132. Holdsworth B, Mossad M (1984) Ellbow function following tension band fixation of displaced fractures of the olecranon. Injury (England) 16/3:182–187

133. Holz U, Thielemann F, Zahedi B (1990) Biomechanik, Operationstechnik und Ergebnisse der Patellafrakturen. H Unfallheilkd 212:142–148

134. Holz U (1994) Die Arthrodese des oberen Sprunggelenkes mit Zugschrauben. In: Stuhler T (ed) Arthrodesen. Thieme, Stuttgart, pp 248–251

135. Hopf T, Brill W (1985) Biomechanische Untersuchungen zur Festigkeit der Trochanterosteosynthese. Orthop Prax 21:110–118

136. Horne G, Tanzer T (1981) Olecranon fractures: a review of 100 cases. J Trauma 21:469–472

137. Horner S, Sadasivan K, Lipka J, Saha S (1989) Analysis of mechanical factors affecting fixation of olecranon fractures. Orthopedics (US) 12/11:1469–1479

138. Houben P, Bongers K, v d Wildenberg F (1994) Double tension band osteosynthesis in supra- and transcondylar humeral fractures. Injury 25:305–309

139. Huberty R (1974) Biomechanische Untersuchung zur Verwendung der Cerclage und Zuggurtung in der Osteosynthese. Dissertation, Homburg

140. Hueter C (1882) Grundriss der Chirurgie, Bd 2. Vogel, Leipzig

141. Hume M, Wiss D (1992) Olecranon fractures. A clinical and radiographic comparison of tension band wiring and plate fixation. Clin Orthop 285:229–235

142. Hung L, Chan K, Chow Y (1985) Fractured patella: operative treatment using the tension band principle. Injury (England) 16:343–347

143. Icart (1775) Lettre en reponse au memoire de M. Pujol. J Med Chir Pharm Roux 44:164–181

144. Ihara H, Megumi M, Takayanagi K (1995) Acute tears of the anterior cruciate ligament treated by early protective motion: second-look arthroscopy after 3-month conservative treatment. Orthopedics 6:475–483

145. Issendorf v W, Ahlers J, Ritter G (1990) Die Drahtzuggurtungsosteosynthese – Untersuchungen zu Spannung und Fixierung des Osteosynthesedrahtes. Unfallchirurgie 16:277–285

146. Jäger R, Blauth W, Schuchardt E (1977) Besondere Indikationen der Zuggurtungsosteosynthese. Hefte Unfallheilkd 129:388–392

147. Jahna H, Wittich H, Hartenstein H (1979) Der distale Stauchungsbruch der Tibia. Ergebnisse von 583 frischen Fällen. Hefte Unfallheilkd 137:1–136

148. Jaskulka R, Ittner G, Raffezeder U (1989) Die chirurgische Versorgung dislozierter Patellafrakturen – Therapie und Ergebnisse. Unfallchirurgie 15:253–260

149. Jaskulka R, Chrysopoulos A, Ittner G (1990) Zur konservativen Therapie der Patellafraktur. Hefte Unfallheilkd 212:152–153

150. Jaskulka R, Harm T (1991) Die konservative Therapie geschlossener dislozierter Olekranonfrakturen im geriatrischen Krankengut. Unfallchirurg 94:424–429

151. Joachimsthal (1902) Ueber Structur, Lage und Anomalien der menschlichen Kniescheibe. Arch Klin Chir 67:342–368

152. Jockheck M, Lang M, Weller S (1994) Langzeitergebnisse nach Arthrodese des oberen Sprunggelenkes. Aktuel Traumatol 24:110–113

153. Jockheck M, Höntzsch D, Brettschneider K (1995) Die Zuggurtungsosteosynthesen bei Olekranonfrakturen Operat Orthop Traumatol 7:156–163

154. Johnson E, Matta J (eds) (1994) Acetabular fractures. A tribute to Emile Letournel. Clin Orthop 305:1–167

155. Johnson R, Roetker A, Schwab J (1986) Olecranon fractures treated with AO screw and tension bands. Orthopedics (US 9/1):66–68

156. Jungbluth K (1983) Frakturen des Actetabulums. Langenbecks Arch Chir 361:179–183

157. Jürgens C, Kortmann H, Schulz J (1990) Die Patellafraktur – eine Operation für den Anfänger? Hefte Unfallheilkd 212:151–152

158. Käch K, Trentz O (1994) Distraktionsspondylodese des Sacrums bei "Vertical-shear-Läsionen" des Beckens. Unfallchirurg 97:28–38

159. Kapandji I (1970) The physiology of joints, vols 1 and 2. Livingstone, Edingburgh

160. Kapandji I (1976) L'ostéosynthese par double embrochage intrafocale. Ann Chir 30:903–908

161. Kasperczyk W, Engel M, Tscherne H (1993) Die 4-

Fragment-Fraktur des proximalen Oberarms. Unfallchirurg 96:422–426

162. Kästner H (1924) Kniescheibenbrüche, ihre Behandlung und Vorhersage. Ergeb Chir Orthop 17:240–307
163. Katthagen B, Müller-Färker J (1979) Indikation u. Spätergebnisse der Patellektomie. Unfallheilkunde 82: 357–363
164. Kaufer H (1971) Mechanical function of the patella. JBJS 53A:1551–1560
165. Kilian H (1980) Meister der Chirurgie. Thieme, Stuttgart
166. Kirschner M (1909) Ueber Nagelextension. Brun's Beitr Klin Chir 64:266–279
167. Kirschner M (1925) Zur Technik der Knochennaht. Zentralbl Chir 52/16:846–852
168. Kirschner M, Nordmann O (1944) Die Chirurgie Bd 4. Urban und Schwarzenberg, Berlin, p 394
169. Kiviluoto O, Santavirta S (1978) Fractures of the olecranon. Acta Orthop Scand 49/1:28–31
170. Klapp R, Rückert W (1937) Die Drahtextension. Enke, Stuttgart
171. Kleinschmidt (1948) Operative Chirurgie. Springer, Berlin Heidelberg New York
172. Kluger P, Gerner H, Trepte C (1989) An unsophisticated improvement in the conventional C1-2 dorsal fusion. 6th annual meeting of the Cervical Spine Research Society, St Gallen, Switzerland, 28.6.–1.7.1989
173. Kluger P, Dickob M, Korge A (1994) Die Verwendung von Drahtseilen an der Halswirbelsäule. In: Matzen K (ed) Die operative Behandlung der Halswirbelsäule. Zuckschwerdt, Munich
174. Knese K (1958) Knochenstruktur als Verbundbau. Thieme, Stuttgart
175. Knese K (1963) Zell- und Faserstruktur des Knochengewebes. Acta Anat 53:396
176. Koch E (1981) Ärzte, die Geschichte machten. Hofmann-Druck, Augsburg
177. Kocher T (1880) Zur Behandlung der Patellafraktur. Centralbl Chir 20:321–326
178. Kölndorfer G, Boszotta H, Prünner K (1994) Langzeitergebnisse nach operativer Versorgung von Patellafrakturen. Unfallchirurgie 20:37–41
179. Konieczny O (1986) Die Koriuminterpositionsplastik in der Gelenk- und Extremitätenchirurgie. Thieme, Stuttgart
180. Konieczny O (1994) Ist die Arthrodese bei Destruktion des oberen Sprunggelenkes immer notwendig? In: Stuhler T (ed) Arthrodesen Thieme, Stuttgart, pp 242–247
181. König F (1886) Lehrbuch der speciellen Chirurgie für Aerzte und Studirende, Bd 3. Hirschwald, Berlin
182. König F (1924) Die operative Behandlung der Knochenbrüche. Verh Dtsch Ges Chir 48. Tagung, pp 380–388
183. König F (1931) Operative Chirurgie der Knochenbrüche, Bd 1. Springer, Wien
184. König S, Kilga M, Kwasny O (1990) Ergebnisse nach Plattenosteosynthese bei der Olekranontrümmerfraktur. Unfallchirurg 93:216–220
185. Kouwenhoven G, Weber B (1969) Zuggurtungs-Osteosynthesen bei Olecranonfracturen. Arch Orthop Unfall Chir 65:244–250
186. Kuechle D, Stuart M (1994) Isolated rupture of the patellar tendon in athletes. Am J Sports Med 22:692–695
187. Kuhn A, Winkler H (1995) Die funktionelle Behandlung einer operativ versorgten beidseitigen Quadricepssehnenruptur beim alten Menschen. Aktuel Traumatol 25:167–170
188. Kullmann E (1975) Fäden und Netze von Spinnen und Insekten. Information of the Institute of Lightweight Structures (IL), University of Stuttgart. IL 8:318–378
189. Kullmann E, Otto F, Braun T (1975) Grundlagen und Ordnung – Übersicht der Netzkonstruktionen der Spinnen. Information of the Institute of Lightweight Structures (IL), University of Stuttgart. IL 8:304–317
190. Kuner E, Siebler G (1987) Luxationsfrakturen des proximalen Humerus – Ergebnisse nach operativer Behandlung. Eine AO-Studie über 167 Fälle. Unfallchirurgie 13:64–71
191. Küntscher G (1940) Die Marknagelung von Knochenbrüchen. Arch Klin Chir 200:443–448
192. Küntscher G (1950) Die Marknagelung. Saenger, Berlin
193. Küntscher G (1962) Praxis der Marknagelung. Schattauer, Stuttgart
194. Kuo R, Sonnabend D (1993) Simultaneous rupture of the patellar tendon bilaterally: case report and review of the literature J Trauma 34:458–460
195. Labitzke R (1975) Neues Prinzip der Zuggurtung. 2. Reisenburger Workshop zur klinischen Unfallchirurgie 18.9.1974. In: Burri C, Rüter A, Spier W (eds) Knochenverletzungen im Kniebereich. Hefte Unfallheilkd 120:76–79
196. Labitzke R (1975) Überlegungen zur Theorie der Zuggurtung. Arch Orthop Unfall Chir 81:179–192
197. Labitzke R (1975) Die laterale Zuggurtung – dargestellt an der Olecranonfraktur. Arch Orthop Unfall Chir 81:193–198
198. Labitzke R (1975) Bipolare interfragmentäre Druckkraftmessung am Modellknochen bei Variierung der Zuggurtung einer Olecranonfraktur. Arch Orthop Unfall Chir 81:199–205
199. Labitzke R (1976) Grundsätzliche biomechanische Probleme bei Osteosynthesen. Arch Orthop Unfall Chir 84:27–37
200. Labitzke R (1977) Patentschrift DE 2754575. Deutsches Patentamt, München
201. Labitzke R (1977) Indikation und Technik der Thoraxwandstabilisierung bei Mehrfachverletzten. Aktuel Traumatol 7:235–241
202. Labitzke. R (1977) Laterale Zuggurtung – sofort belastbare Osteosynthese der Patellafraktur. Arch Orthop Unfall Chir 90:77–87
203. Labitzke R (1979) Biomechanik der Zuggurtung und ihres Osteosynthesematerials. Neukonzipiertes OP-Set mit Drahtseilen, Drahtspanner und Drahtschloß. In: Friedebold G, Kölbel R (eds) Pauwels-Symposium Biomechanik in Orthopädie und Traumatologie, Berlin 18.1.1979. Oscar Helene Heim, Berlin, pp 58–62

204. Labitzke R (1979) Statik und Bewegungsabläufe bei einseitiger Hüftversteifung. Habilitationsschrift, Essen

205. Labitzke R, Towfig H (1980) Operationstechnik und Behandlungsergebnisse nach lateraler Zuggurtung an Patella und Olecranon. Unfallheilkunde 83:450–456

206. Labitzke R (1982) Drahtseile und intraossäre Druckverteilungshülsen in der Chirurgie. Neueinführung eines Implantatsatzes für Seil- und Hülsen-Seilosteosynthesen. Chirurg 53:741–743

207. Labitzke R (1982) Theorie und Klinik der lateralen Zuggurtung am Olecranon, ausgeführt mit Drahtseilen. Hefte Unfallheilkd 155:110–112

208. Labitzke R, Schramm G, Witzel U (1983) "Sleeve-rope-closure" of the median sternotomy after open heart operations. Thorac Cardiovasc Surgeon 31:127–128

209. Labitzke R (1986) "Sleeve-rope-closure". A new method of sternotomy closure. 6th Congress of the Michael DeBakey International Surgical Society, Melbourne 11.–14.3.1986

210. Labitzke R, Witzel U (1986) Biomechanische Grundlagen und Technik der elastischen Hülsen-Seil-Verspannung der Beckenruptur. Hefte Unfallheilkd 181:622–624

211. Labitzke R (1987) Fußamputationen – Alternative zur hohen Absetzung? Vereinigung NWC, Mönchengladbach 8.–10.10.

212. Labitzke R, Witzel U, Upmeyer M (1987) Die Behandlung des "degenerativen Meniskusschadens" durch valgisierende Tibiakopfumstellungsosteotomie. 104. Kongreß der Deutschen Gesellschaft für Chirurgie München 1987. Langenbecks Arch Chir 372:826

213. Labitzke R (1988) Patentschrift DE 3835682 Deutsches Patentamt, München

214. Labitzke R, Upmeyer M (1989) Die "Seilzuggurtung" zur Kompression der kniegelenknahen Umstellungsosteotomie. Orthop Praxis 9:579–584

215. Labitzke R, Upmeyer M (1990) Die Seilzuggurtungs-Arthrodese am Fuß. In: Stahl C, Maaz B (eds) Die Arthrodese an der unteren Extremität. Ecomed, Landsberg, pp 147–156

216. Labitzke R (1992) Bone adaption. Internationales Symposium über das Wolffsche Gesetz und orthopädische Pathophysiologie, Berlin 4.4.1990. In: Regling G (ed) Wolff's law and connective tissue regulation. De Gruyter, Berlin

217. Labitzke R, Fritzsch M (1992) Die transhumerale Fixation der langen Bizepssehne. Operat Orthop Traumatol 4:260–267

218. Labitzke R (1993) Biologische Osteosynthese langer Röhrenknochen durch die Endo-Helix. In: Gahr R (ed) Entwicklungen in der Unfallchirurgie. Springer, Berlin Heidelberg New York

219. Labitzke R (1995) Von der "Knochennaht" zu zeitgenössischen Osteosynthesen – eine Chronologie. Chirurg 66:452–458

220. Labitzke R (1997) Zuggurtungen – Richtiges und Falsches am Beispiel der Patellafraktur. Chirurg 68:638–642

221. Lahm A, Roesgen M (1996) Minimalosteosynthese mit Drahtcerclagen bei dislozierten Humeruskopffrakturen. Aktuel Traumatol 26:22–28

222. Lambotte A (1912) The operative treatment of fractures. Brit Med J 2:1530–1532

223. Lange M (1926) Der Kruppstahldraht als Knochennahtmaterial. Z Orthop Chir 47:519–547

224. Larsen E, Jensen C (1991) Tension-band wiring of olecranon fractures with nonsliding pins. Acta Orthop Scand (Denmark) 62/4:360–362

225. Larson R, Simoian P (1995) Semitendinosus augmentation of acute patellar tendon repair with immediate mobilization. Am J Sports Med 23:82–86

226. Lauterbach H, Kinzl L (1991) Behandlung einer offenen Patellafraktur mit dem Minifixateur externe. Chirurg 62:432–433

227. Lawrence S, Botte M (1993) Jones fractures and related fractures of the proximal fifth metatarsal. Foot Ankle 14:358–365

228. Lehnemann W (1984) 150 Jahre Drahtseile im Bergbau. Bergbau 6:288–289

229. Leitner A, Müller A, Voigt C (1991) Eine modifizierte Behandlung nach primär versorgter Achillessehnenruptur. Aktuel Traumatol 21:285–292

230. Lengsfeld M, Ahlers J, Ritter G (1990) Kinematics of the patellofemoral joint investigations on a computer model with reference to patellar fractures. Arch Orthop Trauma Surg 109:280–283

231. Lennox I, Cobb A, Knowles J (1994) Knee function after patellectomy – a 12- to 48 year follow-up. JBJS 76B:485–487

232. Leser E (1904) Spezielle Chirurgie in 60 Vorlesungen. Fischer, Jena

233. Letournel E (1966) Die operative Versorgung der Hüftgelenkpfannenbrüche. Langenbecks Arch Klin Chir 316:422–437

234. Levack B, Flannagan J, Hobbs S (1985) Results of surgical treatment of patellar fractures. JBJS 67B:416–419

235. Liang Q, Wu J (1987) Fracture of the patella treated by open reduction and external compressive skeletal fixation. JBJS 69A:83–89

236. Lill H, Moor C, Fecht E (1996) Achillessehnenruptur – operative oder konservativ-funktionelle Behandlung? Aktuel Traumatol 26:95–100

237. Lister J (1867) On a new method of treating compound fracture, abscess etc. with observation on the conditions of suppuration (part 1 on compound fracture). Lancet 1:326–329

238. Lister J (1877) A new operation for fracture of the patella. Brit Med J 2:850

239. Lister J (1883) An address on the treatment of fracture of the patella. Brit Med J 11:855–860

240. Lister J (1908) Remarks on the treatment of fractures of the patella of longstanding. Brit Med J 1:849–850

241. Lotke P, Ecker M (1981) Transverse fractures of the patella. Clin Orthop 158:180–184

242. Lugger L, Russe O (1982) Olecranonfrakturen, Ursachen und Formen. Hefte Unfallheilkd 155:83–96

243. Luther R, Schulitz K (1968) Zur Behandlung der Olekranonfrakturen. Monatsschr Unfallheilkd 71:213–220

244. Macko D, Szabo R (1985) Complications of tension-band wiring of olecranon fractures. JBJS 67/9A:1396–1401
245. Maquet P (1974) Biomechanische Aspekte der Femur-Patella-Beziehungen. Z Orthop 112:620–623
246. Maquet P (1976) Biomechanics of the knee. Springer, Berlin Heidelberg New York
247. Marya S, Bhan S, Dave P (1987) Comparative study of knee function after patellectomy and osteosynthesis with a tension band wire following patellar fractures. Ind Surg 72:211–213
248. Matwin B (1984) Stabile Osteosynthese mittels Ankerplatte zur Behandlung von Olecranonfracturen. Unfallheilkunde 87:156–162
249. Maurer C, Ackermann J (1993) Belastungsstabile, minimale Fibulaosteosynthese bei Malleolarfrakturen Weber Typ B durch eine Hemicerclage. Helv Chir Acta 60:235–240
250. Maxwell J (1983) Open or closed treatment of metatarsal fractures. J Am Pod Med Assoc 73:100–106
251. McLaughlin H, Francis K (1956) Operativ repair of injuries to the quadriceps extensor mechanism. JBJS 91A:651–653
252. Meenen N, Balleck M, Jungbluth K (1992) Patellafrakturen – eine historische und aktuelle Übersicht. BG-UMed 79:133–146
253. Meißner A, Fell M, Wilk R (1996) Zur Biomechanik der Symphyse. Unfallchirurg 99:415–421
254. Meißner A, Fell M, Wilk R (1998) Vergleich interner Stabilisierungsverfahren für die Symphyse im multidirektionalen dynamischen Gangsimulator. Unfallchirurg 101:18–25
255. Melzer C (1995) Der Oberarmkopfbruch beim alten Menschen. Aktuel Traumatol 25:136–142
256. Meyer v H (1873) Die Statik und Mechanik des menschlichen Knochengerüsts. Engelmann, Leipzig
257. Meyer-Steineg T, Sudhoff K (1950) Geschichte der Medizin im Überblick mit Abbildungen. Fischer, Jena
258. Mittelmeier H (1975) Draht und Nagel als Osteosynthesemittel. Med Orthop Techn 95/3:49–54
259. Mittelmeier H, Hauser U (1979) Biomechanik der Drahtcerclage. Z Orthop 117:701–705
260. Moehrke T, Hahn F, Mittag-Bonsch M (1993) Die Aalener Rüsselplatte – ein Erfahrungsbericht über 5 Jahre. In: Rahmanzadeh R, Meißner A (eds) Unfall- und Wiederherstellungschirurgie des Schultergürtels. Springer, Berlin Heidelberg New York
261. Mont M, Maar D (1994) Fractures of the ipsilateral femur after hip arthroplasty. A statistical analysis of outcome based on 487 patients. J Arthroplasty 9:511–519
262. Moschinski D, Kleinschmidt F, Klein H (1978) Ergebnisse der operativen Behandlung des Kniescheibenbruches. Hefte Unfallheilkd 81:14–19
263. Müller F (1992) Der Chirurg Johann Friedrich Dieffenbach und sein Einfluß auf die Entwicklung der Plastischen Chirurgie. Chirurg BDC 7:127–131
264. Müller ME, Allgöwer M, Willenegger H (1963) Technik der operativen Frakturenbehandlung. Springer, Berlin Göttingen Heidelberg New York
265. Müller ME (1971) Die hüftnahen Femurosteotomien unter Berücksichtigung der Form, Funktion und Beanspruchung des Hüftgelenkes. Thieme, Stuttgart
266. Müller ME, Allgöwer M, Willenegger H (1970) Manual of internal fixation. Springer, Berlin Heidelberg New York
267. Müller W (1902) Schachtförderung. In: Verein für die bergbaulichen Interessen (ed) Die Entwicklung des Niederrheinisch-Westfälischen Steinkohlenbergbaues in der zweiten Hälfte des 19. Jahrhunderts. Springer, Berlin
268. Müller W (1982) Das Knie. Springer, Berlin Heidelberg New York
269. Müller-Färber J, Müller K (1984) Die verschiedenen Formen der instabilen Beckenverletzungen und ihre Behandlung. Hefte Unfallheilkd 87:441–455
270. Murphy D, Greene W, Gilbert J (1987) Displaced olecranon fractures in adults. Biomechanical analysis of fixation methods. Clin Orthop (US) 224:210–214
271. Murphy D, Greene W, Gilbert J (1987) Displaced olecranon fractures in adults. Clinical evaluation. Clin Orthop (US) 224:215–223
272. Nachtigall W (1974) Phantasie der Schöpfung. Hoffmann und Campe, Hamburg
273. Nagel M, Schober K, Weiß G (1994) Theodor Billroth, Chirurg und Musiker. ConBrio, Regensburg
274. Nast-Kolb D, Betz A, Schweiberer L (1993) Die Minimalosteosynthese der Pilon-tibial-Fractur. Unfallchirurg 96:517–523
275. Naumann T, Kluger P, Wilke H (1993) Unfusionierte Wirbelsäulenaufrichtung im Wachstumsalter bei neuromuskulären Skoliosen vom Typ Duchenne. In: Venbrocks R, Salis-Soglio G (eds) Jahrbuch der Orthopädie 1993. Biermann, Zülpich
276. Neer C (1970) Displaced proximal humeral fractures. Classification and evaluation. JBJS 52A:1077–1089
277. Neumann H, Winckler S, Strobel M (1993) Langzeitergebnisse nach operativer Versorgung von Patellafrakturen. Unfallchirurg 96:305–310
278. Niehaus P, Staudte H (1990) Fixateur oder Zugschraubenarthrodese nach Wagner bei der oberen Sprunggelenkarthrodese? In: Stahl C, Maaz B (eds) Die Arthrodese an der unteren Extremität. Ecomed, Landsberg, pp 101–112
279. Nieländer K, Wolter D (1993) CW Wutzer und B v Langenbeck – die Pioniere des Fixateur externe. Springer, Berlin Heidelberg New York
280. Nonnemann H, Plösch J (1993) Verrenkungsbrüche des oberen Sprunggelenkes. Klassifizierung – Behandlung – Ergebnisse. Aktuel Traumatol 23:183–186
281. Noyez L, Verkroost M, Asten v W (1993) Sternal closure: comparison of two techniques. Cardiovasc Surg 1/6:643–645
282. Ochsner P, Ilchmann T (1991) Zuggurtungsosteosynthesen mit resorbierbaren Kordeln bei proximalen Humerusmehrfragmentbrüchen. Unfallchirurg 94:508–510
283. Oehlecker F (1905) Resultate blutiger und unblutiger Behandlung von Patellarfracturen. Arch Klin Chir 77/3:750–782

284. Oestern H, Tscherne H (1982) Olecranonfrakturen, Therapie und Ergebnisse. Hefte Unfallheilkd 155: 97–109

285. Ogliviert-Harris D, Fitsialos D, Hedmann T (1994) Arthrodesis of the ankle. A comparison of two versus three screw fixation in a crossed configuration. Clin Orthop 304:195–199

286. Orsos E (1925) Über stromerzeugende Knochennähte. Zentralbl Chir 19:1014–1016

287. Otto F (1984) Der Pneu. Arcus 6:286–291

288. Otto F (1985) Natürliche Konstruktionen. Formen und Strukturen in Natur und Technik und Prozesse ihrer Entstehung. Deutsche Verlags-Anstalt, Stuttgart

289. Otto F (1995) Pneu and bone. Information of the Institute for Lightweight Structures (IL), University of Stuttgart. IL 35

290. Pachucki A, Dremsek J, Zifko B (1982) Die Patellektomie-Indikation und Nachuntersuchungsergebnisse. Hefte Unfallheilkd 85:468–472

291. Parker M, Richmond P, Andrew T (1990) A review of displaced olecranon fractures treated conservatively. J R Coll Surg Edinb (Scotland) 35/6:392–394

292. Pauwels F (1935) Der Schenkelhalsbruch. Ein mechanisches Problem. Grundlagen des Heilungsvorganges. Prognose und kausale Therapie, 2. Teil. Beilageheft Z Orthop Grenzgeb 63:96–138

293. Pauwels F (1936) Zur Frage der den Schenkelhals aufrichtenden Kräfte. Beilageheft Z Orthop Grenzgeb 64:361–371

294. Pauwels F (1951) Über die Bedeutung der Bauprinzipien des Stütz- und Bewegungsapparates für die Beanspruchung der Röhrenknochen. Acta Anat 12:207–227

295. Pauwels F (1963) Die Druckverteilung im Ellenbogengelenk nebst grundsätzlichen Bemerkungen über den Gelenkdruck. Z Anat 123:643–667

296. Pauwels F (1965) Gesammelte Abhandlungen zur funktionellen Anatomie des Bewegungsapparates. Springer, Berlin Heidelberg New York

297. Pauwels F (1966) Über die Bedeutung einer Zuggurtung für die Beanspruchung des Röhrenknochens und ihre Verwendung zur Druckosteosynthese. Beihefte Orthop 101:231–248

298. Pels-Leusden F (1910) Chirurgische Operationslehre für Studierende und Ärzte. Urban and Schwarzenberg, Berlin

299. Pennal G, Tile M, Waddell J (1980) Pelvic disruption: assessment and classification. Clin Orthop 151:12–21

300. Perry C, McCarthy J, Kain C (1988) Patellar fixation protected with load-shaving cable: a mechanical and clinical study. J Orthop Trauma 2:234–240

301. Petersen K, Keller J, Jensen J (1989) Fractura patellae. Modificeret tension band osteosyntese Ugeskr. Laeger 151:937–939

302. Pletzer H (1888) Zur Behandlung der queren Kniescheibenbrüche durch die Naht. Dissertation, Bonn

303. Pohlemann T, Krettek C, Hoffmann R (1994) Biomechanischer Vergleich verschiedener Notfallstabilisierungsmaßnahmen am Beckenring. Unfallchirurg 97:503–510

304. Pohlemann T, Tscherne H, Baumgärtel F (1996) Beckenverletzungen: Epidemiologie, Therapie u. Langzeitverlauf. Unfallchirurg 99:160–167

305. Povel J, Paffen P, Busman D (1979) Mechanische Kraftwirkung auf das Ellenbogengelenk bei Olecranonfrakturen. Aktuel Traumatol 9:269–276

306. Povel J, Paffen P, Busman D (1979) Olecranonfrakturen. Aktuel Traumatol 9:347–352

307. Pritchett J (1993) Rush rods versus plate osteosyntheses for unstable ankle fractures in the elderly. Orthop Rev 22:691–696

308. Rabl C (1951) Orthopädische Schuhe und Stützeinlagen. Enke, Stuttgart

309. Rahmanzadeh M, O'Driscall S, An K (1997) Biomechanisch-experimentelle Untersuchungen verschiedener Osteosyntheseverfahren bei unterschiedlichen Olecranonfrakturen. Hefte Unfallchirurg 268:12–13

310. Raschke M, Oedekoven G, Claudi B (1993) Die Behandlung großer Knochendefekte durch Segmentverschiebung. H Unfallchirurg 230:803–808

311. Rasul A, Fischer D (1993) Primary repair of quadriceps tendon ruptures. Results of treatment. Clin Orthop 289:205–207

312. Rauber-Kopsch (1955) Lehrbuch und Atlas der Anatomie des Menschen, vol 1. Thieme, Stuttgart

313. Ray T, Nimityongskul P, Anderson L (1994) Percutaneous intramedullary fixation of lateral malleolus fractures: technique and report of early results. J Trauma 36:669–675

314. Reck T, Landsleitner B, Richter H (1991) Eine neue Methode der transossären Ausziehdrahtfixation bei Bandverletzungen am Daumengrundgelenk. Handchir Mikrochir Plast Chir 23:90–92

315. Regensburger J (1962) Entwicklung und Leistungen der Drahtseilerei in Deutschland. Draht 13/4:148–153 (1962) – pt 1/Draht 13/5:235–240 – pt 2

316. Richli W, Rosenthal D (1984) Avulsion fracture of the fifth metatarsal: experimental study of pathomechanics. AJR 143:889–894

317. Ritter G (1975) Therapie der Patellafraktur. Hefte Unfallheilkd 120:61–67

318. Ritter G, Degreif J (1991) Grundsätzliche Überlegungen zur Problematik der Abbrüche des Trochanter major bei und nach Winkelplattenosteosynthesen. Unfallchirurgie 17:106–110

319. Robinson R (1978) The historical background of internal fixation of fractures in North America. Bull Hist Med 52:354–382

320. Robson M (1889) New method of extraarticular suture of the patella. Brit Med J March 30:743–746

321. Rodgers J (1827) Case of un-united fracture of the os brachii, successfully treated. N Y Med Phys J 6:521–523

322. Roe S (1994) Letter to the editor concerning: tension band wiring of olecranon fractures: a modification of the AO technic by Rowland and Burkhart. Clin Orthop 308:284–286

323. Roesgen M, Koch G (1987) Die Zuggurtungsosteosynthese – eine komplikationsträchtige Methode der operativen Knochenbruchbehandlung? Aktuel Traumatol 17:120–123

324. Rogge D, Oestern H, Gossé F (1985) Die Patellafraktur, Therapie und Ergebnisse. Orthopäde 14:266–280

325. Rommens P, Vanderschot P, De Boodt P (1992) Surgical management of pelvic ring disruptions. Unfallchirurg 95:455–462

326. Rooks R, Tarvin G, Pijanowski G (1982) In vitro cerclage wiring analysis. Vet Surg 11:34–43

327. Rowland S, Burkhart S (1992) Tension band wiring of olecranon fractures. A modification of the AO technique. Clin Orthop 277:238–242

328. Rudig L, Ahlers J, Lengsfeld M (1993) Behandlung und Ergebnisse nach Rupturen des Ligamentum patellae. Unfallchirurgie 19:214–220

329. Rüter A, Burri C (1975) Patellafrakturen – Diskussion und Empfehlungen. Hefte Unfallheilkd 120:91–98

330. Rüter A, Burri C (1982) Olecranonfrakturen – Diskussionsbemerkungen und Empfehlungen aller Teilnehmer (Leitung K Jungbluth). Hefte Unfallheilkd 155:113–116

331. Rüter A, Brutscher R (1989) Die Ilizarov-Kortikotomie und Segmentverschiebung zur Behandlung großer Tibia-Defekte. Operat Orthop Traumatol 1:80–89

332. Salzman C, Goulet J, McClellan R (1990) Results of treatment of displaced patellar fractures by partial patellectomy. JBJS 72A:1279–1285

333. Sambach D (1981) Biomechanik der Olecranonfraktur. Dissertation, Homburg

334. Sattler R, Schikorski M (1987) Patellaquerfraktur – Reposition und Stabilisierung unter arthroskopischer Sicht. Zentralbl Chir 112:1515–1519

335. Savvidis E (1989) Beanspruchung des coxalen Femurendes bei seiner Belastung in der Hüftgelenksbeugestellung. Habilitationsschrift, Aachen

336. Savvidis E, Löer F, Herrboldt U (1989) Die Zugfestigkeit unterschiedlicher Osteosynthesen des instabilen Trochanter major. Unfallchirurg 92:261–265

337. Schäfer A (1906) Beitrag zur Technik der Kniescheibennaht. MMW 53.351–352

338. Scharizer E (1964) Die Entwicklung der modernen Unfallchirurgie. Hefte Unfallheilkd 79:1–76

339. Scharplatz D, Allgöwer M (1978) Ergebnisse der Olecranon-Zuggurtungen. Aktuel Traumatol 8:105–108

340. Schax M, Letsch R, Schmit-Neuerburg K (1990) Indikation, Technik und Ergebnisse der konservativen und operativen Behandlung bei 126 Patellafrakturen. Hefte Unfallheilkd 212:149

341. Schede M (1877) Zur Behandlung der Querbrüche der Patella und des Olecranon. Centralbl Chir 42:657–663

342. Scheuba J, Unger F (1970) Einteilung und Behandlung der Olecranonfrakturen. Monatsschr Unfallheilkd 73:220–224

343. Schmelzeisen H (1977) Olecranonfrakturen. BG-UMed 32:193–198

344. Schmieden V (1915) Der chirurgische Operationskursus. Barth, Leipzig

345. Schmidt R, Meyer-Wölbert B, Gerngroß H (1999) Dynamische Ganganalyse. Mittel zur Qualitätssicherung nach operativ versorgten Sprunggelenkfrakturen. Unfallchirurg 102:110–114

346. Schmit-Neuerburg K, Harting T (1986) Osteosyntheseverfahren am dorsalen Beckenring. Hefte Unfallheilkd 181:566

347. Schmitt E, Schmitt O, Mittelmaier H (1984) Indikation, Technik und Ergebnisse der kniegelenksnahen Umstellungsosteotomie bei hemilateraler Gonarthrose mit Autokompressionswinkelplatte. Orthop Prax 11:903–913

348. Schmotzer H, Fitzpatrick J, Heinze H (1992) Mechanical properties of various multifilament cables and crimps in tensile and elongtion tests. 4th world biomechanic congress, Berlin, 24.4.1992

349. Schneeberger A, Murphy S, Ganz R (1997) Die digastrische Trochanterosteotomie. Operat Orthop Traumatol 9:1–15

350. Schneider R (1982) Die Totalendoprothese der Hüfte. Huber, Bern

351. Schödl C (1996) Ergebnisse der operativen Zuggurtung des Schultereckgelenkes nach Sprengung mittels Labitzke-Drahtseil. Dissertation, Berlin

352. Schröder D, Gall H (1992) Zum biomechanischen Einfluß der Synovialflüssigkeit auf die Funktion der Gelenke. Zuckschwerdt, München, Bern, Wien

353. Schultze F (1924) Was bewirkt die Cerclage der Patella? Hat die Cerclage in der Behandlung der Patellarfraktur eine Berechtigung? Zentralbl Chir 36:1962–1963

354. Schwarzkopf W, Ahlers J, Marburger M (1981) Symphysensprengung mit Verletzung von Rectum und Urogenitalsystem. Chir Prax 28:81–90

355. Schweiberer L, Betz A, Nast-Kolb D, Bischoff B (1987) Spezielle Behandlungstaktik am distalen Unterschenkel und bei Pilonfrakturen. Unfallchirurg 90:253–259

356. Shaw J, Daubert H (1988) Compression capability of cerclage fixation systems. Orthopedics 11:1169–1174

357. Siebel R, Reichelt A (1995/1996) Der diabetische Fuß und seine Behandlung. Chir Prax 50:113–122

358. Siegel A (1987) Endoprothesen im Fußbereich. In: Dahmen G (ed) Der Problemfuß. Verlag CIBA-Zeitschriften, Wehr

359. Slätis P, Karaharju E (1980) External fixation of instable pelvic fractures. Clin Orthop 151:73–79

360. Sourmia, Poulet, Martiny (1982) Illustrierte Geschichte der Medizin, vol 5. Andreas und Andreas, Salzburg

361. Speck W (1921) Beitrag zur Behandlung der Kniescheibenbrüche. Beitr Klin Chir 121:226–233

362. Speck M, Regazzoni P (1997) 4-Fragment-Frakturen des proximalen Humerus. Unfallchirurg 100:349–353

363. Sperner G, Wanitschnek P (1989) Therapieformen und Behandlungsergebnisse der Patellafraktur. Unfallchirurgie 15:247–252

364. Sperner G, Wanitschek P, Benedetto K (1990) Spätergebnisse bei Patellafrakturen. Aktuel Traumatol 20: 24–28

365. Steinmann F (1924) Die operative Behandlung der Frakturen im Dienste der funktionellen Knochenbehandlung. Verh Dtsch Ges Chir 48. Tagung, pp 389–395

366. Storck H (1931) Körperschwere und Gelenke. Arch Orthop Unfall Chir 29:1–25

367. Storck H (1933) Coxa valga, ein Beitrag zur Frage der

den Knochen formenden Kräfte. Arch Orthop Unfall Chir 32:133–228

368. Straub G (1992) Beidseitige subcutane Ruptur der Quadricepssehne durch Bagatelltrauma. Unfallchirurg 95:311–312

369. Stüssi F (1966) Leben und Werk von Othmar H. Ammann. Schweiz Bauztg 84/38:663–672

370. Szyszkowitz R, Seggl W, Schleifer P (1993) Proximal humeral fractures. Management, techniques and expected results. Clin Orthop 292:13–25

371. Tani J, Knoth L (1994) Minifragmentation plating for comminuted distal patella fractures. A report of three cases. Orthop Rev [Suppl] pp 26–31

372. Targonski J (1985/86) Die bewegungsstabile Tenodese der Achillessehne mittels Korium. Chir Prax 35:65–70

373. Teubner E, Gerstenberger F (1992) Die Kinematik des Beckens. Unfallchirurg 95:50–57

374. Thaiss S (1992) Die subcutane Achillessehnenruptur. Chir Prax 45:469–474

375. Thermann H, Zwipp H, Tscherne H (1995) Funktionelles Behandlungskonzept der frischen Achillessehnenruptur. Zweijahresergebnisse einer prospektivrandomisierten Studie. Unfallchirurg 98:21–32

376. Thermann H, Frerichs O, Biewener A (1995) Die funktionelle Behandlung der frischen Achillessehnenruptur. Eine experimentelle biomechanische Untersuchung. Unfallchirurg 98:507–513

377. Thiem C (1905) Über die Größe der Unfallfolgen bei der blutigen und unblutigen Behandlung der einfachen (subcutanen) Querbrüche der Kniescheibe. Arch Klin Chir 77/3:730–749

378. Thiem C (1909) Lockerung des Beckens in seinen Fugen. Monatsschr Unfallheilkd 3:65–70

379. Thorwald J (1972) Das Jahrhundert der Chirurgen. Knaur, München (Taschenbuchausgabe 1972, Bd 3275)

380. Thorwald J (1972) Das Weltreich der Chirurgen. Knaur, München (Taschenbuchausgabe, Bd 3281)

381. Timmes J, Wolvek S, Fernando M (1973) A new method of sternal approximation. Ann Thorac Surg 15:544–547

382. Tönnis D (1970) Die zweifache Zuggurtung mit Kirschnerdrähten – eine verbesserte Technik zur Versorgung von Kniescheibenbrüchen. Monatsschr Unfallheilkd 73:281–284

383. Towfigh H (1982) Entwicklung einer neuen, übungsstabilen Sehnennaht. Unfallchirurgie 8:226–229

384. Towfigh H, Buhl W, Obertacke U (1993) Behandlungserrgebnisse nach konservativer und operativer Versorgung von proximalen Oberarmfrakturen. Aktuel Traumatol 23:354–360

385. Träger D (1985) Gleichzeitige beidseitige Ruptur des Ligamentum patellae. Unfallchirurg 88:547–549

386. Trentz O, Bühren V, Friedl H (1989) Beckenverletzungen. Chirurg 60:639–648

387. Troche A (1953) Grundlagen des Stahlbetonbaues. De Gruyter, Berlin

388. Troell A (1913) Zur Wertschätzung der blutigen Frakturbehandlung (Osteosynthese). Monatsschr Unfallheilkd Invalidenwesen 9:281–295

389. Troidl H, Gaitzsch A, Winkler-Wilfurth A (1993) Fehler und Gefahren bei der laparoskopischen Appendektomie. Chirurg 64:212–220

390. Trupka A, Wiedemann E, Schweiberer L (1997) Dislozierte Mehrfragmentfrakturen des Humeruskopfes. Unfallchirurg 100:105–110

391. Tscherne H, Pohlemann T (1996) Beckenverletzungen: niedrige Inzidienz, aber unbefriedigende Ergebnisse (editorial). Unfallchirurg 99:159

392. Ulrich E (1976) Das Drahtseil als wichtiges Hilfsmittel zur Lösung fördertechnischer Probleme. Bergbau 12:499–502

393. Upmeyer M (1998) Valgisierende Tibiakopfumstellungsosteotomie versus Innenmeniskusektomie. Dissertation, Witten/Herdecke

394. Upmeyer M, Labitzke R (1994) Die Seilzuggurtungsarthrodese am Fuß. In: Stuhler T (ed) Arthrodesen. Thieme, Stuttgart, pp 278–281

395. Verth M zur (1925) Ein Fortschritt in der Technik der Drahtnaht (Ersatz des Drehknotens durch das Lötverfahren). Zentralbl Chir 52/49:1483–1485

396. Vogel O (1926) Die Vorläufer des Albertschen Grubenseiles. Drahtwelt

397. Vogt M, Statz M (1993) Funktionelle Ergebnisse nach Patellektomie. Aktuel Traumatol 23:66–74

398. Volkmann v R (1880) Die Sehnennaht bei Querbrüchen der Kniescheibe. Centralbl Chir 24:385–387

399. Voorhoeve A, Kranz C, Weil E (1981) Die Verwendung von Femurtrichternetzen bei der Totalendoprothese des Hüftgelenkes. Chir Prax 28:489–508

400. Vorschütz J (1925) Die operative Behandlung der frischen Patellarfraktur durch Umschnürung mit einem Streifen der Fascia lata. Zentralbl Chir 52/4:179–182

401. Wagner H, Pock H (1982) Die Verschraubungsarthrodese der Sprunggelenke. Unfallheilkunde 85:280–300

402. Wahl M (1883) Naht einer Patellafractur, pt. 1–3. DMW Nr 18 from 2.5.1883, pp 262–265; Nr 19 from 9.5. 1883, pp 281–284; Nr 20 from 16.5.1883, pp 297–298

403. Wahlheim G, Olerud S, Ribbe T (1984) Mobility of the pubic symphysis. Measurements by an electromechanical method. Acta Orthop Scand 55:203–208

404. Wallenbrock E (1993) Ligamentum-patellae-Ruptur – eine Spätkomplikation nach Entnahme eines Knochen-Sehnen-Knochentransplantats als Kreuzbandersatz. Langenbecks Arch Chir 378:339–340

405. Wapner K, Pavlock G, Hecht P (1993) Repair of chronic achilles tendon rupture with flexor hallucis longus tendon transfer. Foot Ankle 14:443–449

406. Warren G (1997) Conservative amputation of the neuropathic foot – the Pirogoff procedure. Operat Orthop Traumatol 9:49–58

407. Watkins M, Harris B, Wender S (1983) Effect of patellectomy on the function of the quadriceps and hamstrings. JBJS 65A:390–398

408. Weber B (1963) Grundlagen und Möglichkeiten der Zuggurtungsosteosynthese. Chirurg 35:81–86

409. Weber B (1966) Die Verletzungen des oberen Sprunggelenkes. Huber, Bern

410. Weber W (1971) Seile und Seilereimaschinen. Ciba-Geigy Rundsch 1:1–45
411. Weber W (1972/1973) Zur Entwicklung und Herstellung des Drahtseiles. Drahtwelt 58/3:161–167 (1972), pt. I; Drahtwelt 59/3:105–110 (1973), pt. II
412. Weber W (1987) Vitruv und das Drahtseil. Ein Beitrag zur Geschichte. Draht 38:330–331
413. Weber W (1989) Seilerlexikon. Aegis, Ulm
414. Weigand H, Storm H, Birne F (1990) Die temporäre postoperative Sicherung des vorderen Kreuzbandes durch ein transartikuläres Drahtseil. Aktuel Traumatol 20:77–82
415. Weil S, Weil U (1966) Mechanik des Gehens. Thieme, Stuttgart
416. Weller S (1977) Frische Verletzungen der Patella. Langenbecks Arch Chir 345:403–408
417. Weller S (1981) Biomechanische Prinzipien in der operativen Knochenbruchbehandlung. Aktuel Traumatol 11:195–202
418. Weller S (1986) Operative Knochenbruchbehandlung – Osteosynthesen. In: Probst J (ed) Unfallheilkunde 1986. Demeter, Gräfelfing
419. Wenzl H, Krüger P (1971) Transossäre Drahtnaht und Zuggurtung: ideale Osteosynthese der Patellafraktur. Monatsschr Unfallheilkd 74:169–175
420. Wessinghage D (1995) Themistocles Gluck: Von der Organextirpation zum Gelenkersatz. Dtsch Arztebl 92:C1443–1447
421. Willenegger H, Perren S, Schenk R (1971) Primäre und sekundäre Knochenbruchheilung. Chirurg 42:241–252
422. Wilson J, Belloli D, Robbins T (1985) Resistance of cerclage to knot failure. JAVMA 187/4:389–391
423. Winkelbauer A (1925) Erfahrungen mit der Kirschnerschen Knochennaht. Dtsch Z Chir 191:353–360
424. Winter E, Ambacher T, Maurer F (1995) Operative Therapie der Achillessehnenruptur. Unfallchirurg 98:468–473
425. Wissing J, v d Werken C (1991) Die Zuggurtungsosteosynthese aus resorbierbarem Material. Unfallchirurg 94:45–46
426. Witzel U (1980) Untersuchungen über die temperaturabhängige dynamische Tragfähigkeit von Seilendverbindungen mit Aluminium-Preßklemmen. Dissertation, Bochum
427. Wolff J (1891) Ueber eine neues Operationsverfahren bei veraltetem, mit Diastase geheiltem Querbruch der Patella. DMW 20:682
428. Wolff J (1892) Das Gesetz der Transformation der Knochen. Hirschwald, Berlin
429. Wolfgang G, Burke F, Bush D (1987) Surgical treatment of displaced olecranon fractures by tension band wiring. Clin Orthop 224:192–204
430. Wolter D (1991) Wer war Hansmann? In: Wolter D, Zimmer W. (eds) Die Plattenosteosynthese und ihre Konkurrenzverfahren. Spinger, Berlin Heidelberg New York
431. Wondrak E (1967) Beitrag zur Technik der Zuggurtungsosteosynthesen. Chirurg 38:326–327
432. Wozasek G, Moser K, Mousavi M (1993) Klinische Erfahrungen mit dem Lochbohrdraht. Chir Prax 46:647–656
433. Wright R, Barrett K, Christie M (1994) Acetabular fractures: long-term follow-up of open reduction and internal fixation. J Orthop Trauma 8:397–403
434. Ziegler J, Regazzoni P (1991) Behandlungsergebnisse nach Patellafrakturen. Helv Chir Acta 58:949–952
435. Zieren H, Holzmüller W, Rosenberger J (1991) Sind Patellazuggurtungen mit resorbierbaren Materialien möglich? Unfallchirurg 94:634–639
436. Zierold A (1924) Reaction of bone to various metals. Arch Surg 9:365–411
437. Zimmer M, Jansson V (1994) Neues zur Technik der Spickdrahtosteosynthese. Sportverl Sportschad 8:50

438. Hertel R, Leunig M, Ballmer F (1999) In vitro stability of various methods of osteosynthesis of tuberosities in hemiarthroplasty for traumatic conditions. 13. congress of SECEC/ESSE The Hague, 8.–11.9. ·
439. Huhn S, Wolf A, Ecklund J (1991) Posterior spinal osteosynthesis for cervical fracture/dislocation using a flexible multistrand cable system: technical note. Neurosurgery 29(6), 943–946

Subject Index